A.A.O.S.

Symposium on

Tendon Surgery in The Hand

American Academy
of
Orthopaedic Surgeons

Symposium on Tendon Surgery in The Hand

Philadelphia, Pennsylvania
March, 1974

With 385 illustrations

Saint Louis
The C. V. Mosby Company
1975

Printed in the United States of America

Distributed in Great Britain by Henry Kimpton, London

Library of Congress Cataloging in Publication Data

Symposium on Tendon Surgery in the Hand, Philadelphia, 1974.
Symposium on Tendon Surgery in the Hand, Philadelphia, Pennsylvania, March, 1974.

At head of title: American Academy of Orthopaedic Surgeons.
Includes bibliographical references and index.
1. Hand—Surgery—Congresses. 2. Tendons—Surgery—Congresses. I. American Academy of Orthopaedic Surgeons. [DNLM: 1. Hand—Surgery—Congresses. 2. Tendons—Surgery—Congresses. WE830 S988s 1974]
RD559.S87 1974 617′.474 75-37577
ISBN 0-8016-0046-4

CB/CB/B 9 8 7 6 5 4 3 2

CONTRIBUTORS

Robert W. Beasley, M.D.

Professor of Surgery, New York University School of Medicine; Director, Hand Service, Institute of Reconstructive Plastic Surgery of New York University Medical Center, New York, New York

William Blythe, Ph.D.

Professor and Chairman, Department of Civil Engineering and Applied Mechanics, San Jose State University, San Jose, California

Joseph H. Boyes, M.D.

Emeritus Clinical Professor of Surgery, University of Southern California, Los Angeles, California

James D. Cahill, Jr., M.D.

Research Fellow, Orthopaedic Surgery, Duke University Medical Center, Durham, North Carolina

Howard S. Caplan, M.D.

Fellow, Hand Surgery Research, Thomas Jefferson University Hospital, Philadelphia, Pennsylvania

Josephine Cohen, M.A., O.R.T.

Assistant Professor in Occupational Therapy, School of Allied Medical Professions, University of Pennsylvania, Philadelphia, Pennsylvania

Myles J. Cohen, M.D.

Beverly Hills, California. Former Christine Kleinert Fellow in Hand Surgery, University of Louisville School of Medicine, Louisville, Kentucky

James H. Dobyns, M.D.

Assistant Professor of Orthopaedic Surgery, Mayo Medical School, Department of Orthopaedics, University of Minnesota, Rochester, Minnesota

James R. Doyle, M.D.

Assistant Clinical Professor of Orthopaedic Surgery, University of California Medical Center, San Francisco, California

Robert J. Duran, M.D.

Clinical Associate Professor and Co-director of the Hand Service, Department of Surgery, Division of Plastic Surgery, Ohio State University College of Medicine, Columbus, Ohio

Martin A. Entin, M.D., C.M., M.Sc., F.R.C.S.(C), F.A.C.S.

Associate Professor of Surgery, Department of Surgery, McGill University, Montreal, Quebec; Chief of Plastic Surgery, Royal Victoria Hospital; and Consultant in Hand and Plastic Surgery, Shriners Hospital, Montreal, Quebec, Canada

Frank C. Forshew, M.D.

Akron, Ohio. Former Christine Kleinert Fellow in Hand Surgery, University of Louisville School of Medicine, Louisville, Kentucky

J. Leonard Goldner, M.D.

Professor and Chairman, Division of Orthopaedic Surgery, Duke University Medical Center, Durham, North Carolina

Robert G. Houser, M.D.

Clinical Assistant Professor, Department of Surgery, Division of Plastic Surgery, Ohio State University, College of Medicine, Columbus, Ohio

James M. Hunter, M.D.

Associate Professor of Orthopaedic Surgery, Jefferson Medical College of Thomas Jefferson University, Philadelphia, Pennsylvania

François Iselin, M.D.

Chief of Hand Surgery Unit, Department of Surgery, Hospital of Nanterre, University of Paris-Nanterre, Paris, France

Scott H. Jaeger, M.D.

Resident and Research Fellow in Orthopaedic Surgery, Jefferson Medical College of Thomas Jefferson University, Philadelphia, Pennsylvania

Harold E. Kleinert, M.D.

Clinical Professor of Surgery, University of Louisville School of Medicine, Louisville, Kentucky; and Clinical Professor of Surgery, Indiana University-Purdue University School of Medicine, Indianapolis, Indiana

Joseph E. Kutz, M.D.

Assistant Clinical Professor of Surgery, University of Louisville School of Medicine, Louisville, Kentucky

Norman S. Levine, M.D., Major, MC

United States Army Institute of Surgical Research, Brooke Army Medical Center, Fort Sam Houston, Texas

Evelyn Mackin, L.P.T.

Director of Hand Therapy, Hand Rehabilitation Center, Ltd., Philadelphia, Pennsylvania

Daniel W. McKeel, Jr., M.D., Major, MC

United States Army Institute of Surgical Research, Brooke Army Medical Center, Fort Sam Houston, Texas

Robert J. Merklin, M.D.

Associate Professor of Anatomy, Jefferson Medical College of Thomas Jefferson University, Philadelphia, Pennsylvania

Lee Milford, M.D.

Associate Clinical Professor of Orthopaedic Surgery, Department of Orthopaedics, University of Tennessee, Memphis, Tennessee

Frederick V. Minkow, M.D.

Department of Orthopedic Surgery, St. Joseph–Mercy Hospital and Pontiac General Hospital, Pontiac, Michigan; Consulting Hand Surgeon, Pontiac State Hospital, Pontiac, Michigan

Rod A. Mortenson, M.D.

Resident, Department of Orthopaedic Surgery, Duke University Medical Center, Durham, North Carolina

Edward A. Nalebuff, M.D.

Clinical Assistant Professor of Orthopaedic Surgery, Department of Orthopaedic Surgery, Harvard University School of Medicine, Chief of Hand Surgery, Robert B. Brigham Hospital, Boston, Massachusetts

Austin D. Potenza, M.D.

Sierra Orthopaedic Group, Las Vegas, Nevada

Basil A. Pruitt, M.D., Col., MC

United States Army Institute of Surgical Research, Brooke Army Medical Center, Fort Sam Houston, Texas

R. Guy Pulvertaft, C.B.E., M.D.(Hon.), M.Chir., F.R.C.S.

Orthopaedic Surgeon Emeritus, Derbyshire Royal Infirmary and Honorary Civil Consultant, Royal Air Force, Derby, England

Patrick R. Robins, M.D.

Orthopaedic Surgeon, Missoula, Montana

Spencer A. Rowland, M.D.

Clinical Associate Professor, Department of Surgery, Division of Orthopaedics and Consultant to the Hand Service, University of Texas Health Science Center, San Antonio, Texas

Roger E. Salisbury, M.D., Major, MC

United States Army Institute of Surgical Research, Brooke Army Medical Center, Fort Sam Houston, Texas

Lawrence H. Schneider, M.D.

Assistant Clinical Professor of Orthopaedic Surgery, Jefferson Medical College of Thomas Jefferson University, Philadelphia, Pennsylvania

Richard J. Smith, M.D.

Chief of Hand Surgery Service, Department of Orthopaedic Surgery, Massachusetts General Hospital, Associate Clinical Professor of Orthopaedic Surgery, Harvard Medical School, Boston Massachusetts

Morton Spinner, M.D.

Clinical Professor of Orthopaedic Surgery, Department of Orthopaedic Surgery, Albert Einstein College of Medicine, New York, New York; and Chief of the Hand Surgical Service, Brookdale Hospital Medical Center, Brooklyn, New York

Alfred B. Swanson, M.D., F.A.C.S.

Chief, Orthopaedic Research Department, Blodgett Memorial Hospital; Chairman, Orthopaedic Training Program, Blodgett Memorial Hospital and Butterworth Hospital, Grand Rapids, Michigan; Clinical Professor of Surgery, Michigan State University College of Human Medicine, East Lansing, Michigan

Genevieve deGroot Swanson, M.D.

Grand Rapids, Michigan

James R. Urbaniak, M.D.

Associate Professor, Department of Orthopaedic Surgery, Duke University Medical Center, Durham, North Carolina

Claude E. Verdan, M.D.

Professeur à la Faculté de Médecine, Chef du Service de Policlinique Chirurgicale Universitaire et Clinique de Longeraie, Lausanne, Switzerland

Clarence W. R. Wade, Ph.D.

Biomaterials and Evaluation Division, United States Army Medical Bioengineering Research and Development Laboratory, Fort Detrick, Frederick, Maryland

PREFACE

The papers contained in this symposium are representative of the efforts of the faculty who participated in the Philadelphia Hand Symposium, March 16-17, 1974, entitled "The Hand: A Decade of Tendon Surgery." This program was sponsored by the Committee on Musculoskeletal Diseases of the American Academy of Orthopaedic Surgeons.

Ten years earlier, on March 11-13, 1964, Drs. Ramsey Straub, the late Herbert Conway, and James Smith of the New York Hospital (Cornell Medical Center) organized an International Hand Symposium focused on tendon surgery in the hand. In the keynote address, Dr. Joseph H. Boyes summarized the problems of tendon surgery. The works of Bunnell, Koch, Mason, Mayer, and others were reviewed and their contributions were related to the knowledge and understanding of hand surgery at that time. Mr. R. Guy Pulvertaft concluded the meeting with his view of tendon surgery of the future. Significantly, those present at the 1964 meeting were impressed by the fact that although surgery of the hand had advanced, especially since World War II, great gaps still existed between our knowledge and successful clinical application. Hand surgery was noted to be progressing toward a regional specialty affording boundless opportunities for future progress. At the termination of the meeting, all agreed that a reassessment 10 years in the future would be a worthwhile project. Papers from the 1964 meeting were published in the *American Journal of Surgery* in March, 1965.

The 1974 Philadelphia meeting was attended by over 500 surgeons and therapists with special interests in hand surgery. Together with a distinguished faculty of 40, they shared a 3-day in-depth study of the tendon problems in the hand. As in 1964, the decision to publish came at the end of the meeting, representing an appeal to preserve for those present, and those not able to attend, the essence of the program.

This symposium contains up-to-date contributions from the research and clinical areas as they relate to tendon surgery in the hand. Tendon nutrition, tendon healing, tendon and tendon sheath anatomy, the status of tendon grafting, preserved tendon homografts, tenolysis, staged reconstruction, artificial tendons, the changing concepts of immediate and delayed tendon repairs, considerations for preoperative and postoperative management, and the hand therapist's view of rehabilitation of the hand after tendon surgery are included. The authors were given freedom to express their viewpoints without editorial restriction. In that respect, this publication represents a departure from the traditional textbook format and is in keeping with the original purposes of the 1974 symposium.

It is a privilege to add as an appendix one paper not presented at the 1974 symposium: "Repair of Tendons in the Fingers" by Sterling Bunnell, reprinted from *Surgery, Gynecology, and Obstetrics* 35:88-97, 1922. All should read this historical paper and ask "How much have we really progressed in the past 50 years?" and "How can we best help those with hand tendon disabilities in the future?"

Finally, we wish to thank the many helping hands that made the 1974 symposium a success and, hence, this publication possible.

James M. Hunter, M.D.
Lawrence H. Schneider, M.D.

CONTENTS

1. The philosophy of tendon surgery

Joseph H. Boyes, M.D.

From the title of this presentation, you might well ask: "Is it possible for a surgeon to be a philosopher?" Yes, it is, if you will accept the definition of a philosopher as one who seeks after the truth. He does not claim to be wise, but only hopes to be wise enough to keep the truth when he finds it.

A surgical philosophy is best called pragmatism. In other words, is it practical? Does it work? In the early days of surgical therapy the knowledge of the treatment of the results of trauma was based on empirical methods that, if they produced results that were satisfactory and that could be obtained by others, were continued and passed on directly from teacher to pupil. In the nineteenth century, knowledge spread widely when the university system of medical schools developed; but a greater influence was felt when surgical journals and periodicals began to be published. Many students were then able to benefit from the writings of the great teachers.

Sir Isaac Newton who, when complimented on his discovery of the law of gravity, replied, "If I have been able to see further, it is because I stood on the shoulders of giants." We have all stood on other's shoulders who have allowed us to see further—Ambroise Paré, Paget, Jones, Little, Adams, Stromeyer, Volkmann, Ollier, Thiersch, Lange, Mayer, Steindler, and Bunnell. We should remember and honor these men who have shown us the way. Let us not be smug about our presumed superior knowledge. René Dubos has said that a simple cure for this deceit is to take a large dose of history. We must consider the time in which they lived and the facilities they had.

William Heberden, the first to describe coronary thrombosis, did not have a stethescope; there was no clinical thermometer. He did not have a clinical laboratory; there was no x-ray machine and no electrocardiogram. Yet he described the symptoms and made the diagnosis, proven at the autopsy done by John Hunter. Duchenne had a little black box with a battery in it; he roamed the wards of the Paris hospitals and made fundamental observations, which we rely on even today. Have we done much better?

Ten years ago there was a meeting, similar to this, in New York. This symposium is called "A Decade of Tendon Surgery" because it follows somewhat the format of that meeting. At that time, I was given the topic "The Problems of Tendon Surgery." I asked for more studies on the normal tendon, its physical structure, its tensile strength, and its blood supply; and the blood supply in various areas and age groups. I asked for more studies on the control of adhesions in tendon repair as well as in grafts. The need for any further study on the use of homogenous or heterogenous grafts was questioned. The idea that we might someday have an artificial tendon was discussed. The value of tenodeses was noted and the old, accepted principles of tendon transfer were reported. These were the problems 10 years ago. I urged our colleagues in the laboratories to develop puzzles that could be solved in an experimental method that would answer some of these questions. When recently reviewing the paper, presented in 1964, I was impressed that many of the questions posed still remain unanswered.

When Scaglietti, the Italian orthopaedist, visited Hong Kong, an elderly Italian missionary nun very proudly showed him the school she had built, the children she was educating, and the hospital she was directing. His response was, "This is wonderful, Sister, but what have you done for Sicily lately?" What have we done for tendon surgery lately?

I want to take you back, not just the one decade to the New York meeting, not three decades to the publication of Bunnell's book, nor even the five decades when his first articles were written. I want to go back 70 years, at a time when most of us were not yet born.

It was in 1903, just 72 years ago, that a symposium, "The Current Status of Tendon Surgery," was held at a meeting of the German Orthopaedic Congress. Professor Vulpius of Heidelberg was the main speaker and was followed by the famous Fritz Lange of Munich. Vulpius said that tendon surgery consisted of procedures for lengthening, shortening, and transplanting tendons. He also said the other part of tendon surgery was the filling of defects. In that day, the term *tendon transplant* was used to describe the procedure we now call *tendon transfer.*

Lengthening of tendons was well known. Lorenz in Vienna had done probably the first Achilles tenotomy for club foot and Delpech of Toulouse had published his work on it about 1816. He lost enthusisam for this operation because of complications from infection. Later he was shot and killed by a patient on whom he had operated for a varicocele and who claimed that he became impotent as a result; a rather severe judgment for alleged malpractice. Stromeyer in Hanover popularized the subcutaneous tenotomy, and in 1836 corrected the crippled foot of W. H. Little. Little returned to England, founded the Royal National Orthopaedic Hospital and trained Adams, who introduced subcutaneous fasciotomy for Dupuytren's contracture.

The healing process in tendons was being argued even then. Sir Stephen Paget, using a rabbit, decided that the ends of the severed tendon united by what he called "nucleated blastema," but Adams used the material from Little's own patients and recorded findings at various times after operation to eventual autopsy. He believed that all healing took place from tissues outside the tendon itself. Does that sound familiar?

Vulpius had hedged. He said he thought that the tendon healing came from what he called the peritendineum, both internal and external. Dr. Lindsay reported earlier at this meeting that perhaps Mason and Shearer in 1932 had seen something in their slides that he is seeing now, that is, some regenerative process from the tendon itself, or at least from the epitenon. Vulpius also described what he called the "mirror-shine" as the smooth glistening appearance of tendon as compared to scar. Dr. Madden showed us a severed flexor carpi radialis tendon that had regenerated into what was clinically effective tendon. But it was a pearly gray color and lacked the typical "mirror-shine." Vulpius in his review described other methods of lengthening a tendon by turning flaps from each end, but said these healed by massive scar tissue.

Tendon shortening procedures consisted of excision with suturing of the ends together. Already the plain over-and-over suture, the simple bite, was considered obsolete. It was agreed that it was necessary to make multiple passes through the tendon. All preferred to bury the knot. Lange used a puckering suture for shortening a tendon, which he described as being similar to that closing a tobacco sack. Codivilla showed that tendon to bone was a much more efficient attachment than tendon to periosteum or tendon to tendon.

What we today call tendon transfers, were referred to as transplantations or grafting. The accepted principle was to reduce the deformity first, then to supply additional motor power by transposing an active muscle-tendon unit. Some made the new attachment side-to-side but often the donor tendon was divided and laid over the recipient tendon where it was sutured in place. Vulpius believed that a donor tendon could be split into two strands that could be inserted separately to provide two distinct functions. Lange disagreed and later Bielsalski was able to show that this was not feasible.

Leo Mayer worked with Bielsalski in Berlin just before World War I, and they authored the 1914 classic on tendon transfers. It was interesting that Vulpius described, as a common procedure, the passage of transferred tendons beneath the fascia and through the interosseous membrane. He had begun to use an aluminum bronze wire suture for the tendons. He said that when formerly using silk, he had much difficulty with the silk being extruded. He agreed that tendon to bone was a strong union and noted that Wolff had passed the tendon deep into the bone and Mueller had passed the tendon through the bone and back, suturing it to itself.

The problem was how to prolong a tendon to obtain a better insertion. Lange had used silk sutures to do this, expecting fibroblasts to grow along these strands and make a new tendon. When Leo Mayer came to work in Lange's clinic, he tried in many ways to prevent the scarring and adherence of these "tendons." He has described in his biography how he experimented with various substances to act as a barrier, using veins, vaseline gauze, cargile membrane—almost anything he could think of. Had silastic been available, I am sure he would have tried it also. It was the failure in this attempt that led him to the association with Bielsalski in Berlin.

The audience was familiar with the work of Franke whose original transfers were done for radial palsy. They knew about Tubby's operation for redirection of the pronator teres. The accepted the principle that a transferred muscle-tendon unit functions whether you call it a synergist or an antagonist.

Free grafts, autogenous and homogenous, had been tried but failed. Lange said the biggest problem was the foreign body reaction to the silk being used. He called attention to a report of 400 tendon repairs on Vulpius' service, in which 25% later had extrusion of the silk. His results of only 2% of this complication, he felt, were better because of a technical difference and not because of sepsis. He said that although Vulpius used only a cap and cotton gloves while he used a cap, mask, and rubber gloves, the fact that he drained his wounds with a gauze wick dipped in 1:1,000 bichloride of mercury solution made the difference. He gave credit to a young assistant for a technical trick you have seen used. When a plaster dressing is to be applied over a wound in which there is a drain, fasten a long suture to the drain and let it come out above the plaster. The drain can then be withdrawn from the wound without disturbing the dressing or the immobilization.

That was a meeting 72 years ago. What do we do today? We have better suture material, better control of sepsis, and more success with free grafts. The concept of the bridge graft contributed by Bunnell has helped in lengthening of tendons, but are we not using essentially the same technics? If those surgeons had our materials and our facilities, their results would undoubtedly equal ours.

As was said 10 years ago, we need to know more about the normal tendon and particularly its blood supply. We need to know more about the healing process, how to promote the good aspects of it such as the union of the ends, and how to prevent the bad parts of it such as the formation of dense scar that binds the tendon and interferes with the gliding mechanism. This knowledge can only come from the experimental surgeons, men who have the imagination and skills to set up programs with proper controls and arrive at logical conclusions. But we in the clinical field can contribute also. It was the cumulative experience of clinical surgeons at the turn of the century that gave us the basis for what we are doing today. We can follow their example by making accurate observations, recording our findings and results carefully and in detail, and arriving at our conclusions honestly and logically. Dr. Steindler said there was no place for partisanship and bias in surgery or in surgical writings. Every detail may be an important factor in the solution of a problem. Let us stop publishing the propaganda articles.

There is a period in the early stages of a science when the literature consists of the description of phenomena, of recorded observations, and of case reports.

This clinical period is then succeeded by a period of unifying theories and setting up the hypotheses to be tested. Fortunately we have a few men who have passed to this second level, but are not most of us still in that early clinical period? Are not most of our journals full of descriptions of things we see, case reports, and anecdotal and unquantitated testimonials? There is no objection to the writing of these reports. The value is in the writing, as the author learns the most. It's a marvelous exercise for your residents because it is a form of education, but the report does not have to be published. The collection of data, the careful argument, and logical conclusions reached tell us when the writer has matured. In Dr. Steindler's library there were over 50 unpublished manuscripts.

Ten years ago Mr. Pulvertaft, speaking on the future of tendon surgery, quoted Lord Byron who said the best prophet of the future is in the past. We have looked over a little of the past and found its problems to be still with us. Perhaps we can now embark on the second phase of our special field, and with the clinical findings we have collected develop the hypotheses to be tested. It is not a scientific experiment when you do an operation or modify someone's procedure just to see what will happen. But if you study the problem thoroughly, being familiar with what has been done before, and if you feel that a certain change might be beneficial and most important, that it has no chance of doing harm, then do it under the best conditions and with proper control of all possible factors. You now have a prospective study that will be of value to others when it is reported honestly and without bias. From reports like these, it is then possible that the experimental surgeon in the laboratory will be able to develop the necessary puzzles, the hypotheses, to test and we will see some progress in our search for the truth.

A philosophy may be said to consist of four parts—ethics, logic, aesthetics, and metaphysics. Ethics means the aim, which for our purposes implies providing the best care for our patient by promoting the ideal healing of the damaged tendons. Logic is the approach to that aim by the best methods available. Aesthetics means an appreciation of the beauty and function of the parts. What is more remarkable than this hand of ours with its intricate design, marvelous mechanism, and exquisite sensibility? Metaphysics, from the Greek *meta* meaning beyond, can be interpreted as something beyond the physical, something beyond our present state of knowledge. It is the unknown that we seek, and though each small success seems only to show us that there is more beyond, we must keep trying. And that is what philosophy is; seeking, seeking, always seeking.

2. The decades of tendon surgery

Claude E. Verdan, M.D.

Tendon surgery is as old as surgery itself. Instead of speaking of decades, we ought to say centuries and even millenia for it is clear that the Aesculapii of all times had to treat this kind of wound.

In modern literature we find thousands of papers referring to tendon surgery, confirming the rule existing in science: the more papers written on a certain subject, the less we know about that subject. When something is definitely clear, one does not need to have more than one or two papers to bring the fact into evidence.

During the period of World War I, which so tremendously stimulated the development of modern surgery, two great American schools, one at San Francisco with Sterling Bunnell and his disciples like Boyes and Howard, the other one in Chicago with Kanavel, Sumner Koch, Mason and their followers, called the world's attention to the importance of hand surgery. These pioneers had to fight against old habits and outdated techniques. They understood that we had to avail ourselves of new instruments, a peculiar technique, smooth movements—what Bunnell called atraumatic surgery—for this both delicate and powerful organ, the hand. Even today, atraumatic surgery is not always achieved by all those who work in hand surgery.

But knowledge blooms because of the hundreds and thousands who precede us. The course of this scientific development shows a tremendous acceleration. For us hand surgeons, that has been made manifest by the ever-growing number of members of the International Federation of Societies for Surgery of the Hand.

One of the major problems concerning us has always been and continues to be the repair of flexor tendons in the digital canal. There are, of course, many other problems involving tendon surgery, particularly in regard to the delicate extensor apparatus. But compared with the flexors, unsatisfactory results of these other conditions have not so many serious issues. A failure in repairing flexor tendons may be equivalent to an amputation.

Upon considering the fact that primary flexor tendon sutures in the digital canal, performed as an emergency procedure was nearly always a failure, Bunnell and his followers gave us the following rules:

1. When both flexors are severed in the so called no-man's-land, close the skin and let the wound heal. After 3 weeks, perform a *secondary procedure* consisting of removing the two flexor tendons. Abandon the proximal sublimis stump, or use it as a graft. Graft the profundus alone (generally with a palmaris longus, plantaris, or toe-extensor) from far above in the palm, at the lumbrical level, to the digital tip in order to avoid any callus formation in the narrow digital theca, where the tendon must glide like a piston in its cylinder. If the proximal profundus stump is not mobile, use the sublimis as a motor, perhaps from the wrist level to the digital tip.

2. If the profundus alone has been severed, never sacrifice an intact sublimis to repair the profundus. Carry out a tenodesis of the distal stump or an arthrodesis at the distal interphalangeal (DIP) joint, to shun instability and hyperextension of the distal phalanx.

3. If the profundus has been severed near its distal insertion (up to 1.5 cm.), perform an advancement procedure, removing the short-end stump, and reinsert the proximal stump onto the bony terminal phalanx, using a pull-out wire.

I very conscientiously applied these rules during the earlier years of my career. The results were often disappointing. Some results were good, some bad, with success and failure being unpredictable. However, as a general rule, if collateral nerves and arteries are severed together with the tendons, the dystrophic changes and vascular disorders will be an important cause of failure. The same is true, of course, in cases where associated lesions are present, such as fractures, the opening of a joint capsule, combined lesions of the extensor apparatus, crushed skin, any impairment of the suppleness and flexibility of the finger, or any injury that demands a long period of immobilization and ensuing stiffness.

It should be remembered that a tendon wound is not to be considered as a mere division of a tendon, but as a whole trauma. Tidy, clean cuts are considerably different from crushed and torn injuries, toward which particular rules must be applied.

Over 25 years have elapsed since the time when I thought it was in fact possible, under specific circumstances, to make primary sutures of flexor tendons inside the digital synovial canal, thus taking a stand against the recommended usage of always doing secondary tendon grafts within the famed no-man's-land.

My first paper was presented in Chicago, 1959.[8] Michael Mason was entrusted with the discussion that followed. Unexpectedly, his comments were rather favorable, though that paper looked to many like a terrorist bomb! Two years later, in the main report presented at the French Society for Orthopaedic Surgery in 1961,[10] in Paris, I proposed with Michon to abandon the too exclusive denomination of no-man's-land and to introduce seven topographic surgical zones, no-man's-land corresponding since then to zone 2.

I would like to try to judge the results connected with that stand of mine and to draw up its various consequences:

1. Those among my colleagues who were the fiercest in fighting my opinions became, and have remained, my best friends. Joseph Boyes, Guy Pulvertaft, William Littler, and Eric Moberg were tenacious defenders of the graft and did not accept the suture.

2. My experiences occurred in very peculiar conditions in a private department, receiving patients from nearby areas and frequently within minutes after an accident.

3. The wounded were first operated upon by myself; I was living in the building containing the Emergency Service, and so was available at any time following the arrival of the patient.

Later on, after outstanding young associates were formed, such as Simonetta, Narakas, Cantero, and others, we were able to disperse several teams of hand surgeons sharing the days and nights of vigil, so that operations could be performed in emergency by people trained for such delicate surgery.

4. The postoperative follow-up and rehabilitation periods were watched over by the same surgeon in our own department of physical therapy and functional rehabilitation.

5. The kind of injury—and I have emphasized this point since the beginning—was mainly the cutting, tidy, and sharp type, rather than the crushing, bursting, or lacerating type, that is so frequently seen in big industrial centers.

6. Those who adopted our standpoint, like Michon in Nancy, Duparc in Paris, Iselin father and son, Bolton in England, and above all, Kleinert in Louisville, Kentucky, have worked within similar circumstances. Our and their results have come to point this out: a *suture*, correctly performed with an adequate technique can bring results equivalent to or slightly better than those of a *graft*, at a lower cost. Time can be saved for the patient, the period of disability shortened, and hospitalization reduced or even eliminated.

7. Nevertheless, I must admit that when these specific operations are performed in a poorly furnished emergency room by young residents, less trained, less supervised, less accurate, less demanding, the final outcome also tends to be far less gratifying. I have also observed that when the first repair has been performed badly, it compromises and jeopardizes the whole future of the digit. I have wondered, therefore, if I was altogether right in creating that new dogma of the primary suture. On those occasions, I remember all the points set up in their defense by Boyes and Pulvertaft. They become like living reproaches, and I feel that I ought to beg their pardon.

Actually conditions sine qua non of such surgery are: perfect anatomical knowledge, good anesthesia, soft and fine technique, intact tissues, very exacting suture comparable with that of a nerve, good hemostasis, very well-fitted dressing, excellent postoperative care, and preciseness of functional rehabilitation. In short, one needs everything that has rendered hand surgery what it is or aims at being: a complete specialty.

Maybe it will become mandatory in future years to utilize magnifying glasses or even the microscope to ensure technical exactitude, which too many still consider of little importance and a sort of wild talk by old dotards! We have witnessed the same trend in the field of peripheral nerve surgery.

That being said, a surgeon working upon a tendon ought to realize several basic principles, which have always been true but have taken a clearer shape and a deeper meaning through these last decades:

1. Whoever is confronted with a tendon repair should never be content with a strong and firm suture, for the main characteristic of a tendon is *gliding*.

2. A tendon is a living organ; no one should be deceived by its whitish hue and its smooth and gleaming appearance. Flexor tendons are provided with an extremely delicate system of nutrition, as shown by James Smith[1] and Howard Caplan (Chapter 5). It affords their gliding within a fibrous sheath, as perfectly fitted as a piston in its cylinder, along a surprisingly long distance, ranging from 4 cm. at the base of the fingers to 8 cm. at the wrist.

3. This nutritional system is ensured by mesotenons and vincula whose wounding is tantamount to a tendon infarct. Actually arterial and venous blood is relatively scarce within a tendon, but the lymphatic network—as I have shown with Setti[7] of Parma—is abundant. That perhaps explains the maintenance of a low but constant cellular metabolism, preserving the life of the rare tenocytes we can see.

4. The masterful experiment of Peacock[5] has shown that nutrition brought about by mesotenons is far more important than that produced by the musculotendinous junction or the osseotendinous distal insertion. This accounts for the phenomenon that when a tendon segment is deprived of blood supply along a certain length, it can only recover its nutrition, which is its life, by being invaded with connective tissue, full of newly created capillaries coming from the sheath, or from adjacent tissues if the sheath is wounded or absent.

The same is true for callus formation, which cannot be expected from the tendon ends, but only from the surrounding tissues. In other words, the so-called unsatisfied fibers are not growing out of the tendon ends, but rather are growing into them. The capillary buds try to connect themselves with the intratendinous blood and lymph network, either by means of what remains of the mesotenon (as has been experimentally shown by Potenza), and of course in that case gliding is better preserved, or by pushing massively across the epitenon along a much greater length. We have then the vessel-carrier adhesion that blocks any further gliding.

Can we imagine a more tragic destiny for a tendon, whose genius is in gliding? It has but one alternative; either it dies or it lives, but remains blocked by its adhesions. Therefore, as it must first live ("primum vivere"!), we must accept the inevitable adhesions. We have, then, two possibilities:

1. To excise part of the fibrous sheath in order to constrain adhesions to grow from as many soft tissues as possible and permit their gradual reabsorption by physical exercises.

2. To make a secondary tenolysis, which can be a very effective procedure. This is true for both sutures and grafts.

There is an important moment from the clinical and therapeutic standpoint. When the cast has been removed, the surgeon should be concerned with breaking recent fibrous adhesions. The surgeon should not only ask the patient to flex and extend alternately the digit at each joint, gently restrained by the examiner's hand, but he should himself perform a number of careful passive motions, designed to detach the adhesions. A little noise may be perceivable, as of crumpled paper. The patient is then able to actively move that phalanx better than before. It is a somewhat painful contrivance, but surely worthwhile. We have no more than one or two weeks, namely the fourth and fifth postoperative weeks, to free the digit from this kind of fresh adhesion. Then the rehabilitation begins, entrusted to good physical therapists and afterwards to the patient himself, when he has resumed his daily job, usually in 5 or 6 weeks instead of several months as in grafting.

Summing up, if the operative act is paramount, the postoperative care is no less important in this succession of therapeutic acts and controls.

I do not adhere exclusively to the procedure of primary suture I have described. If other techniques are inspired by the same principle, I gladly accept them.

Kleinert's idea, one of the new elements that have been developed in the last decade, has been realized thanks to the new advances made with suture material.

A primary, modified, Bunnell lacing suture, completed with a 7-0 continuous epitendinous nylon suture, is needed that is strong enough to dispense with having to block up the tendon for longer than the few minutes necessary for performing the suture. But too powerful and too long a movement by the tendon should be prevented with a device controlling posture through splinting. The wrist is half flexed, and the finger is flexed with an elastic band fixed through the fingernail and fastened to the immobilizing cast in the palm. Therefore the patient can perform only a very weak active flexion with the injured finger (just try it yourself!). On the other hand, and chiefly when he actively extends the finger, the respective flexor muscle is forcefully relaxed, thus slackening the sutured tendon so that its suture will be submitted to a minimum of traction. The same would have been sufficient, however, to break my own tiny sutures. With the fine but firm material utilized by Kleinert, there is no rupture and no gap. The two stumps are likely to be facing each other with less precision than with my technique, but something else is probably gained, and that is *immediate motion.*

Here we are meeting with one of the most controversial topics of all tendon surgery of these last decades. It came up even before Mason's and Allen's experiences[4]: should we use a system of strong sutures, to mobilize early, without any risk of tearing them out, or should we put our sutures to rest during the first 3 weeks, and wait until the tendinous callus becomes steady enough to resist rupture and so avoid any gap?

This essential alternative is true for both sutures and grafts. For the latter, Pulvertaft has demonstrated that results were nearly the same, nonetheless slightly in favor of the immobilized cases.

As for the sutures, Mason and Allen had drawn the conclusion, from their experiments upon animals, that early mobilization was not only useless but harmful. It actually accounted for an exuberant tendon callus and more adhesions. So the ideal time of immobilization was about 3 weeks because of various changes of structure inside the healing tendon.

Now, is the truth from the decade 1940-1950 still in force for the decade 1970-1980? I am personally tempted to think that the truth is to be found halfway between the two opposite stands.

If our techniques enable us to avoid the gaps observed by Lindsay on tendons of the chicken, it also seems logical that some slight movement can become useful. They may cause the vessel-carrier adhesions to arrange themselves in a more orderly fashion. Shortly after being formed, the adhesions that lie on the anterior and lateral aspects of the tendon will keep breaking gradually, as the mobilization continues. But the connective buds originating on the dorsum, chiefly along the posterior track, where the mesotenons penetrate, will probably be lengthened, allowing the necessary blood and lymph vessels to unite with their intratendinous fellows. Practically speaking, these vessel-carrier adhesions are reconstructing mesotenons at their strategic anatomical locations.

Yet, another side of that problem still remains to be considered. When both flexor tendons are divided within zone 2, we take for granted that the superficialis will have to be removed in order to give more room to the profundus, and that the latter alone will be sutured. That is also the way we generally proceed with grafts of the profundus (on condition, of course, that the superficialis has also been severed, since if one finds it intact, he will never destroy it on behalf of a hypothetical profundus repair).

Now, the mesotenons and vincula that supply the profundus at the level of the proximal phalanx cross the superficialis. If the latter is resected, precious vincula are being torn away, thus depriving the profundus of its supplies. Potenza has shown experimentally that by grafting the profundus, the results were better when the distal stump of the sublimis was left in place rather than excised. That is also why we have set out in Lausanne to repair *both* flexor tendons in emergency situations. The premises being theoretical, we were very anxious to know the outcome. Well, these last results have been the best of all our series.[9]

So, after a long way round, our present philosophy for clean, sharp, and tidy wounds, seen under good general and local conditions in very plain and straightforward language is *to immediately repair every severed structure,* namely the *tendons,* the *nerves,* and in the future maybe also *collateral vessels,* if one has the indispensable training in microsurgery.

If the wound is crushed, if the general and local conditions are bad, or it no specialized surgeon is available, gently excise the wound margins, close the skin, and let somebody *who knows how* do a secondary procedure.

An important thing that happened during the decade 1960-1970 is the possibility, demonstrated by Peacock and Madden,[6] and confirmed by Hueston,[2] of transplanting, from cadavers, composite tissue allografts of the whole flexor mechanism—the intact sheath with both tendons. The practical consequence would be the creation of tendon banks from lyophilized material.

During the present decade, I have searched for really new ideas and new possibilities. I found 71 papers from 1971 to 1973 dealing with:

Barbwire and immediate mobilization
Injection of fluid silicone
Enveloping tendon suture with millipore sheaths
Silicone rubber sheaths
Pedicled tendon transfer
Delayed primary suture
Primary tendon grafting
Freeze-dried homografts and allografts

There is also an interesting paper by Wilson and Hueston[11] on the intratendinous anatomical architecture of flexor tendons. Different approaches to our problem are now on the way, especially chemobiologic and experimental studies.

But the biggest step taken in our *present decade* concerns the reconstruction of a new tendon sheath,[3] by means of artificial implants, or the implantation of a definitive tendon prosthesis. These new techniques bring us a great hope in this type of surgery, and that is the salvage of badly wounded digits, for which we formerly would have had to admit defeat. To paraphrase your astronaut Armstrong: "A little step for a man; a giant step for tendon surgery."

So we see that what is too frequently called minor surgery, what is still looked upon with some disregard by surgical teams of general surgeons, this surgery is actually a difficult and highly specialized field. It cannot be left to young interns, so that they may make their first campaign. This surgery is designed for the more skilled among us. It has to be taught with competence and order and it has to be sternly learned! It comes within the scope of a most desirable specialization, resulting in a title of Specialist in Surgery of the Hand or a Board of Hand Surgery, for the sake of which the *coming decade* will have to fight.

References

1. Conway, H., Smith, J. W., and Elliott, M. P.: Studies on the revascularization of tendons grafted by the silicone rod technique, Plast. Reconstr. Surg. **46**:582-587, 1970.
2. Hueston, J. T., et al.: Homografts of the digital flexor tendon system, Aust. N. Z. J. Surg. **36**:269-274, 1967.
3. Hunter, J. M., Salem, A. W., Steindel, C. R., and Salisbury, R. E.: The use of gliding artificial tendon implants to form new tendon beds, J. Bone Joint Surg. **51A**:790, 1969.
4. Mason, M. L., and Allen, H. S.: The rate of healing of tendons; An experimental study of tensile strength, Ann. Surg. **113**:424-459, 1941.

5. Peacock, E. E.: A study of the circulation in normal tendons and healing grafts, Ann. Surg. **149**:415-428, 1959.
6. Peacock, E. E., Jr., and Madden, J. W.: Human composite flexor tendon allografts, Ann. Surg. **166**:624-629, 1967.
7. Setti, G. C., and Verdan, C. E.: A study of the lymphatic circulation in flexor tendons. In Proceedings of the 12th Congress of the Sicot. Tel Aviv, Oct. 9-12, 1972. Amsterdam, 1973, Excerpta Medica.
8. Verdan, C.: Primary repair of flexor tendons, J. Bone Joint Surg. **42-A**(4):647-657, 1960.
9. Verdan, C. E., and Crawford, G. P.: Flexor tendon suture in the digital canal. In Fifth World Congress of Plastic and Reconstructive Surgery, London, 1971, Butterworth & Company (Publishers) Ltd.
10. Verdan, C., et Michon, J.: Le traitement des plaies des tendons fléchisseurs des dogits, Rev. Chir. Orthop. **47**(3):285-425, 1961.
11. Wilson, J. S. P., and Hueston, J. T.: Personal information, Melbourne, 1971.

3. A finger points toward tomorrow

Lee Milford, M.D.

A finger points toward tomorrow with the hope that tomorrow may bring an expanded, yet a more clearly defined identification of the hand surgeon. Hand surgery has *always* been in our midst in one form or another, but the surgeon has not *always* been called a hand surgeon.

He may have been responsible for treating the amputated fingers drawn on the cave walls in Altamira and Lascaux some 5,000 years B.C.; that treatment may have been a mud cake dressing or cauterization with charcoal from the family campfire. He was possibly a chieftain, a priest, and a doctor combined. These individual roles had not been separated nor defined. Even during the time before Christ, the priest made decisions concerning health problems. One such decision related to leprosy; the inquirer was advised, concerning a possible skin lesion, that he must be shut up for 7 days and after this quarantine be examined again for complete healing before again joining his tribe and family. Leprosy is still the greatest crippler of hands today. When a cure, "miracle," was accomplished the person was directed to go and show himself to the priest first. He could then be accepted in their community once again through the authority of the priest who declared him healed: just as now, you as a hand surgeon may report that a patient may return to work safely and take his productive place in our society earning a living again for his family.

Over 100 years ago the hand surgeon, and still unnamed as such, performed such things as tendon transfers for paralysis, skin grafts for surface defects, and appreciated at times the tremendously prolonged disability of an apparent simple fracture in a capital joint such as the base of the thumb. These all took place before the 20th century. It was later that Kanavel realized the enormity of the destruction of function of the hand by infection, and how this was accentuated by the unfortunate severance of nerves and tendons by the unknowing surgeon attempting to drain these infections without sufficient knowledge of anatomy. These people were all acting as hand surgeons but were not identified as such by *name*. A name implies identification with those qualities or values and characteristics to which one ascribes.

Between birth and death, an Indian may have four different names, these names being changed at critical times of life such as birth, puberty, a notable feat, and retirement. At birth, he may have been known as just "Boy." He may have obtained a more identifying name when he had assumed some characteristics suggesting something fitting such as "Brave Warrior." It is interesting to note that the name may be mistranslated. A name given after battle may be properly translated "Recklessly Brave" but is frequently incorrectly translated "Crazy Brave." The leader of the Creek opposition was officially named "Crazy Snake." Misconception also makes for poor understanding such as the name "Tahaibadal," which is literally translated "Stinking Saddle Blanket." It is not a perverse name, but honorable since it really means that the brave was on the warpath so continuously that he did not have time to take off his saddle blanket. This change of name implied a past accomplishment or feat that earned him the honor of his name. It did identify him, but it did not give him authority. Now what about authority?

God charged Moses to go back to his people and lead them out of Egypt; then Moses said to God, "If I came to the people of Israel and said to them 'The God of your father sent me to you,' and they asked me 'What is his name that sends you?'—What shall I say to them?" God said to Moses "I am who I am and I am what I am and I will be what I will be." This answer of identity implies eternity with both past and future, and enjoins unlimited authority. He also pointed out that he was the same in the past, the same God of Abraham, Isaac, and Jacob but his name was now Yahweh.

Historically, the surgeon has been performing hand surgery but not under the name of hand surgeon. Historical advances have been made in this specific area that helped to better identify these proficient area specialists, but further identification is necessary. Authority cannot be presumed. By what authority can one who performs surgery on the hand and its more proximal dependent parts be called a hand surgeon? The authority comes in part from the heritage of special accomplishments. Certainly in the immediate past the need for such a specialty surgeon was recognized by some as exemplified by the formation of hand surgery centers during World War II. These centers were staffed by those persons especially interested in hand surgery. Because of the special problems, and the interest and efforts necessary to solve these problems, experience and knowledge were gained and they were eventually recognized as authorities; yet they were still not called hand surgeons except by a few. The formation of an organziation by these experienced authoritative few helped to identify hand surgery more than any other single feat—the American Society for Surgery of the Hand.

During the past 25 years, special interest by this group promoted, in the large field but small geographic area such ideas as the neorovascular island skin flaps, which at the time of their resurrection were considered avant-garde. This single stage graft of skin and fat with a built-in blood and nerve supply was dramatic and remarkable. The appreciation of the exquisite sensibility of the hand has been slow in diffusion, but none is better prepared to comprehend it as thoroughly as the hand surgeon. The revelation of the importance of sensibility helped to explain the extremely poor results from tendon transfers and tendon grafts in an anesthetic finger or hand.

The development of special instruments and the borrowing of a few from other groups such as the ophthalmologists has made surgery easier to perform in this field of low tolerance for surgical trauma. The application of the production assembly line technique to our surgical technique, by studying time and motion engineering, has resulted in lowering the operative time by more than 50%. Most of you will not remember that it was not unusual to spend 3½ hours doing a complicated Dupuytren's contracture, neither was it unusual to spend more than 3 hours doing a tendon graft. The ideal sitting height, lighting, and stabilization of the operative field all have diminished the surgeon's fatigue and increased operative efficiency tremendously. The mere emphasis of learning detailed anatomy and especially functional anatomy has enabled more accurate surgery and more accurate diagnosis.

Hand surgeon as an identifying name is now emerging in the eyes of medical colleagues and the American public, for advancements have now been made in this type of surgery. For these advancements, the hand surgeon receives due credit and respect. Recently such accomplishments as internal prostheses for tendons and joints, chemical surgery, and microsurgery have placed the hand surgeon in an authoritative role. This is not obtained by one who just has a special interest, but he must also have the special training. Such technique as microvascular surgery enabling limb reattachment was a natural for the hand surgeon. He soon became an expert since he already had the necessary basic training for this technique.

More than a dozen countries outside the United States have national organizations oriented toward advancement of hand surgery. These are now organized under an International Federation of Hand Surgical Societies. This has enabled the production of many modes of communication that permit a more easily understood transference of knowledge and information. A booklet on standard nomenclature is one of these, enabling better understanding in functional anatomy; another is the universal evaluation of disability due to lost function.

Now what are the dreams and the future roles of the hand surgeon with this impressive past history? Will we ever solve the lacerated tendon problem in the critical areas? I think we will. Will we be able to immediately close a wound from top to bottom without pain and swelling? Will we be able to hold a fracture with unquestionable stability that enables immediate movement and avoids stiffness but permits natural healing? Will we be able to promote growth by transferring a living epiphysis from the same individual or even from another individual? This epiphyseal transfer would be in the province of microvascular surgery. It is only one step further down the line from the already possible procedure of taking a free composite graft from the lateral thigh to the hand in only one stage, reattach its blood vessels, and obtain immediate continued viability and coverage.

Will the hand surgeon ever fully realize and evaluate the psychological impact that the patient has when suddenly being wrought with a severe hand injury? The patient soon realizes the severe personal and social implications this carries for him. Very little has been written concerning the patient who becomes psychotic following this impact. I have personally had three that were rendered overt or borderline psychotic. This is just as important a consideration as an insulin dosage in the diabetic about to undergo major surgery.

These are all in the domain of the hand surgeon. The finger that points toward tomorrow is the finger of the hand surgeon. He has identified himself well by his accomplishments in the past, his exciting activities of the present, and his dreams of the future.

4. Concepts of tendon healing and repair*

Austin D. Potenza, M.D.

Flexor tendon injuries in the hand are among the most potentially serious and troublesome problems a surgeon is called upon to treat. They often result in severe and permanent functional disability. The results of their surgical treatment are highly variable and relatively, if not absolutely, unpredictable with regard to an individual case. The postoperative care of such injuries requires the continuing and utmost attention to detail on the part of the surgeon, and an unfailing and untiring effort on the part of the patient in performing arduous active exercises, often for many months. The emotional burden on the patient and the family, as well as the financial burden imposed by inability to work, can wreak havoc on their entire social and economic well-being.

Any unified and logical approach to the management of flexor tendon injuries must be based on a thorough understanding of the mechanisms of flexor tendon healing and the various factors that influence those mechanisms. Over the last 15 years, extensive experimental studies have been conducted on the mechanisms of flexor tendon healing within the flexor digital sheath. These studies have been conducted in the dog and have been correlated with clinical observation and surgical application of the principals adduced from these studies.

EXPERIMENTAL METHODS AND TECHNIQUES

The results reported in this paper and the conclusion drawn from those results are based on extensive experiments on the mechanisms of healing of digital flexor tendons within the canine digital flexor sheath. The dog was selected as the experimental subject since the flexor-tendon mechanism in the canine forefoot is comparable to that in the human hand. Each digit contains both a flexor digitorum profundus tendon and a flexor digitorum sublimis tendon, which are enclosed in a synovial sheath that extends from a point in the paw immediately proximal to the metacarpophalangeal joint to the insertion of the profundus tendon into the distal phalanx. The sublimis tendon divides into two slips that are inserted into the base of the middle phalanx. Each tendon is enclosed

*All figures in this chapter courtesy Medical Audio Visual Dept., Walter Reed Army Institute of Research, Washington, D. C.

in an inelastic osseofibrous tunnel at the metacarpophalangeal joint quite comparable to the pulley mechanism found at this level in the human finger. Two further distinct annular ligaments or pulleys are contained within each flexor digital sheath, one at the level of the midpoint of the proximal phalanx and the other at the level of the proximal third of the middle phalanx. Within the digital sheath the tendons are not connected to the synovial layer of the sheath by a continuous mesotenon; rather, the profundus and sublimis tendons have vincula comparable to those of the human finger. One triangular vinculum brevum connects the dorsal surface of the profundus tendon to the synovial membrane overlying the distal phalanx at the insertion of the tendon. Two more vincula breve join the two slips of the sublimis tendon to the synovial membrane overlying the bony phalanx. The single remaining vinculum-like connection of either tendon is found at the proximal end of the flexor sheath in the paw, where the synovial layer of the sheath is reflected onto the sublimis tendon and the profundus tendon is enfolded within the sheath. The profundus tendon is thus attached to the synovial membrane of the digital sheath only at the extreme ends of the latter. It otherwise lies free of any connections within the sheath.

In each experiment, an atraumatic technique[8] was used to manipulate and divide the flexor profundus tendons. No tendon was ever held by forceps or other piercing or crushing instruments except in those experiments related to the effects of trauma to the surface of the tendon in regard to the mechanisms of tendon healing. A standard wound was employed throughout, a fact attested to by the consistent reproducibility of results.

BASIC HEALING MECHANISMS OF FLEXOR PROFUNDUS TENDONS

Digital flexor tendons (profundus tendons) divided and repaired within the flexor digital sheath (no-man's-land) are healed by the cellular activity of the sheath and surrounding tissues and not by any instrinsic tenoblastic response of their own; rather, they heal by the proliferative cellular (fibroblastic) and vascular response of surrounding tissues whose own integrity has been violated either by accidental injury or by surgery (another, although specific, form of injury). The tenocytes of tendon proper play no active role in the repair of tendon. As the healing process begins after the division and repair of the tendon, the synovial layer of the digital sheath in the immediate vicinity of the wound disrupts by cellular proliferation. Granulation tissue derived from the synovial sheath grows between the ends of the severed flexor tendons and into the suture tracts in the tendons as well. This disruption of the synovial layer of the sheath in the vicinity of the tendon wound is complete by the fourth or fifth postoperative day. Thereafter, the synovial cell layer of the sheath is gradually restored. This latter process begins on approximately the fourteenth postoperative day and reaches completion by the twenty-first postoperative day. At this point, a new synovial gliding surface surrounds the tendon except for persistent filmy adhesions to the tendon at the immediate site of tendon repair.

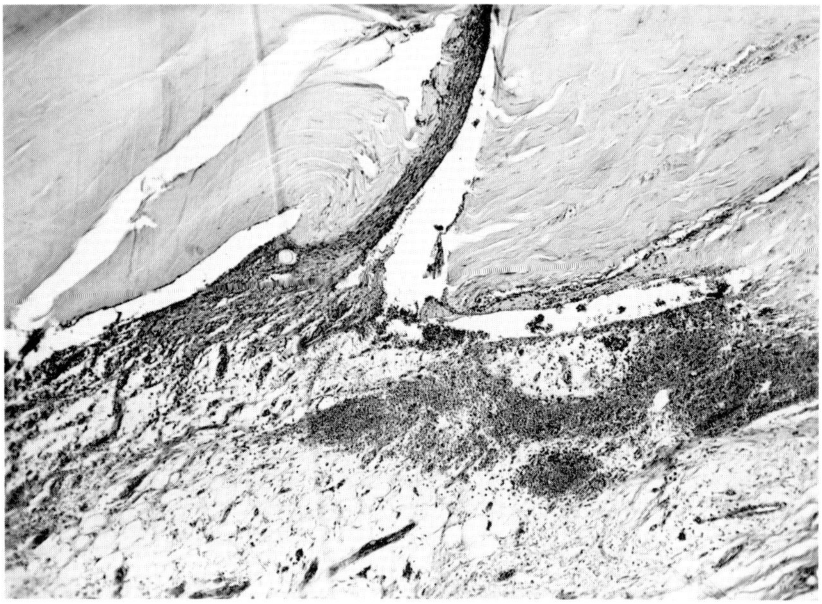

Fig. 4-1. Longitudinal microscopic section of primarily repaired profundus tendon within the flexor sheath at 9 days postoperatively showing growth of fibroblasts from the sheath between the tendon ends (hematoxylin and eosin ×21).

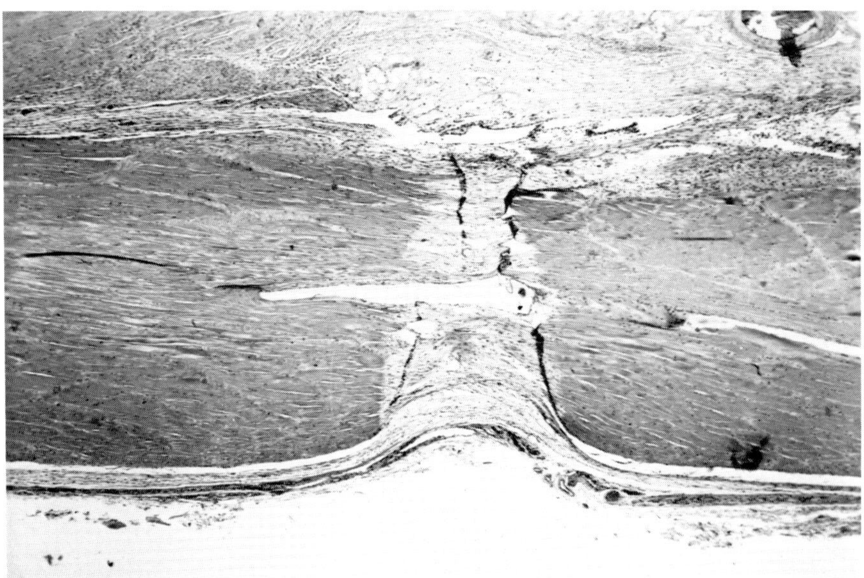

Fig. 4-2. Longitudinal microscopic section of repaired profundus tendon within the flexor sheath at 28 days postoperatively showing longitudinal oriented wound collagen and very sparse adhesions at anastomosis site (hematoxylin and eosin ×29).

Granulation tissue

The formation of reparative granulation tissue (capillary buds and fibroblasts) begins on the fourth postoperative day, following proliferation of the synovial cells of the flexor sheath. This granulation tissue engulfs the tendon wound and ultimately grows between the tendon ends and into the suture tracts in the tendon. Fine, young collagen fibers appear in this granulation tissue on or about the seventh postoperative day, and by the tenth postoperative day this granulation tissue has a distinct fibroblastic character (Fig. 4-1). The fibroblasts that initially grow into the wound between the tendon stumps lie in a plane perpendicular to the long axis of the tendon, and the collagen fibers that they produce are similarly oriented. In contrast, the collagen fibers laid down in granulation tissue on the surface of the tendon are deposited parallel to that surface. By the twenty-first postoperative day, the fibroblasts in the wound scar between the tendon ends begin to orient themselves in line with the longitudinal axis of the tendon, and by the twenty-eighth postoperative day this process is complete so that all the fibroblasts, as well as the new collagen fibers in the tendon wound, are aligned with the long axis of the tendon (Fig. 4-2).

Collagen fiber formation

The newly deposited collagen fibers in the tendon wound scar remain separate, though parallel, fibers until approximately the ninetieth postoperative day, when collagen bundle formation begins. This formation continues so that by 112 days after division and repair of the tendon, the collagen in the former scar between the tendon ends is now in the form of bundles identical microscopically with those of the original tendon.

Wound maturation

Although ultimately there is complete maturation of the collagen in the tissue between the repaired tendon ends, so that one can no longer discern a true tendon wound, the collagen in the persisting filmy adhesions attached to the line of tendon repair remains sparse, delicate, and loose, and does not interfere with the functional integrity of the tendon.

From the above it is clear that digital flexor tendons are apparently passive in the matter of their own healing after division. The synovial sheath tissues and/or the subcutaneous tissues, by giving rise to fibroblasts and capillary buds, are the active healing agents.

USE OF BLOCKING MATERIALS OR "CUFFS" ABOUT SITES OF FLEXOR TENDON REPAIR

The results noted above and the conclusions derived from them were further vertified by experiments[10] in which flexor tendon wounds were excluded from intimate contact with the synovial sheath and other surrounding tissues by poly-

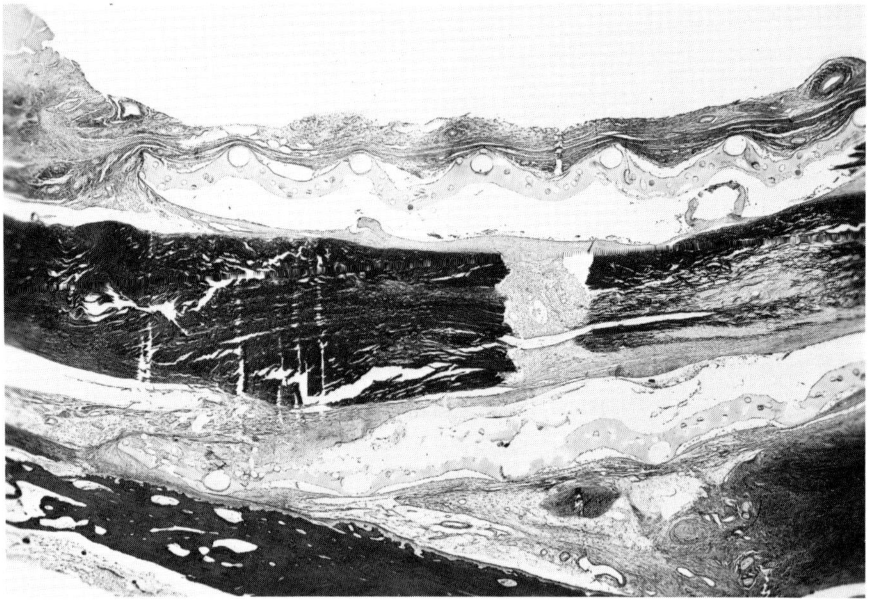

Fig. 4-3. Longitudinal microscopic section of repaired profundus tendon within millipore tube at 30 days postoperatively showing that the granulation tissue necessary for tendon healing has grown beneath the edges of the tubing along the tendon surfaces to finally reach the wound site (Reinhart's ×10.4).

ethylene and/or millipore* tubes. When a repaired profundus tendon was blocked from contact with the sheath and other surrounding tissues, the tendon would not unite until reparative granulation tissue from the sheath and surrounding tissues grew beneath the ends of the interposition or blocking tube, along the tendon surface, finally to reach the wound site (Fig. 4-3). Tendon healing was thus delayed precisely by the time required for the granulation tissue to reach the area of repair, regardless of whether polyethylene or millipore tubes were employed. Moreover, there was no detectable intrinsic tenoblastic response on the part of the repaired tendon within the tubes. The ultimate filmy adhesions normally expected at sites of repair when no such blocking tubes are used, were replaced instead by thick, restrictive, vascular adhesions at the ends of the tubing. These adhesions were, of necessity, thick and vascular because they provided the vascular, nutritional support for the healing granulation tissue as it traversed a course between a synthetic barrier impervious to blood vessels on one side and the tendon on the other.

FORMATION OF ADHESIONS

In another series of experiments[9] designed to determine the effect of associated trauma on the healing of divided profundus tendons, it was shown that ad-

*Millipore Filter Corp., Bedford, Massachusetts.

hesions to the tendon occur at each point at which the physical integrity of the surface of the tendon is disturbed. Adhesions form quantitatively in proportion to the number of puncture wounds inflicted or the extent of a crushing injury, as well as at each point at which the tendon surface is broken by a suture. The propensity for resolution of these adhesions by restoration of the synovial layer of the sheath is remarkable, but limited quantitatively by the extent of trauma to which the tendon surfaces have been subjected. It was thus determined that one of the single most important factors in the etiology of adhesions to repaired digital flexor tendons is physical trauma to the tendon surfaces. Such adhesions can be prevented or minimized only by the most meticulous and painstaking surgical technique. Such technique includes the avoidance of the use of any instruments to handle tendons. Surgical exposure must be adequate enough to permit manipulation of the tendon ends by the surgeon's moistened glove finger tips. Surgical trauma must be limited to the passage of fine sharp suture needles needed for effecting tendon repair. Furthermore, no heavy knots in the suture material should press against and further traumatize tendon surfaces during healing.

DAMAGE TO THE DIGITAL FLEXOR TUNNEL

Another extensive series of experiments[11] was undertaken to determine what effect damage to the tissues surrounding the healing flexor tendon would have on the process of tendon healing. It was found that the anatomical integrity of the digital flexor tunnel is an essential factor in the effort to minimize tendon adhesions following flexor tendon repair. Excision of the flexor digital synovial sheath following primary flexor tendon repair with preservation of the superficial tendon has no adverse effect on tendon healing or on the ultimate functional result, since a new gliding sheath mechanism forms. In stark contrast, however, if the integrity of the bony floor of the digital canal is violated, as in total excision of the superficial tendon, a profound inflammatory response is produced that results in adhesions that are broadly based upon the rigid ungliding bony phalanges of the digit. Flexor tendon healing is then accompanied by the formation of dense restrictive adhesions that assure an unacceptable functional result (Fig. 4-4). If the superficialis tendon is excised by transverse division immediately proximal to its vinculum, the anatomic integrity of the periosteal floor of the digital canal is preserved and the healing profundus tendon remains free of any adhesions to that bony floor (Fig. 4-5).

TENDON GRAFTS

Mechanisms of healing and fate of fresh autogenous flexor tendon grafts

Another extensive series of experiments[12] was designed to determine the fate of autogenous tendon grafts within the digits and the factors that influence that fate. Once again a special standard experimental wound was designed so that the normal anatomic field of the digit was preserved as best as possible. As in the

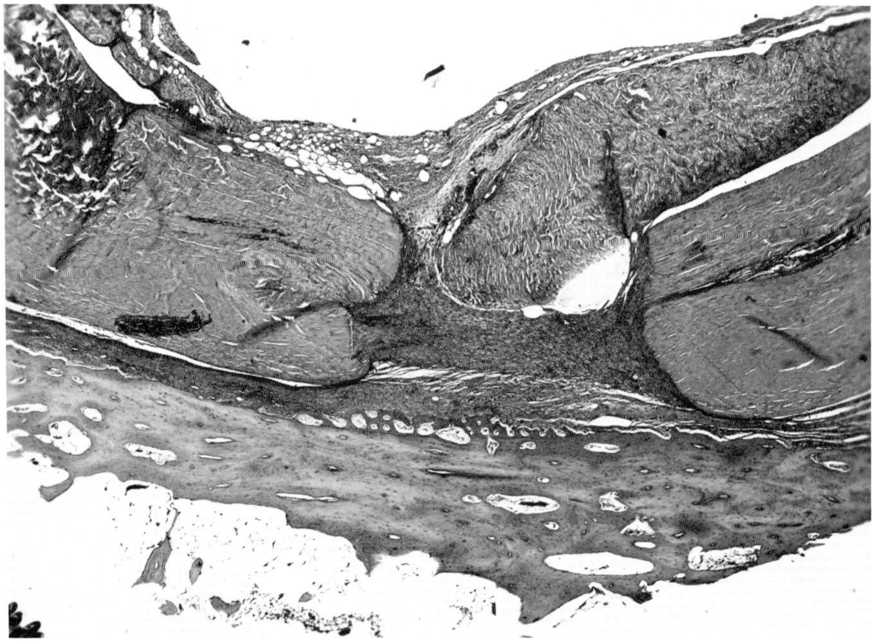

Fig. 4-4. Longitudinal microscopic section of healing profundus tendon within the flexor sheath following total sublimis tendon excision. Note that the surgically disturbed periosteum of the underlying bony phalanx, as well as the synovial sheath, contribute to the healing of the tendon resulting in dense restrictive adhesions to the phalanx (hematoxylin and eosin ×19).

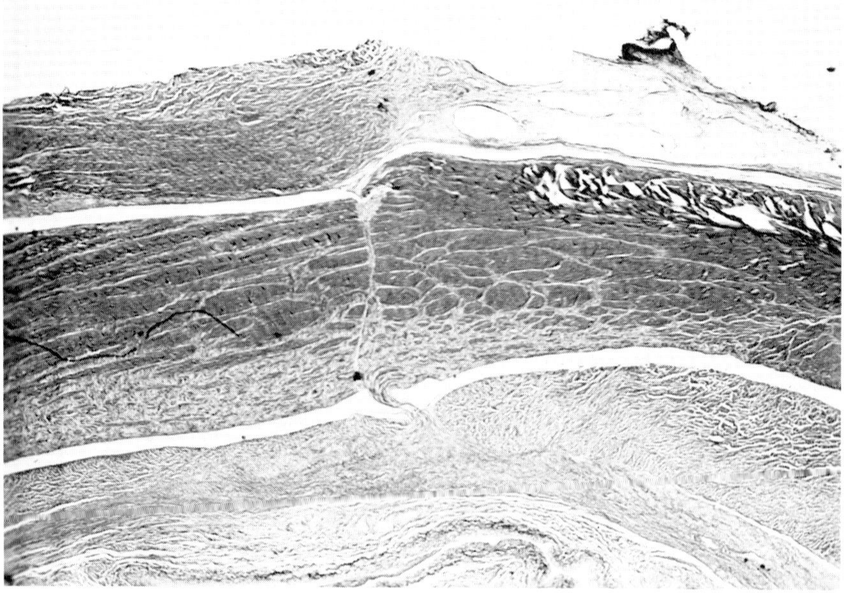

Fig. 4-5. For legend see opposite page.

preceding experiments, nonreactive stainless steel suture was used throughout. In performing these experiments, profundus flexor tendons were completely removed from their digital sheaths, completely divided of all soft tissue and bony attachments, and then returned to their previous anatomic site within the flexor digital sheath, preserving intact the annular ligaments, the superficialis tendons, and the sheath, except for necessary openings in the sheath at its extreme ends both proximally in the palm and distally at the level of the distal phalanx. The digital sheaths over the proximal and middle phalanges remained intact as did the sublimis tendons and annular ligaments; thus, no-man's-land was preserved as anatomically intact as possible. Profundus flexor tendon grafts were placed through intact sublimis tendons, pulleys, and sheaths.

Careful study of these free autogenous flexor tendon grafts showed that the proximal and distal tendon-graft anastomosis sites were healed solely by the proliferative cellular activity of the paratenon (in the palm) and synovial sheath, respectively. These tissues gave rise to a granulation tissue of fibroblasts and capillary buds that invaded the spaces between tendon stumps and laid down new collagen, ultimately effecting tendon-tendon graft union. The highly vascular adhesions, formed at the wound sites and at the points where the integrity of tendon surfaces had been broken by suture tract or by undue suture pressure upon tendon, gradually resolved, becoming filmy and loose. No intrinsic reparative tenoblastic activity was observed in either the proximal or distal tendon stumps or in the grafts.

The tendon grafts remained completely viable by all histologic criteria. Tendon cells retained their normal staining and cytologic characteristics throughout the entire period of study when compared to normal, viable, undisturbed sublimis tendons in the same digital flexor sheath (Fig. 4-6). There was no evidence of a general pattern of collagen swelling, degeneration and/or replacement in the grafts. When damage to tendon caused by undue focal pressure was present, focally specific tendon degeneration occurred. These specific areas were repaired by the growth of fibroblasts from the surrounding granulation tissue into the traumatized areas of tendon. These cells laid down delicate, fine, new collagen fibers that were clearly identifiable and easily distinguished from the collagen bundles of the tendon graft by staining sections with special connective tissue stains. No other areas in the grafts showed these changes. Similarly, areas of increased cellularity in the grafts occurred in or in direct proximity to suture

---

Fig. 4-5. Longitudinal microscopic section of repaired profundus tendon within the flexor sheath from which the sublimis has been excised by subtotal transverse division immediately proximal to its vinculi, thus not disturbing the periosteum of the underlying bony phalanx. Note that there is no periosteal reaction and no adhesions to the phalanx. The tendon has healed and the adhesions at the wound site are sparse, loose, and filmy (hematoxylin and eosin ×19).

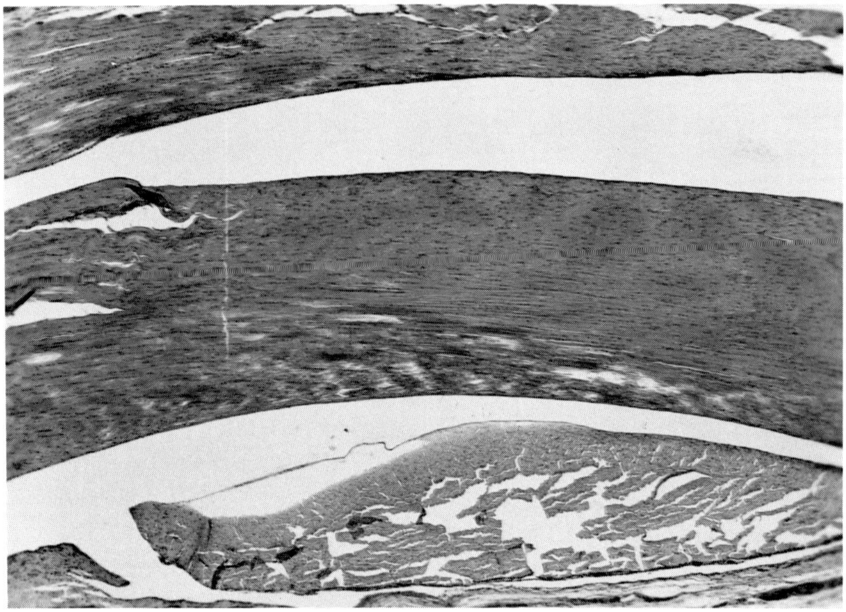

Fig. 4-6. Longitudinal microscopic section of a free autotopic profundus tendon graft within the flexor sheath in its normal anatomic position with respect to the sublimis tendon (above) and annular ligament (below). Note normal collagen structure, normal cellular content, structure, and staining characteristics (hematoxylin and eosin ×22.3).

tracts and were the direct result of fibroblast invasion along the same suture tracts. No evidence of proliferation of tenocytes proper was present.

Adhesions to tendon stumps and tendon grafts beyond immediate wound site occurred only at those discrete points at which the integrity of tendon surfaces had been broken by sutures. These adhesions ultimately became filmy and loose. Since no trauma had been sustained by those portions of the grafts in no-man's-land, nor by any other normal structures of this portion of the flexor digital sheath, no adhesions formed between any of these anatomic elements.

Comparative study of the healing and fate of paratenon-covered and nonparatenon-covered tendon grafts

In this series of experiments the mechanisms of healing and the fate of autogenous (profundus) flexor tendons used as free flexor tendon grafts in the digits were compared with free paratenon-covered canine flexor carpi ulnaris tendons used as free flexor tendon grafts within the digit.

The mechanisms of healing and their rate of progress were the same in the two groups of tendon grafts. These processes were identical to those already described for the healing of free autogenous profundus tendon grafts. As with the latter, the tendon grafts studied in this new series of experiments remained viable and normal by all histologic criteria upon detailed study of their cells and collagen. There was no evidence of graft "death" or necrosis. Adhesions to the autogenous profundus grafts occurred as previously described; there were no adhesions to these grafts in no-man's-land. The situation was quite the reverse with the autogenous paratenon-covered flexor carpi ulnaris grafts.

The paratenon-covered flexor carpi ulnaris autogenous grafts were involved in diffuse adhesions to surrounding structures throughout their length in the palm and in the digital flexor sheath. Their surfaces were irregular with many loose tags and areas of hyperemia throughout the full time period of this experiment that was terminated at 77 days. These irregular and diffuse adhesions appeared microscopically to have several sources of origin. In many areas, the paratenon covering the grafts appeared to be proliferating and attaching itself to the surrounding tissues, particularly the synovial layer of the sheath. In other areas, the surrounding tissues in contact with the paratenon of the grafts were apparently stimulated to proliferate and form adhesions to the paratenon. This phenomenon was observed throughout the length of the synovium-lined digital sheath and was particularly noticeable in the region of the annular ligaments and the vincula breve of the untraumatized sublimis tendons. In addition to these findings, the granulation tissue produced by the adventitial tissues of the palm appeared to grow along the paratenon of the flexor carpi ulnaris grafts and extend well out into the digital sheaths. The paratenon appeared to provide a fertile and, in some way, attractive biologic bed for this proliferating tissue so that it extended itself along the length of the grafts rather than simply taking part in sealing off the sheath ends as was observed with the profundus grafts in these experiments. This tissue also occasionally attached itself to areas of the grafts microscopically denuded of paratenon, atlhough to a much lesser degree.

These various adhesions to the flexor carpi ulnaris grafts, while extensive in their relative distribution, did not contain significant quantities of collagen and would, therefore, not be expected to restrict motion of the graft significantly under the conditions defined in these experiments; this is in keeping with the rigidly atraumatic techniques employed throughout these studies. However, in the presence of significant surgical trauma to the grafts or surgery on contiguous anatomic structures within the digital sheath, adhesions would be expected to be more florid and invasive and would, therefore, probably restrict graft motion significantly.

From this series of experiments, contrary to popular belief, paratenon does not appear to be essential to the survival of free autogenous tendon grafts. Moreover, its very preservation on such grafts results in greater adhesion formation than if it is not present, and may significantly compromise the ultimate functional result. These conclusions agree with the clinical impression of experienced hand surgeons that the preservation of paratenon on a free tendon graft often produces poorer results than if it is meticulously removed prior to transplantation. Paratenon appears to actively form adhesions to surrounding tissues and to stimulate the adhesion-producing potential of such tissues. It also appears to serve as a fertile recipient bed for adhesion-producing granulation tissue. Thus it would appear wise to meticulously remove all paratenon prior to performing a free autogenous tendon grafting procedure within the digital flexor mechanism. While there is still a tendency to adhesion formation to paratenon-covered tendons after the paratenon is removed, this tendency is considerably less than with the paratenon preserved.

Healing and fate of lyophilized homologous tendon grafts within the flexor digital sheath*

The series of experiments described above strongly suggests that there is but one ideal replacement substitute for an irreparably injured profundus tendon—another atraumatically obtained autogenous profundus tendon. Since there could be little justification for removing a normal profundus tendon from a healthy digit to repair a damaged one, it was decided to experiment with preserved profundus tendons.

Methods and techniques

Fresh flexor digitorum profundus tendons were aseptically obtained from canine donors by the atraumatic techniques previously described in this chapter. They were attached by their ends, at normal length, on annealed, hooked Pyrex rods for atraumatic handling throughout processing and subsequent experimentation. Immediately upon removal from donors and placement between the hooks of the glass rods, all grafts were stored in a sterile nutrient medium for no longer than 45 minutes. During this time they were taken to the Tissue Bank Department, United States Naval Medical School, Bethesda, Maryland, where they were freeze-dried by a standardized technique. They were not treated chemically in any way for sterilization or for any other purpose either before or after freeze-drying.

Immediately prior to transplantation of the desiccated, mummified freeze-dried homografts to new dogs, they were immersed in sterile saline, without antibiotics or antiseptics, for one half hour. This hydrated them sufficiently to make them flexible enough to insert and suture. They were then atraumatically transplanted into the flexor digital sheaths, annular ligaments, and sublimis tendons under aseptic operating room conditions. The host profundus tendons were used as guides to which the freeze-dried tendons were attached distally. They were then drawn into the normal anatomic digital bed by removal of the host profundus tendons through the palm. Proximal and distal anastomosis was then accomplished by the Bunnell pull-out technique using No. 36 stainless steel surgical suture.

After placement and suture of grafts, skin incisions were closed with con-

*This series of experiments has not been previously published and so is presented here in detail.

tinuous sutures of No. 36 monofilament surgical stainless steel wire. Sterile, fluffed, compressive dressings were applied and, after release of tourniquets used at surgery, wire-reinforced, padded plaster casts were applied from the digits to the brachia of all extremities (one in each dog) with the paws in the relaxed position. Sutures and casts were left undisturbed (with the exception noted below) until each animal was sacrificed.

Seventeen dogs, each with two freeze-dried grafts in one paw were sacrificed at the following times: one each at 7, 10, 14, 18, 21, 22, 35, 42, 56, 59, 63, 70, 93, 126, and 160 days; and two at 180 days postoperatively. One of the animals sacrificed at 180 days had had the cast and sutures removed 8 weeks before sacrifice; the two freeze-dried tendons were thus subjected to full functional use for 56 days.

Immediately prior to sacrifice, all animals were anesthetized by the same technique used at initial surgery. The brachial arteries in the operated extremities were cannulated and injected with a 25% (by volume) suspension of barium sulfate (Micropaque*) in sterile saline injected under physiologic pressure over a period of 15 minutes. This was done to assist in the identification of blood vessels in the later histologic analysis. Digits for study were then removed en bloc by sharp ray amputation after skin excision. In one specimen from each paw, the digital sheath was opened in the midlateral line for gross photographic documentation and then immediately fixed in 10% buffered Formalin. The remaining digit of the experimental pair in each paw was immediately fixed in 10% buffered Formalin after amputation. After fixation, flexor mechanisms were freed of all bone by sharp subperiosteal dissection. Each specimen was divided into four separate subspecimens for individual processing, imbedding, and study as follows: (1) the proximal host tendon stump–tendon graft wound for longitudinal sections, (2) the distal host tendon stump–tendon graft wound for longitudinal sections, (3) a segment in no-man's-land for cross sections, and (4) a segment in no-man's-land for longitudinal sections. Separate tissue sections for each subspecimen were stained with hematoxylin and eosin, Wilder's silver stain, and Reinhart's modification of Hale's colloidal iron stain.

Gross findings. The gross findings following transplantation of freeze-dried flexor tendon homografts into the flexor digital sheath were quite remarkable. No adhesions were observed between the freeze-dried grafts and host digital sheaths, annular ligaments, or sublimis tendons in any specimen (Fig. 4-7). There was no gross evidence of graft degeneration or replacement. In point of fact, at scheduled re-exploration, the freeze-dried grafts could not be distinguished from normal in situ profundus tendons by competent but unsuspecting fellow surgeon-observers.

Histologic findings. The histologic findings were divided into two categories:

*Micropaque is a product of Damancy & Co., Ltd., England.

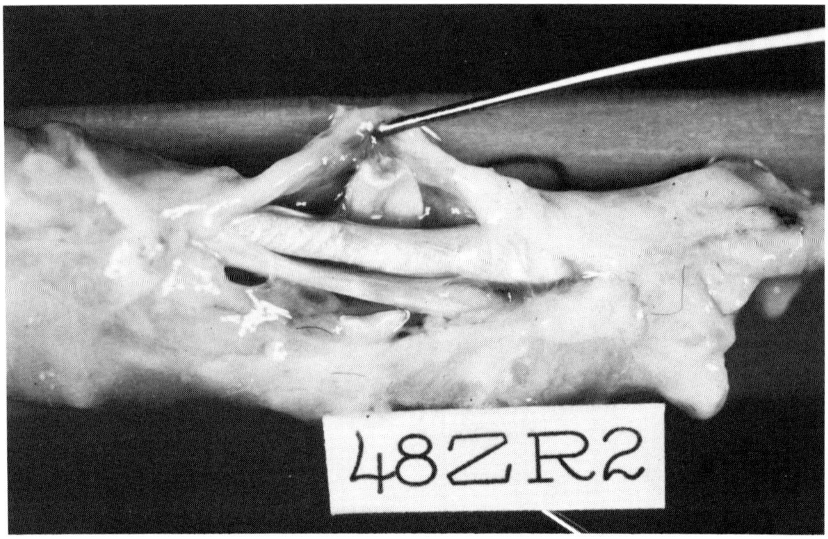

Fig. 4-7. Gross photograph of freeze-dried profundus tendon homograft with the flexor sheath, and in normal anatomic position with respect to the sublimis tendon and annular ligaments 49 days following implantation. Note normal appearance of the graft, lack of any degenerative changes, and lack of any adhesions.

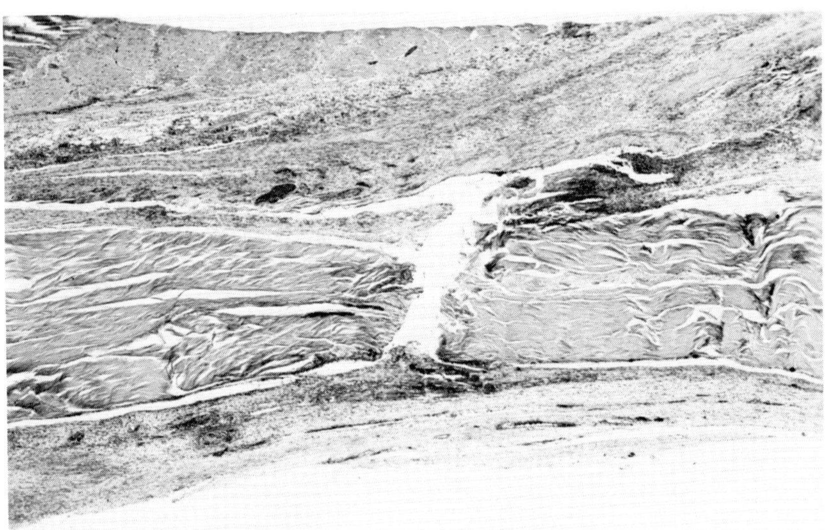

Fig. 4-8. Longitudinal microscopic section of host tendon stump-freeze-dried graft wound at 7 days postimplantation. Note the early inflammatory reaction of healing with edema and exudation of blood elements about the wound. Note the normal appearance of the graft collagen bundles seen on the right when compared with the host stump (hematoxylin and eosin ×19).

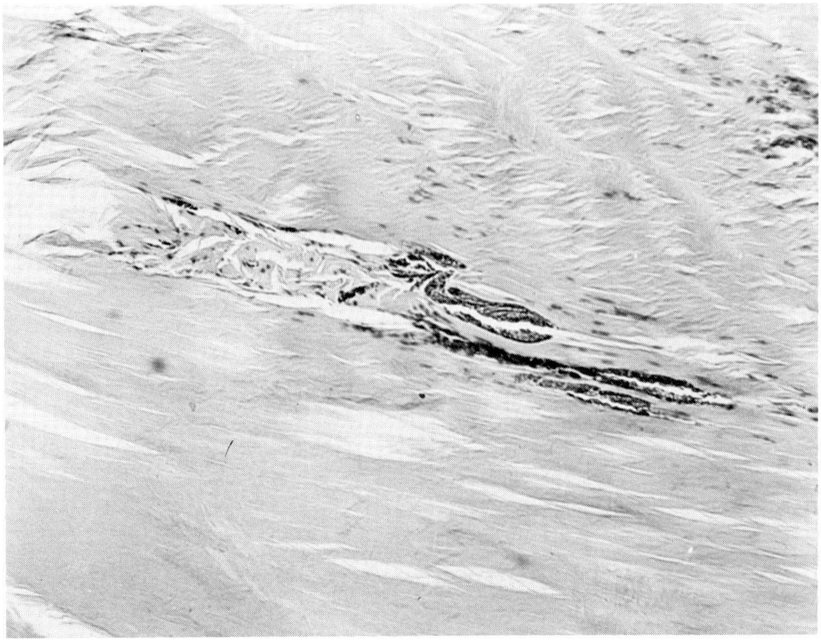

Fig. 4-9. Longitudinal microscopic section of freeze-dried profundus 21 days postimplantation showing a suture tract along which host fibroblasts and vascular elements have grown resulting in local recellularization and revascularization of the graft in the region of the palmar anastomotic wound (hematoxylin and eosin ×79).

(1) the findings at the proximal (in the palm) and the distal (over the distal phalanx) host tendon stump–tendon graft anastomosis sites and (2) the findings within the flexor digital sheath. It is possible to discuss the anastomotic wounds from the proximal and distal sites together since the processes at both sites were essentially identical.

Part I· Anastomosis wounds. During the first week, the connective tissues surrounding the host-graft wounds manifested the usual acute inflammatory reaction of early healing, with exudation of blood elements and moderate edema (Fig. 4-8). The wounds were soon surrounded by a highly cellular and vascular granulation tissue of new blood vessels and fibroblasts. This tissue invaded the wounds between the cellular host tendon stumps and the acellular freeze-dried grafts. It also invaded the host stumps and grafts along suture tracts in these respective structures (Fig. 4-9).

By the fourteenth day, fine new collagen fibers had been deposited in the tendon-graft wounds by the fibroblasts in the invading granulation tissue. Collagen was sparse at this time and randomly arranged in the wounds, which were highly cellular and vascular. Round cells in the wound granulation tissue also invaded the cut ends of the freeze-dried grafts and began to recellularize the grafts by migrating longitudinally along the collagen bundles. Recellularization

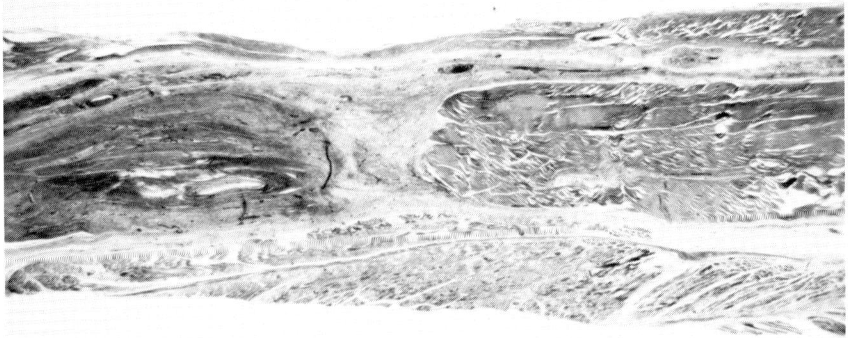

Fig. 4-10. Longitudinal microscopic section of host tendon stump-freeze-dried graft wound in the palm 28 days postimplantation showing deposition of collagen in the vascular and cellular wound scar (hematoxylin and eosin ×11).

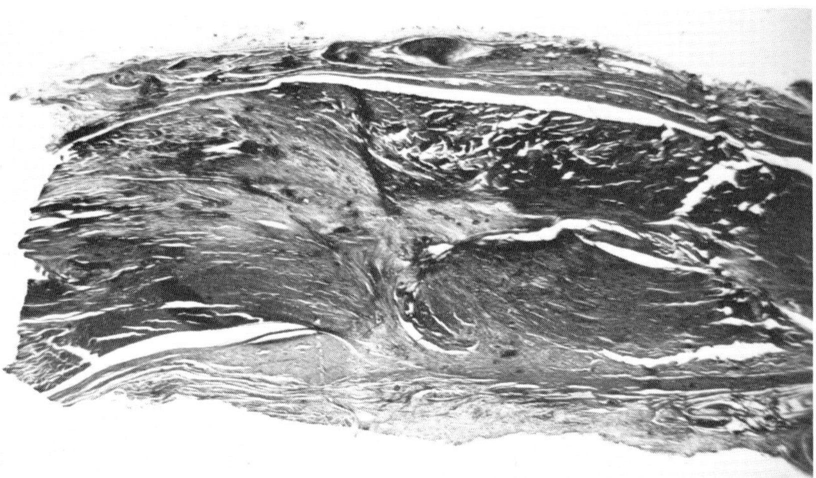

Fig. 4-11. Longitudinal microscopic section of host tendon stump-freeze-dried graft wound at 42 days postimplantation. Note the advanced state of wound maturation with resolution of adhesions to surrounding tissues. Note the similarity between the collagenous structure of the graft seen on the right and the host tendon stump (Wilder's ×19).

of the grafts was also begun by cells associated with the fine blood vessels and fibroblasts that grew into suture tracts; the areas of the grafts around such tracts showed early recellularization while more remote areas in the grafts remained acellular for a longer period of time (Fig. 4-9).

A moderate amount of collagen in the tendon-graft wounds, evident by 21 days and through 28 days postoperatively, was largely oriented in the longitudinal axis of the tendons (Fig. 4-10). The edema of surrounding tissues had receded and considerably less vascularity was present in the tissues, which had given rise to the healing granulation tissue. The tendon-graft wounds were attached to surrounding tissues by loose vascular adhesions, but there were no other significant adhesions except at suture tract sites where granulation tissue had invaded either the freeze-dried grafts or the host tendon stumps.

The wounds matured progressively over the next several weeks so that by 35 and 42 days, union was moderately advanced to a degree roughly comparable to that observed with fresh autotopic profundus tendon grafts.

All microscopic signs of acute inflammation in and about wounds had subsided by 6 weeks (Fig. 4-11). There were loose adhesions to the tendon-graft units only at wound sites. The cellularity and vascularity of the wounds had decreased and there was considerably more collagen oriented longitudinally in the wounds. Recellularization of the freeze-dried grafts in the areas up to 1 cm. from the wounds was complete. However, the wounds could still be easily identified histologically.

Wound maturation progressed through the next several weeks so that by 93 days the wounds could be identified histologically only with difficulty by noting residual areas of increased cellularity and slightly increased vascularity in the reconstituted tendon-graft units. The cellularity of the freeze-dried grafts and the host tendon stumps were identical in the area of the wounds. Adhesions

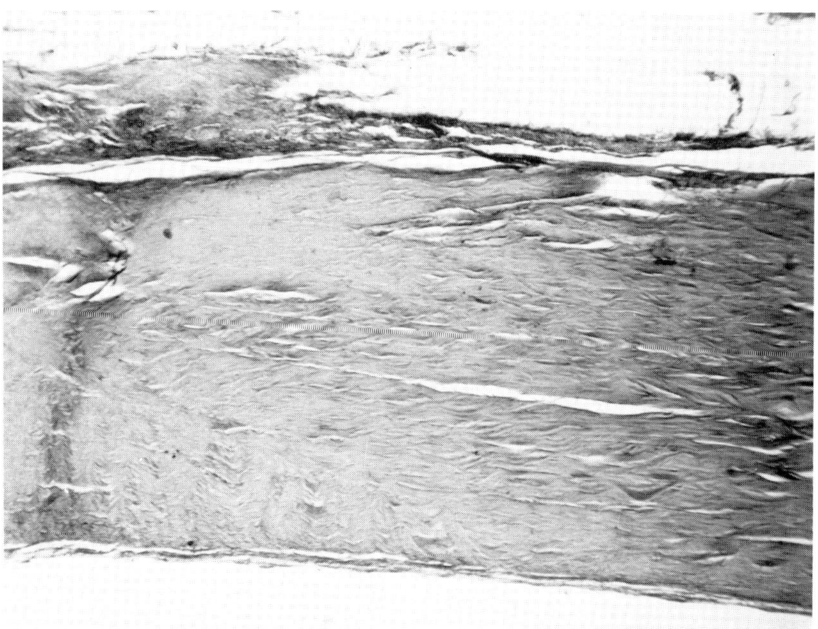

Fig. 4-12. Longitudinal microscopic section of host tendon stump-freeze-dried graft wound at 180 days postimplantation showing that the wound collagen has been formed into bundles identical to those of the normal tendon so that the wound can no longer be identified by the presence of a scar (Reinhart's ×16).

to wound sites had become very loose and filmy and separation between the reconstructed tendon and surrounding tissues could be seen histologically with ease.

In the 160-day and 180-day specimens, the anastomotic wounds could no longer be identified histologically, since the collagen in the wounds had formed bundles, identical with those of tendon proper, across the wound sites (Fig. 4-12). This collagen blended perfectly with the host tendon stumps and the freeze-dried grafts. Since the cellularity of the latter was identical with that of the former, it was not possible to distinguish grafts from host tendons by cellular morphology.

Throughout this entire sequence of events there was no evidence of degeneration of any of the collagen in the freeze-dried grafts (Figs. 4-1 to 4-7). The staining characteristics of the grafts remained identical to those of the host tendon stumps with each of the three staining techniques used in this study. There was no suggestion of any process that could be interpreted as degeneration of the grafts. Similarly, there was no evidence of replacement of the freeze-dried collagen grafts by the host tissues. It appeared merely that host cells recellularize the grafts, migrate along, and then take their permanent places among the collagen bundles of the grafts.

Part II: Fate of grafts within the flexor digital sheaths. Within the flexor digital sheaths remote from the anastomotic wounds, in the area classically known as no-man's-land, the acellular freeze-dried grafts were carefully studied by en bloc histologic sections of the entire digital flexor mechanism. The experimental design employed provided a unique opportunity to critically assess the fate of the freeze-dried grafts since they could be accurately compared histologically to the normal untraumatized host sublimis tendons seen in longitudinal section and in normal host annular ligaments seen in cross section in each longitudinal field. Moreover, the subspecimens used for cross sections presented the freeze-dried grafts enfolded within the normal host sublimis tendons.

The acellular freeze-dried grafts remained intact with no evidence of degeneration of their collagen (Fig. 4-13) from 7 days postoperatively through the end of this study at 180 days. There was no evidence of collagen swelling, fragmentation, or degeneration in the grafts when they were compared with host sublimis tendons and annular ligaments. The staining characteristics of the freeze-dried grafts, except for initial acellularity, remained identical with those of the host sublimis tendons and annular ligaments following use of the three histologic stains used in this study.

Cellular changes within the flexor digital sheaths presented an unexpectedly unique process. Areas of cellular proliferation appeared in the synovial cell layer of the sheaths apposing the freeze-dried grafts. This also occurred on the apposing surfaces of the host sublimis tendons in the region of origin of their extensive, synovium-covered vincula. Serial histologic sections of each specimen revealed a proliferation of the synovial layer of the sheath with seeding of the

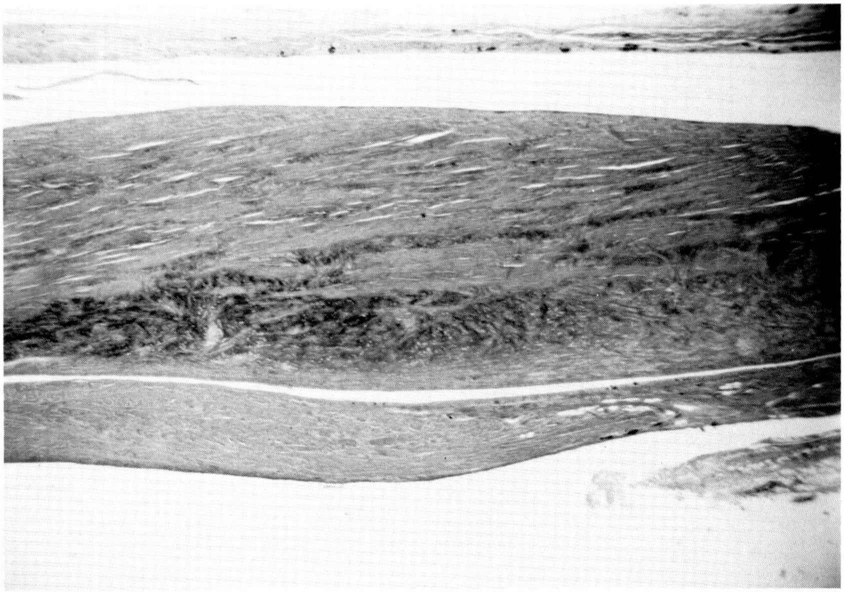

Fig. 4-13. Longitudinal microscopic section of a freeze-dried graft within the flexor sheath 14 days postimplantation showing intact collagen bundles with no evidence of swelling, fragmentation, degeneration, or replacement. The collagen structure of the graft (above) is identical with that of the sublimis tendon (below) (Reinhart's ×19).

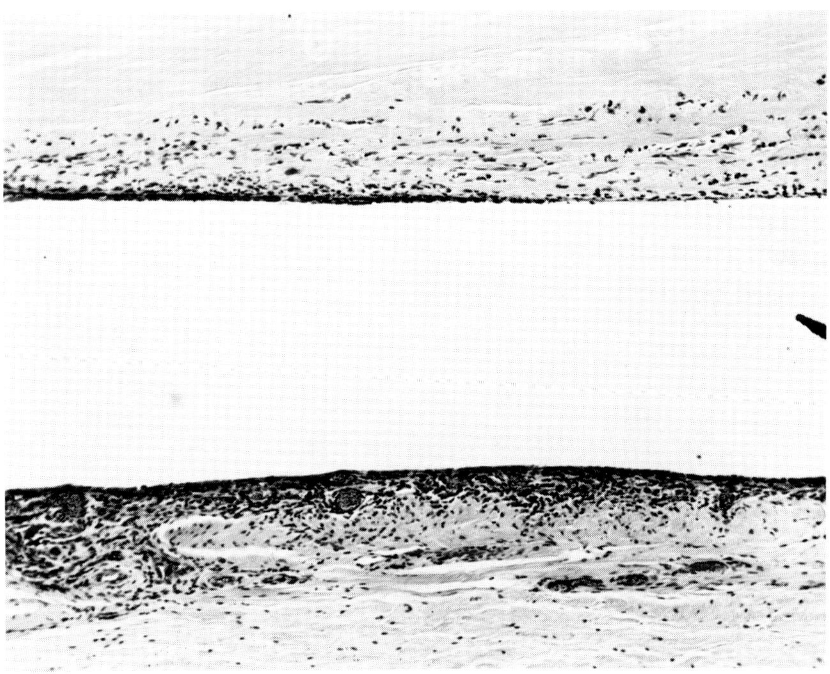

Fig. 4-14. Longitudinal microscopic section of freeze-dried profundus homograft within the flexor digital sheath 14 days postimplantation. Note the area of extensive cellular proliferation (with many blood vessels) in the sheath seen below. This is matched by an area of surface and subsurface recellularization of the freeze-dried graft seen above. Note lack of blood vessels in the graft (hematoxylin and eosin ×79).

underlying freeze-dried tendons with cells from this source (Fig. 4-14). These proliferative cellular changes were accompanied by focal increases in the vascularity of the sheaths. The large areas of synovial cellular proliferation were observed to be perfectly matched by collections of similar cells opposite them on the surfaces of the otherwise acellular freeze-dried grafts (Fig. 4-14). These latter collections of cells apparently arose from the synovium, invaded the grafts, and proceeded to recellularize them by migration from these focal areas. This cellular seeding of the freeze-dried grafts occurred across the potential space between the grafts and digital sheaths. While these structures were contiguous in situ, the en bloc histologic sections showed that the freeze-dried grafts remained separate from the sheaths, sublimis tendons, and annular ligaments (Figs. 4-13 and 4-14).

In some hematoxylin and eosin sections, it appeared that the sheaths and grafts were united by intensely cellular adhesions. This finding was inconsistent with the gross observation that there were no adhesions to the grafts in no-man's-land. Special stains (Reinhart's and Wilder's) resolved this seeming difficulty by demonstrating that there had been no collagen deposited in the cellular masses that arose from the sheaths and seeded the grafts by bridging the sheaths' space (Fig. 4-15). The cells did not lay down collagen during the seeding process and,

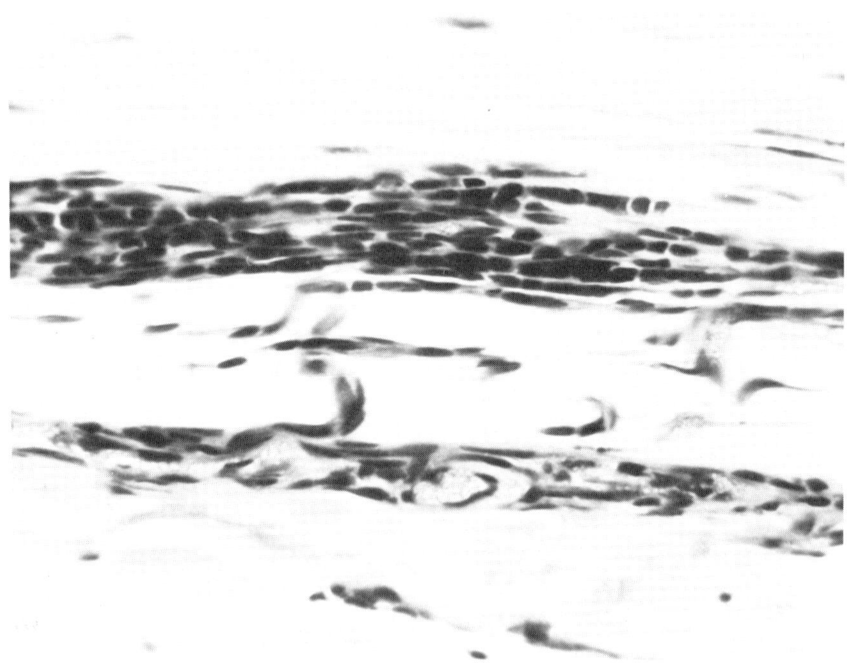

Fig. 4-15. Longitudinal microscopic section of freeze-dried profundus homograft (above) within the flexor sheath (below). Note the extensive cellular seeding of the graft that has taken place from the sheath across the space between them without the formation of collagenous adhesions.

therefore, no adhesions were produced between the freeze-dried grafts and the other structures of the flexor mechanism.

This process of cellular seeding of the grafts from the sheaths' synovium without the formation of collagenous adhesions proceeded until the grafts were progressively recellularized. However, by the end of this experiment, 180 days postimplantation, all those grafts that had been immobilized throughout the postoperative period were incompletely recellularized since they had central longitudinal cores of relative or absolute acellularity within the flexor digital sheaths. The remaining peripheral graft areas had normal cellularity by 42 days. There was one exception to this; the two grafts harvested at 56 days had been completely recellularized and histologically presented the appearance of normal tendon (Fig. 4-16). This probably represents an instance of biologic variability in regard to the entire series of animals. Similarly, the two grafts subjected to 8 weeks of functional use before sacrifice at 180 days postoperative were totally recellularized while the pair of tendons held immobile until that time had central longitudinal cores of relative acellularity.

It is important to note that while there was sheath, synovial and vascular proliferation during the process of cellular seeding of the freeze-dried grafts, no blood vessels could be detected in the freeze-dried grafts histologically (Figs.

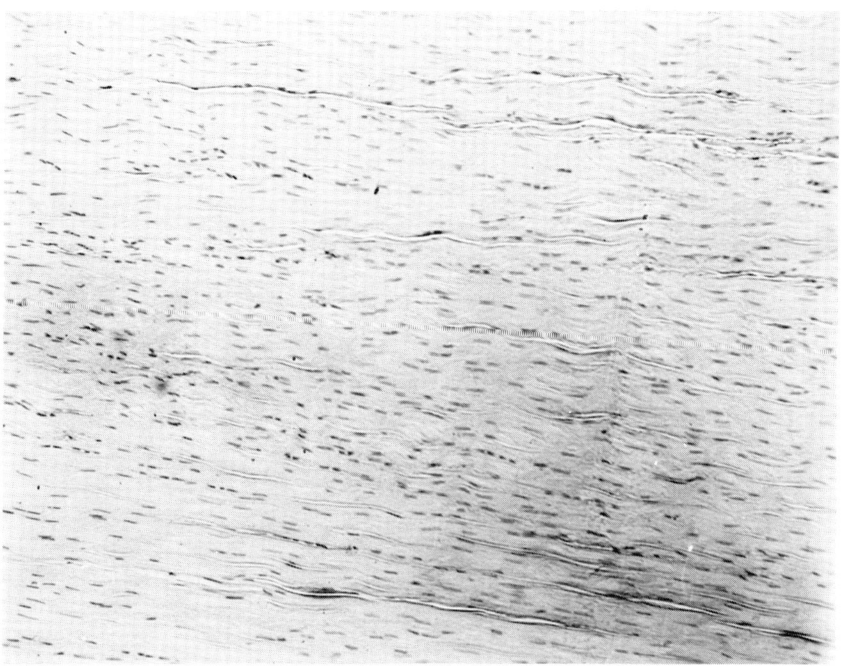

Fig. 4-16. Longitudinal microscopic section of a freeze-dried profundus homograft within the flexor sheath 56 days postimplantation showing complete recellularization of the graft with normal collagenous structure (hematoxylin and eosin ×79).

4-13 to 4-16), and with the aid of the vascular-injected Micropaque, within the flexor digital sheaths during the duration of the experiment (180 days). This observation further supports the conclusion that the sheaths' synovium provided the sole basis for recellularization of the freeze-dried grafts within no-man's-land.

At no point in this study was there any suggestion of a homograft-rejection phenomenon. The inflammatory cells of healing present in the wounds disappeared as normal healing progressed. They did not appear at areas remote from the wounds or about the grafts within the digital sheaths. Rather, the entire process described above was one of complete host acceptance of the freeze-dried homografts.

Discussion. This is by no means the first experimental study devoted to investigating the possible use of preserved tendons for implantation as tendon grafts; the detailed history of these and others has been reviewed by Cordrey et al.[1] Relatively few investigators, however, have studied freeze-dried tendon grafts.

The unique results described here are particularly provocative when one considers that they were achieved within the canine digital flexor mechanism, a test system not employed by others who have studied freeze-dried tendon grafts. It is within the flexor digital sheaths that the severest clinical problems in tendon injury and repair occurs; thus it is here that our experimental efforts should be focused. Carpal flexor and extensor tendons and tendo Achillis present neither the anatomical peculiarities nor the clinical problems seen in the digits. The freeze-dried homografts implanted in the studies reported here were fully accepted by their hosts without degeneration or replacement of the collagen of the homografts. Rather, host cells accepted and recellularized the grafts by a unique cellular-seeding process originating in the synovial layer of the digital sheath. This was accomplished without the formation of collagenous adhesions. The process was one of complete host acceptance of the freeze-dried grafts for incorporation into the host canine digital flexor mechanism.

Flynn and Graham,[2] in a study of lyophilized heterogenous (not homogenous as in this series of experiments) tendon grafts in the canine ulnar carpal extensor reported complete replacement of the transplants by host cells after complete ischemic necrosis of all the transplants. Their photomicrographs clearly support this conclusion. Significantly, however, they reported "there was no anatomic evidence of antibody reaction. . . ." Cordrey et al.,[1] in a study of variously preserved homogenous tendon grafts in the rabbit tendo Achillis, found that lyophilized tendon homografts were soon surrounded by marked "scarring" that later resolved somewhat. They noted that host tendon-graft joints were well healed by 7 weeks, but there were areas of collagen fiber fragmentation and foci of necrosis in the grafts. They were unable to resolve the question of whether or not the collagen of the grafts remained "alive" or "died" and was replaced.

While the results of Flynn and Graham appeared diametric to those of this report, it is essential to emphasize that they used freeze-dried heterografts, not homografts. Further, they used calf extensor tendons and not flexor profundus tendons as we used in this study. Finally, the tendon grafts were washed in saline for 5 days and then chemically sterilized with betapropiolactone before freeze-drying, while the tendons studied in this report were never subjected to chemical denaturants. Each or all of these differences in our respective experimental methods may account for the differences in our results. Although Cordrey et al.,[1] did use lyophilized homografts, they were not digital flexor tendons, but rather tendo Achillis, and these investigators used silk rather than nonreactive suture material for tendon anastomosis.

Peacock[6] has suggested, on the basis of experiments with refrigerated trypsin-treated heterografts that such structures may primarily represent homostatic collagen transplants. The results of the experiments recorded in this report present no data contrary to Peacock's hypothesis.

Too often and too easily, perhaps, investigators have thought of nonautogenous (homologous and heterogenous) tendons as "dead" grafts. While their cells may be dead because of processing, or may die after implantation, the word "dead" is meaningless in regard to the collagen of the grafts. Since collagen, a protein, is per se an extracellular product of cellular activity, it can have neither "life" nor "death." The essential question concerning it in regard to transplantation is whether or not it has been denatured. If it has not been denatured, and presents no clinically significant immunologic competence (as indicated by this study as well as those by Peacock, Flynn and Graham) there is no compelling reason why it should be rejected or undergo a process of necrosis and replacement. In fact, as demonstrated in this study, it may be completely accepted by the host and become an integral and apparently normal anatomic component of the host after recellularization. It would appear that this favorable sequence would be least likely to be adversely affected by the freeze-drying technique of preservation. Indeed, various proteins, enzymes, viruses, bacteria, and protozoa have been preserved by freeze-drying. Upon reconstitution they have proven to be stable and to manifest again their biologic and immunologic competence; the freeze-drying process apparently causes minimal if any permanent protein denaturation in these biologic specimens.[4] Preservation of tendons in chemical disinfectants that act by denaturing essential protein complexes of microorganisms may also denature the collagen of the grafts to a degree that stimulates a prolonged host inflammatory response resulting in graft necrosis and replacement. Moreover, residual disinfectants in the grafts may cause irritation and destruction of local host tissues assuring a more profound host inflammatory response. This factor may have been responsible for the marked and persistent hyperemia about tendon homografts preserved in 1:1,000 aqueous thimerosal (Merthiolate) by Cordrey et al.

Thus it appears that there may be important potential usefulness for preserved tendon homografts. Extensive experiments in the dog have revealed that digital flexor profundus tendons are the best tendons for fresh autografts within the digital flexor mechanism; they are far superior to autogenous paratenon-covered tendons. Freeze-dried profundus homografts appear to be the second best to (indeed, if not just as good as) fresh profundus autografts. Freeze-dried grafts must be obtained, processed, and handled atraumatically. Avoidance of their exposure to protein denaturants appears to be an important factor in their successful use if one is to avoid necrosis and replacement of the grafts. The freeze-dried process is probably the least traumatic procedure for preserving tendon grafts and the one least likely to cause protein denaturation. Properly obtained and properly implanted, such grafts are fully accepted by the host within the canine flexor digital sheath. The latter, far from acting as an inert barrier about the grafts, recellularizes the grafts by an active proliferative cellular-seeding process without the production of collagenous adhesions.

General discussion

Flexor digitorum profundus tendons divided and repaired within the flexor digital sheath are healed by the reparative cellular response of the sheath and surrounding tissues and not by any intrinsic response of their own. This was confirmed by the experiments dealing with the initial standard wound study of the mechanisms of flexor profundus healing. It was further confirmed by the experiments using polyethylene and millipore blocking tubes about repaired flexor tendons; such tubes delayed tendon healing by precisely the time it took healing granulation tissue from the sheath to grow beneath the tubes to the tendon repair sites. That flexor tendons possess no intrinsic reparative response of their own was further confirmed in the experiments in which the subtotally divided sublimis tendons failed to give rise to any fibroblastic granulation tissue from their cut ends. Had this not been so, the profundus tendon wounds would have been firmly united by adhesions to the sublimis stumps. Here, after subtotal sublimis excision, the repaired digital flexor sheath provided the only source of a reparative granulation tissue for profundus tendon healing. After total sublimis excision, which of necessity disturbs the periosteal floor of the digital canal, the granulation tissue arose not only from the repaired synovial sheath, but from the disturbed bony floor of the digital canal as well. The cut tendon ends per se never produced a reparative tenoblastic response.

The oft-repeated clinical impression that flexor tendons repaired within the flexor digital sheath manifest postoperative swelling and undergo necrosis unless the digital sheath and sublimis tendon are excised is not confirmed by the series of experiments reported. No such reaction or series of events was ever seen.

It is generally accepted that trauma to tendons can result in extremely poor functional results after their repair. It has not been generally appreciated, however, that adhesion formation in response to tendon trauma is a discrete and specific phenomenon. Adhesions form at each point at which the surface integrity of tendon is disrupted. Adhesion formation in response to tendon trauma is directly proportional to the degree of tendon-surface trauma. This is a predictable and semiquantitative phenomenon.

Trauma to contiguous anatomic structures is also of extreme importance in the matter of tendon adhesions. When the sublimis tendon is totally excised, the disturbed periosteal floor of the digital canal gives rise to a florid fibroblastic response that takes part in the profundus tendon healing processes. The broad, bone-based adhesions so formed can tether the healing profundus tendon within the digit, effectively destroying all hope of useful function. A flexor tendon requires an extrinsic source of granulation tissue for its healing. Therefore, it will become adherent to any contiguous structure that is capable of producing a fibroblastic granulation tissue response when injured. Thus, an uninjured sublimis tendon should not be sacrificed in order to repair a damaged profundus tendon in the same finger; profundus repair in the presence of an intact sublimis tendon will not result in adhesions between the two tendons provided the sublimis is not traumatized. If the sublimis tendon is badly damaged so that its excision is required, it should be subtotally excised by sharp transverse division immediately proximal to its vincula. The vincula should not be injured or disturbed in removing the sublimis as described.

The surgeon must meticulously avoid iatrogenic injury to all structures in the fingers. Normal anatomic structures should be preserved uninjured whenever possible. It is injudicious, to say the least, to excise or unnecessarily disturb normal structures within the flexor digital mechanism. The price of such action is greater adhesion formation with resultant compromise of delicate digital flexor function.

The experiments with tendon grafts described above clearly demonstrated that paratenon-covered tendons are relatively unsatisfactory as free tendon grafts within the digital flexor mechanism with regard to the experimental parameters defined. Paratenon serves both as a source of adhesions and as an excellent recipient bed for adhesion-producing granulation tissue from other structures. Tendons normally covered by paratenon make better free tendon grafts for the digital flexor mechanism if their paratenon is first carefully removed by dissection taking care not to injure the surface of the tendons. It is well to emphasize, however, that there is no better substitute for a flexor tendon than a free graft of another flexor tendon. If an untraumatized profundus tendon or sublimis tendon is available for grafting, as in the case of amputation, it should be used as a free graft in preference to any other tendon.

The cells of the fresh tendon autografts, both profundus and the paratenon-covered flexor carpi ulnaris, survived free transplantation into the flexor digital sheath and remained intact. There was no evidence of cell death. Similarly, the collagen of the grafts remained intact with no evidence of degeneration except at sites of trauma.

The results of the experiments dealing with the use of freeze-dried profundus tendon homografts are unique and provocative. Such grafts are fully accepted by their new hosts and undergo a process of recellularization effected by an active cellular seeding of the grafts by the host digital sheaths. This recellularization occurs without the formation of adhesions within the area of the flexor digital sheath popularly known as no-man's-land. The excellent anatomic results following the use of these grafts are equaled only by fresh autotopic profundus grafts; remarkably, the freeze-dried profundus homografts produced better anatomic results than fresh paratenon-tendon autografts. It would certainly appear that the time has arrived for us to consider using such grafts clinically where indicated.

Clinical application

Flexor tendons are not healed by an intrinsic tenoblastic response of their own to injury, but rather by the proliferative fibroblastic and vascular reaction of all surrounding tissues whose own integrity has been violated either by accidental injury or surgery. The tissues that surround or lie in proximity to flexor tendons and provide the fibroblastic and vascular basis for flexor tendon healing include the flexor digital sheath (synovium) and periosteum of the bony phalanges as well as the subcutaneous tissue in the fingers, the deep adventitial tissue and palmar fascia in the palm, the synovial tissue and transverse carpal ligament in the carpal canal, and the deep adventitial tissue and antebrachial fascia in the forearm. Of these various tissues, the palmar fascia, the transverse carpal ligaments, the antebrachial fascia, and the osseous floor of the digital flexor tunnel covered with periosteum are tough, unyielding, nongliding structures. An appreciation of this fact is essential to understanding many of the problems of flexor tendon injury and repair. Any of these tissues that contribute to flexor tendon healing become attached to the tendon by adhesions, which provide the cellular and vascular support for the healing tendon wound. As the tendon wound scar (collagen) matures, these adhesions, under ideal circumstances, become loose and filmy. They will not restrict tendon gliding unless they are derived from rigid or unyielding structures (bone, palmar fascia, thick ligaments, or antebrachial fascia). In the latter instance, the tendon is tethered to an unyielding structure and tendon gliding is severely restricted or prevented entirely.

Thus, if a healing flexor tendon is not to become adherent to the bony floor of the digital tunnel, the periosteum of the underlying phalanx must not be traumatized at surgery. If a healing tendon wound is not to become adherent to the palmar fascia in the palm or the antebrachial fascia in the forearm, local palmar fasciectomy or local resection of the antebrachial fascia respectively should be performed at the time of tendon repair.

Because trauma to the tissues surrounding a divided flexor tendon is extremely important to the type and extent of adhesions formed between the tendon and surrounding tissues, so too is the extent of specific trauma to the tendon. The surgeon must employ meticulously atraumatic techniques in order to minimize adhesions to the surface and wound of the healing tendon.

In 1970, I had published the rationale of my approach to flexor tendon injuries as well as the specific techniques employed, based upon my experimental and clinical experience. The reader is encouraged to review that article.[13] Since that time my approach to flexor tendon injuries within the flexor digital sheath has undergone considerable modification and shall be reviewed here in detail.

Injuries to flexor tendons within the digital flexor sheath. In general, three types of tendon injury can occur in this area:

1. Laceration of the superficialis tendon with the profundus left intact
2. Laceration of the profundus tendon with the superficialis left intact or partially intact (one slip of insertion) so that active flexion of the proximal interphalangeal joint as well as the metacarpophalangeal joint is still present
3. Laceration of both flexor tendons

If the superficialis tendon alone is severed, no tendon repair is required since the intact profundus can fully flex the proximal interphalangeal and distal interphalangeal joints.

If the profundus tendon alone has been divided and the superficialis tendon is intact, providing full proximal interphalangeal joint flexion, there are several surgical approaches possible: (1) distal interphalangeal joint volar tenodesis[13] in mild flexion for stability, (2) distal interphalangeal joint arthrodesis[14] in mild flexion for stability, (3) primary flexor (profundus) tendon repair, or (4) free flexor tendon grafting. I now consider primary profundus tendon repair to be the treatment of choice. The rationale for this approach and its indications shall be considered later.

When both flexor tendons are lacerated, again several choices of surgical treatment may be considered:

1. Excision of the lacerated tendons and primary insertion of a free tendon graft
2. Primary repair of the severed profundus tendon with excision of the superficialis tendon
3. Primary repair of both flexor tendons
4. Wound debridement and simple primary closure of the skin to be followed after an appropriate interval by either excision of both severed tendons and the insertion of a free tendon graft as a secondary procedure, or delayed primary repair of one or both tendons

I now consider primary repair of both flexor tendons and certainly at least the flexor profundus tendon where the superficialis may have been irreparably damaged, the treatment of choice. Similarly, where it has not been possible to perform primary flexor tendon repair either because of severe contamination of the original wound or lack of appropriate surgical facilities or skills at the time of primary wound care, I consider delayed primary repair or even early (up to 21 days) secondary repair of both flexor tendons and certainly at least the flexor profundus tendon to be the treatment of choice.

The experimental work presented in previous publications[8-12] and in this paper as well as the superb results achieved clinically by Verdan[15, 16] and Kleinert[3] show that not only is primary repair of flexor tendons in no-man's-land now feasible, but when performed under appropriate circumstances and with proper indications can produce exceedingly gratifying results. Those results are often far superior to primary or secondary flexor tendon grafting.

Primary flexor tendon repair has one supreme advantage over all other techniques devised for dealing with flexor tendon injuries: it restores the flexor muscle-tendon dynamic unit to its ideal functional length. By performing primary or delayed primary repair, the flexor muscle-tendon unit is neither too long nor too short as so frequently occurs with free flexor tendon grafting. By accurately and meticulously repairing the flexor tendon, the entire flexor functional unit is restored to its normal and, therefore, ideal length for optimal flexor function (with no need to sacrifice lumbrical in that finger). I know of no other way of achieving this optimal restoration of functional length following flexor tendon injury. Certainly every method devised to decipher the appropriate length of a free flexor tendon graft is at best an estimate. Primary or delayed primary flexor tendon repair removes all doubt as to whether or not the flexor muscle-tendon unit has been restored to normal or optimal functional length. Secondly, with the proper skills, primary or delayed primary flexor tendon repair effects re-anastomosis of the flexor mechanism with a minimum of dissection and therefore minimizes the possibility of iatrogenic trauma to the other structures of the digital flexor mechanism. As seen in the studies reported above, this is an extremely important consideration in terms of the functional results to be expected following restoration of the flexor mechanism.

When both flexor tendons are severed, both should be meticulously and atramatically repaired if at all possible, even though they may then heal attached to each other by adhesions. If the repair has been meticulous, these adhesions will be loose and filmy and will lyse spontaneously on active use. If the repair has been less than ideal, they can be readily lysed surgically at an appropriate interval after the original primary repair. The essential factor here is that by repairing both tendons, at the very least, the repaired superficialis tendon restores a smooth gliding surface beneath the repaired profundus tendon and effectively prevents any unyielding restrictive adhesions between the latter and the traumatized bony floor of the flexor tunnel. The reader is referred to the work of Verdan[15, 16] and Kleinert[3] for the specific techniques of primary flexor tendon repair.

When primary flexor tendon repair fails because of scar tissue or adhesion formation, the scarring is often so extensive that heretofore it has been felt that all scar tissue had to be excised from the digital flexor sheath along with the extensively scarred tendons so that the finger could be prepared for free tendon grafting. In the experience of many hand surgeons who have treated such fingers, it was found that the results in such cases were often far worse than had the original flexor tendon injury simply been treated by debridement and closure of the wound and by delayed secondary tendon grafting. However, I have found that most primary repair failures can be salvaged without excising the repaired tendons, by employing a special technique of tenolysis. Before discussing this technique, it must be emphasized that primary repair of flexor tendons should be performed for relatively sharply incised, clean wounds in which there is a minimum of trauma to surrounding structures. The surgeon must employ the utmost skill in performing meticulous atraumatic surgery. Following such repair, the hand must be appropriately immobilized disallowing any attempt at active motion of the repaired tendon for at least 3 weeks, at which time gentle active flexion is started. After 4 weeks, full active flexion with maximum strength is allowed. These patients may require dynamic splinting as well as intensive formal physiotherapy and rehabilitation to achieve the optimal results. If that result has not been achieved by 6 months then tenolysis should be considered.

Technique for flexor tendon tenolysis. The digital flexor sheath is exposed in the finger by either a midlateral incision or the Brunner volar zig-zag incision. The flexor sheath is removed in the area of scarred primary tendon repair, while carefully preserving the essential annular ligaments at the base of the proximal phalanx and at the middle of the middle phalanx. These should be preserved even though they are scarred. They can be freed of the underlying scarred tendons by meticulous sharp dissection. Once this has been achieved, regardless of how much thickened dense scar tissue may be present and regardless of whether the flexor profundus and flexor superficialis tendons are densely scarred to each other or even inseparable, they are not excised. Rather, again using meticulously sharp scalpel dissection the surgeon literally carves out of this mass of scar tissue a new tendon so that there is both profundus and superficialis tendon continuity. One should be very careful not to decrease the width or diameter of the tendons lest they be so weakened that they rupture in the postoperative period. When this part of the dissection has been completed, two tendons will be left in continuity even though their surfaces may be irregular and ragged. Next, a very fine thin sheet (0.005 in.) of medical grade silastic, cut to appropriate length and width, is wrapped about the profundus tendon so that it completely, though loosely, encloses the ragged tenolyzed area of the tendon. The silastic sheath is thus converted into a semiclosed tube whose ends are tacked at either end to the proximal and distal annular ligaments with fine 5-0 nylon suture. This effectively separates the profundus tendon from the underlying sublimis tendon or raw bony floor of the digital canal, as the case may be, as well as the scarified subcutaneous tissue. The skin incision is then closed appropriately and a bulky fluff dressing is applied. Of course, if there is not full mobility of the proximal interphalangeal joint at the time this dissection is carried out, appropriate surgical mobilization of the joint should be carried out prior to wound closure.

Immediately postoperative when the patient awakens, active flexion and extension exercises of the finger are begun. On the third or fourth postoperative day, the bulky dressing is removed, a light sterile spray plastic dressing is applied, and active flexion and extension exercises are continued. The patient usually achieves optimal functional restoration of active motion by the fifth or sixth postoperative day. The active range of motion of the joints in all cases so treated has been limited only by the passive range of motion of the joints at the time surgery was completed.

I have performed such tenolysis on a number of cases of failed primary flexor tendon repairs and have been able to convert each of those failed cases into what would be considered an excellent result by any standard. In each case done so far, I have re-explored the finger to remove the silastic membrane several months after the tenolysis. At each exploration, the tenolyzed tendon or tendons have been perfectly smooth* and enclosed in a smooth gliding flexor sheath. Indeed, except for the presence of the silastic and the suture material used to achieve primary repair, one would not be able to determine that the tendons had indeed been injured. Thus even grossly failed primary flexor tendon repairs can be salvaged with remarkable functional results.

The use of a silastic "blocking" membrane here is not a violation of principles laid down earlier in this paper proscribing the use of "adhesion blocking" tubes or membranes about sites of tendon repair. At the time of tenolysis, there is tendon continuity albeit badly scarred, with no tendon wound with a requirement for granulation tissue from without for healing. The use of such materials here to "block" adhesions to a segment of intact tendon therefore has no contraindication.

The discussion above concerning primary flexor tendon repair must not be interpreted as a rejection of free flexor tendon grafting. There is no question that free flexor tendon grafting is still a very essential part of the hand surgeon's armamentarium, but we should be performing a higher proportion of primary flexor tendon repairs. Where primary flexor tendon repair has not been possible and too long a period of time has elapsed for restoration of normal flexor muscle-tendon continuity or where primary flexor tendon repair has failed and for whatever reason tenolysis is not possible, then one must resort to free flexor tendon grafting. Very often such fingers will require prior treatment with the Hunter tendon prosthesis as described elsewhere in this volume. I still perform flexor tendon grafting procedures, but in terms of the modified approach to flexor tendon injuries described above, I find that fewer and fewer free flexor tendon grafts are necessary. The reader is referred to an earlier article[13] for the technique of flexor tendon grafting.

*This observation provides some index of the capacity for structural remodeling on the part of flexor tendons under the stress of functional use.

References

1. Cordrey, L. J., McCorkle, H., and Hilton, E.: A comparative study of fresh autogenous and preserved homogenous tendon grafts in rabbits, J. Bone Joint Surg. **45B**:182-195, 1963.
2. Flynn, J. E., and Graham, J. H.: Lyophilized heterogenous and autogenous tendon transplants, Surg. Gynecol. and Obstet. **116**:345-350, 1963.
3. Kleinert, H. E., et al.: Primary repair of lacerated flexor tendons in "no man's land," J. Bone Joint Surg. **49A**:577, 1967.
4. Kreuz, F. P., Hyatt, G. W., Turner, T. C., and Bassett, A. L.: The preservation and clinical use of freeze-dried bone, J. Bone Joint Surg. **33A**:863-872, 1951.
5. Mason, M. L.: Primary tendon repair, J. Bone Joint Surg. **41A**:575-577, 1959.
6. Peacock, E. E., Jr., and Petty, J. M.: Biological reactions to collagen transplants, Surg. Forum **9**:815-819, 1958.
7. Peacock, E. E., Jr.: Morphology of homologous and heterologous tendon grafts, Surg. Gynecol. and Obstet. **109**:735-742, 1959.
8. Potenza, A. D.: Critical evaluation of flexor tendon healing and adhesion formation within artificial digital sheaths, J. Bone Joint Surg. **45-A**:1217-1233, 1963.
9. Potenza, A. D.: Effect of associated trauma on healing of divided tendon, J. Trauma **2**:175-184, 1962.
10. Potenza, A. D.: Flexor tendon injuries, Orthop. Clin. North Am. **1**:355-373, 1970.
11. Potenza, A. D.: The healing of autogenous tendon grafts within the flexor digital sheath in dogs, J. Bone Joint Surg. **46A**:1462-1484, 1964.
12. Potenza, A. D.: Prevention of adhesions to healing digital flexor tendons, J.A.M.A. **187**:187-191, 1964.
13. Potenza, A. D.: A technique for arthrodesis of finger joints, J. Bone Joint Surg. **55A**:1534-1536, 1973.
14. Potenza, A. D.: Tendon healing within the flexor digital sheath in the dog; an experimental study, J. Bone Joint Surg. **44A**:49-64, 1962.
15. Verdan, C. E.: Primary and secondary repair of flexor and extensor tendon injuries, In Flynn, J. W., editor: Hand surgery, Baltimore, 1966, The Williams & Wilkins Co.
16. Verdan, C. E.: Primary repair of flexor tendon, J. Bone Joint Surg. **42A**:647-657, 1960.

5. Intrinsic vascularization of flexor tendons

Howard S. Caplan, M.D.
James M. Hunter, M.D.
Robert J. Merklin, Ph.D.

INTRODUCTION AND HISTORICAL BACKGROUND

Several studies dealing with the extrinsic blood supply to tendons have been published during the last half century. These have included postmortem injection studies and in vivo studies utilizing intravital microscopy and radioassays. Only a few of these studies have actually dealt with human material and none have included detailed microscopic investigations.

Mayer[6] pointed out the segmental sources of the extrinsic vasculature. These are: (1) musculotendinous junction as a continuation of the perimyseal vessels, (2) paratenon vessels, (3) plical and vincular vessels (mesotenon) in sheathed areas, and (4) tendinosseous junction as a continuation of the periosteal vessels. Within the tendon, Mayer[6] described that "vessels travel in the hilum of the tendon, in the epitenon, and in the connective tissue septa between the tendon bundles (the endotenon)" and these vessels "anastomose freely by transverse and oblique branches." Edwards[3] further defined the intrinsic pattern as simple and uniform throughout the tendon. Each tendon fascicle is surrounded by endotenon carrying a series of longitudinally oriented vascular bundles (an arteriole and two larger venules). These vessels are fed from surface vessels by transversely oriented vessels of the same size that thread their way around and between the fascicles, linking the longitudinal system into a uniform plexus. All vessels and capillary loops are interfascicular and none penetrate into the collagen bundles. Brockis[2] and Smith[8] confirmed this interfascicular pattern in human flexor tendons and made an additional observation peculiar to the flexor digitorum profundus (FDP) in the area of the proximal (PIP) and distal (DIP) interphalangeal joints. At these points, the longitudinal system is "upset by an artistic grouping of peculiar vertical loops originating from the dorsal channel or the vinculum longae (VL) and brevae (VB)." Peacock[7] showed that in dogs the longitudinal circulation through intrinsic vessels was nonexistent for distances greater than one third the length of isolated tendons. Young and Weeks,[10] studying monkeys, concluded that within the digital sheath (1) the FDP, at the proximal end of the sheath, was less well perfused than distally, (2) the distal portion of the FDP was perfused by the VB, (3) the proximal portion was perfused by the palmar vessels, and (4) the VL alone could not maintain normal levels of perfusion.

Since healing in vascularized tissues is governed by its blood supply, it is our goal to investigate in detail the intrinsic microcirculation of human flexor tendons.

MATERIALS AND METHODS

Twenty fetal upper extremities were utilized in this project. The fetuses ranged in gestational age between 7 and 9 months and in weight between 1 and 4 kilograms. Hand controlled injections were made through angiocaths placed in the largest available artery—umbilical in the smaller specimens and axillary in the larger. The vascular system was flushed with physiologic saline solution until clear fluid exited from the venous system and then a diluted India ink latex solution (3:1 through 15:1) was injected. The injection was continued until the India ink solution appeared in the venous system. A tourniquet was applied when possible and 50 to 100 ml. more material was injected to obtain maximal filling at the capillary level. The specimens were then dissected and/or sectioned, dehydrated in ethanol, cleared in a 2:11 solution of tributyl phosphate and tricresyl phosphate, and photographed by transillumination. Selected specimens were processed and serially sectioned for microscopic study.

OBSERVATIONS

Intrinsic vascularization

Paratenon system. The flexor sublimis and profundus tendons, from their musculotendinous origin to the level of the proximal portion of the flexor digital sheath, have a uniform intratendinous vascular pattern as previously described by Edwards,[3] Brockis,[2] and Smith.[8] The basic unit of tendon vascularization, the fascicle, consists of multiple collagen bundles and their investing connective tissue, the endotenon. Within the interfascicular connective tissue, in a uniform cross-sectional distribution, is found the basic vascular unit—a single arteriole and one or two venules (Figs. 5-1 to 5-3). This system is oriented longitudinally, paralleling the longitudinal course of the tendon fascicles; however, there are frequent cross connections between the intratendinous vessels and between the segmental vessels of the surrounding paratenon. This system ends at the point where the palmar vessel branches on the volar surface of the sublimis (FDS) and profundus (FDP) tendons with their investing mesotenon become intratendinous, forming the prepucial fold. Anatomically, this occurs at the base of the proximal phalanx under the proximal pulley (Figs. 5-4 and 5-5).

Vincular system. In the digital sheath, a separate, more elaborate, dorsally-

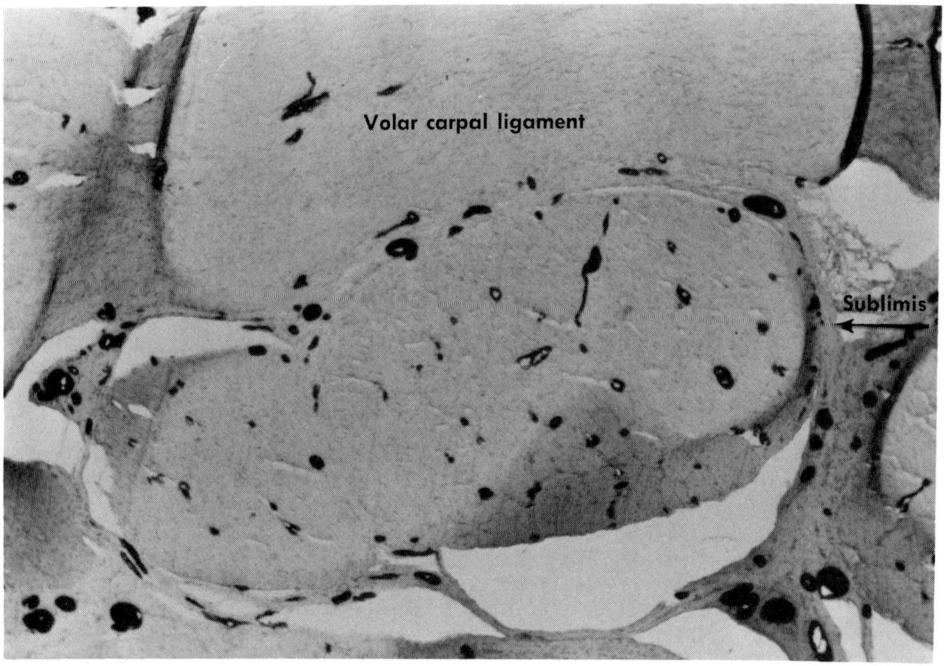

Fig. 5-1. Flexor digitorum sublimis under volar carpal ligament in carpal tunnel (cross section hematoxylin and eosin).

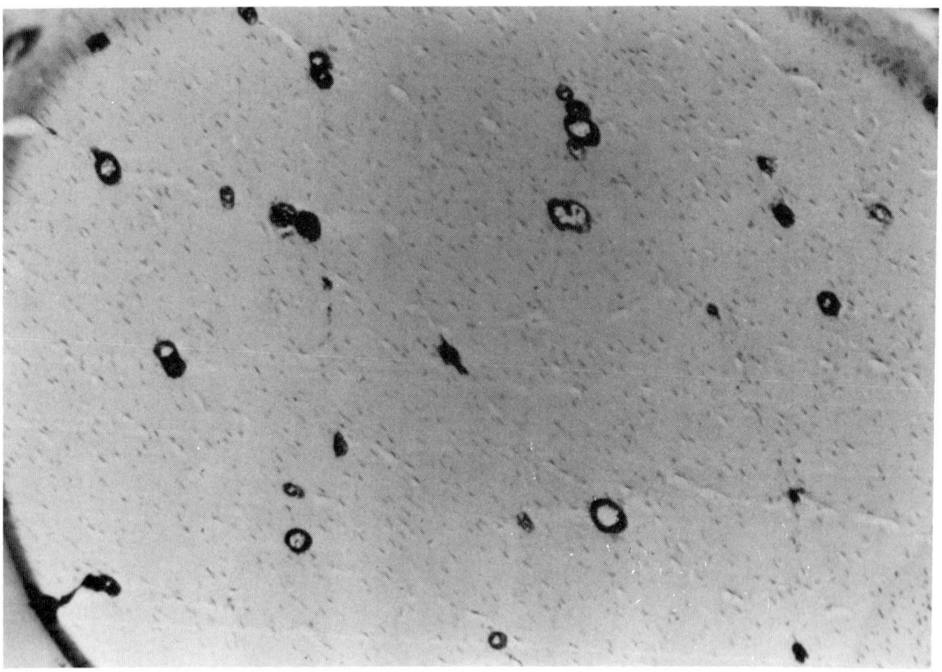

Fig. 5-2. Flexor digitorum profundus at same level as Fig. 5-1 (cross section hematoxylin and eosin).

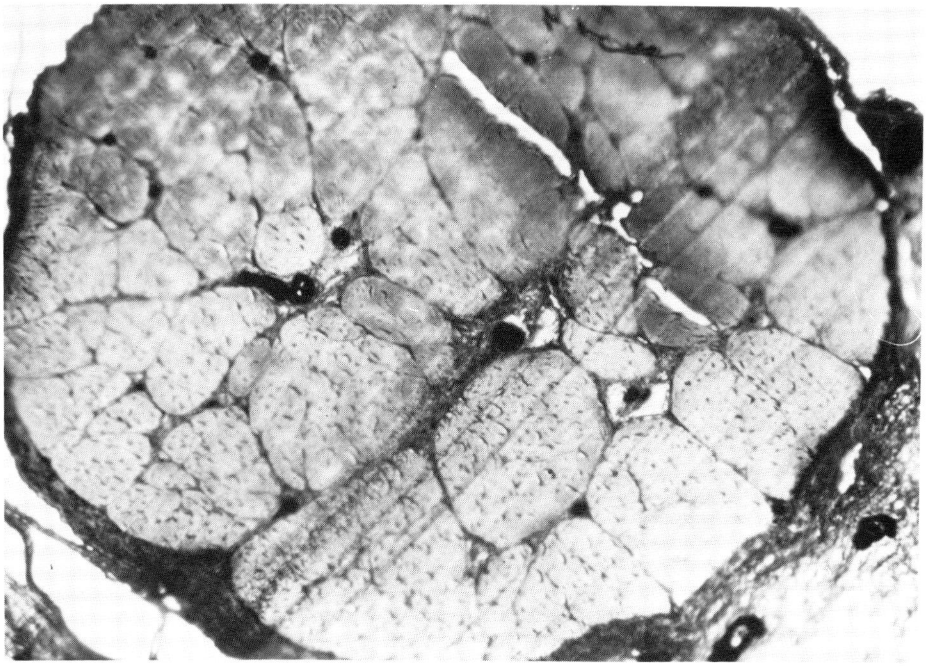

Fig. 5-3. Flexor digitorum profundus at level of origin of lumbricals (cross section hematoxylin and eosin).

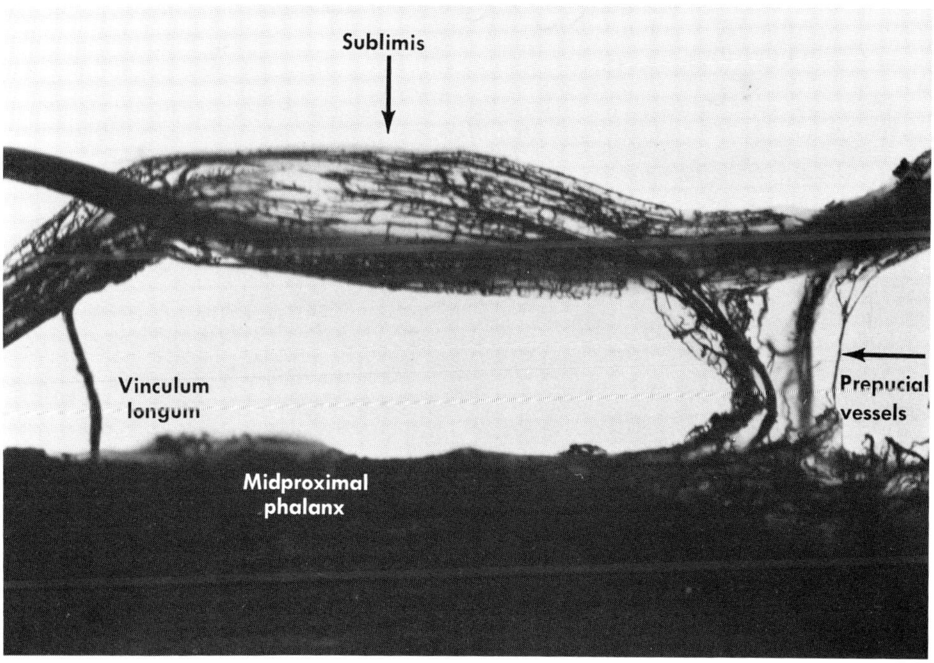

Fig. 5-4. Flexor digitorum sublimis and flexor digitorum profundus in digital sheath. Prepucial fold with termination of palmar vessels is on the right. The termination of the vinculum longum coursing across inferior surface of flexor digitorum sublimis onto the flexor digitorum profundus is at the left. Note the lack of communication of longitudinal vessels in crossover area at the midproximal phalanx level.

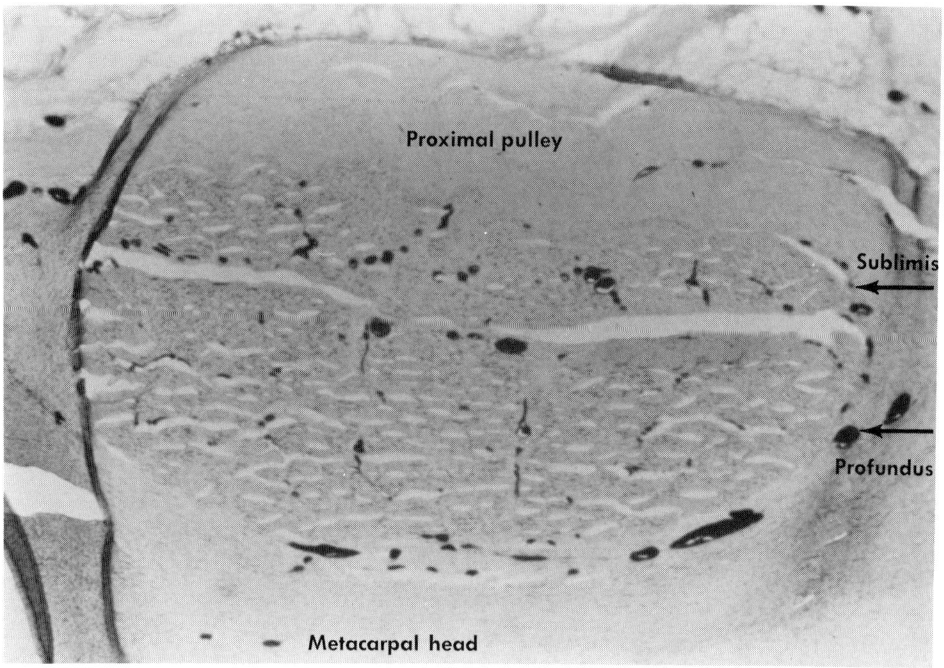

Fig. 5-5. Flexor digitorum sublimis and flexor digitorum profundus at the level of the base of the metacarpal head (cross section hematoxylin and eosin).

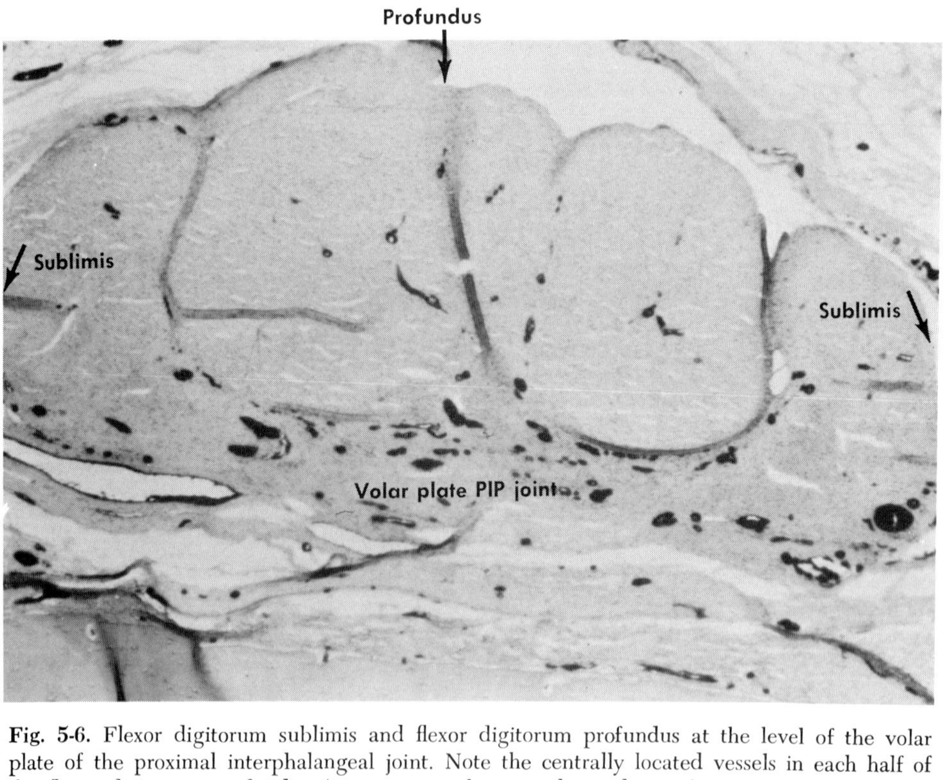

Fig. 5-6. Flexor digitorum sublimis and flexor digitorum profundus at the level of the volar plate of the proximal interphalangeal joint. Note the centrally located vessels in each half of the flexor digitorum profundus (cross section hematoxylin and eosin).

based system exists. The major extrinsic vessels, the vinculae, form a single longitudinal system on the dorsal surface of the FDP and each slip of the FDS to a level a few cms. proximal to the decussation of the sublimis. Similarly, the intratendinous vasculature has a predominantly dorsal distribution except for the insertional slips of the FDS, which are covered by a highly vascularized synovium. In the sublimis, the intratendinous vessels are concentrated in the central portion of the tendinous slips while the more peripherally located fascicles are relatively avascular (Fig. 5-6). The interface between the dorsally-based vincular system and the uniform paratenon system occurs proximal to the decussation of the sublimis at the midportion of the proximal phalanx. In the profundus, this predominantly dorsal distribution of the intratendinous vascularization is more obvious. The main vascular channel of the FDP lies surrounded by loose areolar tissue on the dorsal surface of the tendon in the central groove.[5] It arises as the vinculum brevum (VB) and is supplemented by the vinculum longum (VL) at the PIP joint (Fig. 5-7). Radiating from this central channel are three groups of vessels oriented perpendicularly to the long axis of the tendon. These interconnecting vessels, in the form of vascular loops, connect into the longitudinal intratendinous system. The intrinsic system in cross section is restricted to the central por-

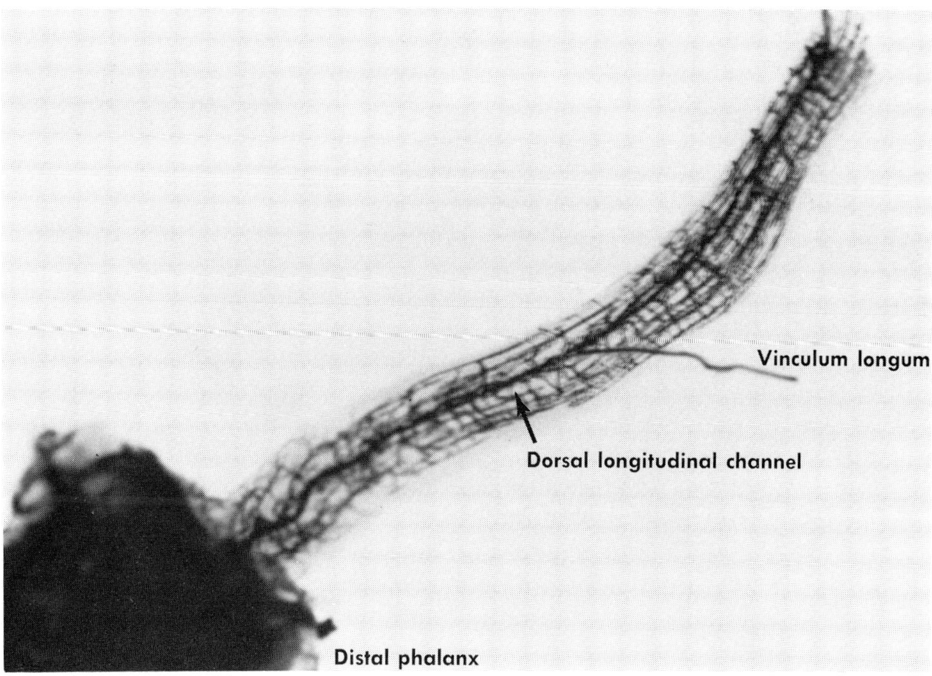

Fig. 5-7. Dorsal aspect of the flexor digitorum profundus showing the dorsal longitudinal channel and vinculum longum. Insertion of the flexor digitorum profundus onto the distal phalanx is on the left.

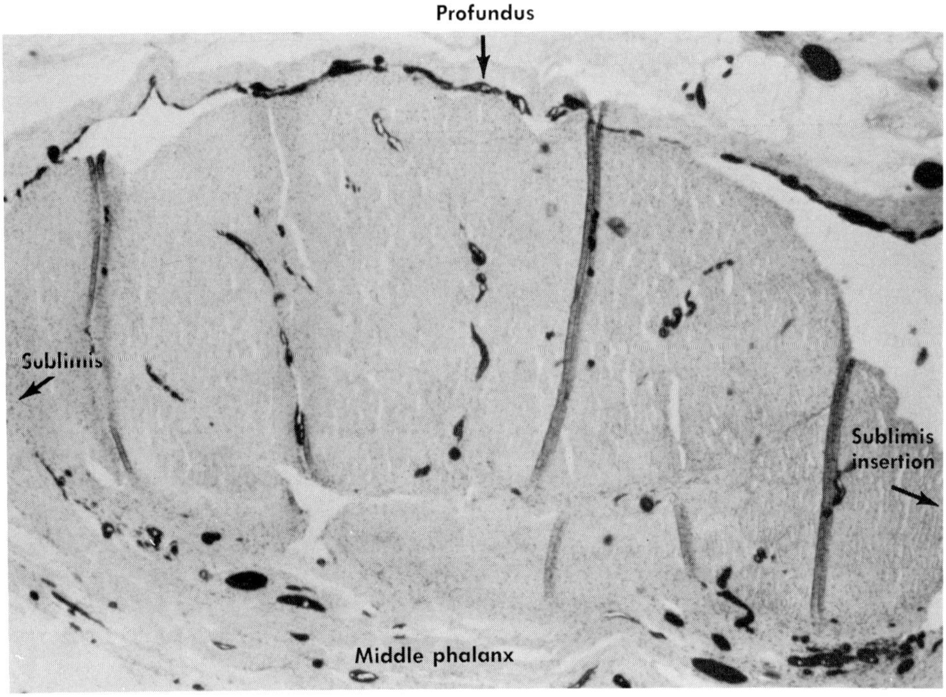

Fig. 5-8. Flexor digitorum profundus at insertion of the flexor digitorum sublimis on the middle phalanx; note concentration of vessels in central portion of flexor digitorum profundus and centrally in each half of the flexor digitorum profundus.

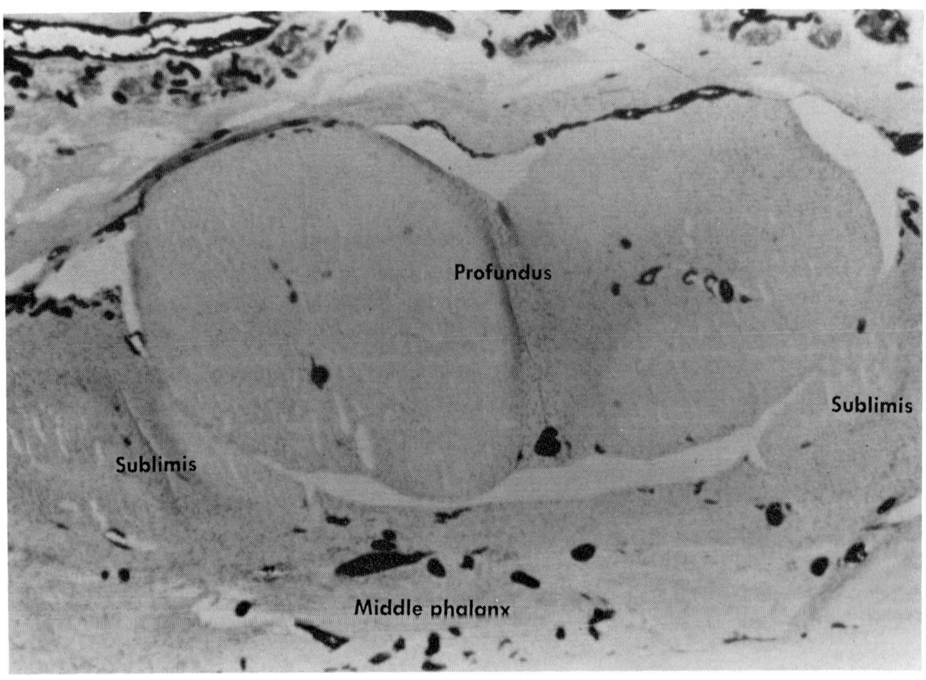

Fig. 5-9. Flexor digitorum profundus at the distal interphalangeal joint vessels in central portion of each half of the flexor digitorum profundus and dorsal longitudinal channel.

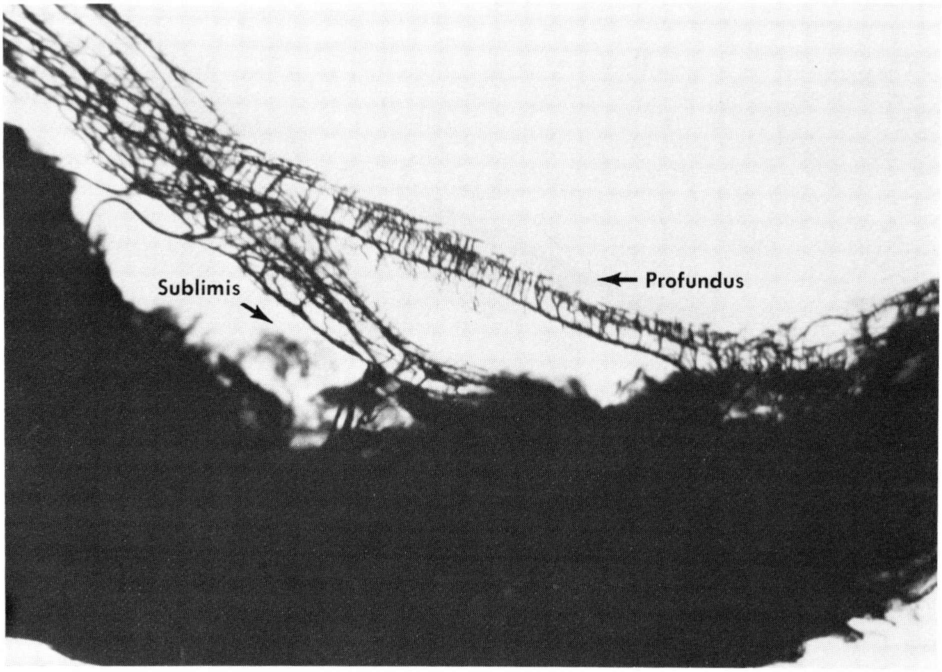

Fig. 5-10. Midportion of proximal phalanx (on the left) and insertion of the flexor digitorum sublimis and flexor digitorum profundus (on the right). Note vascular loops and vinculum longum of the flexor digitorum profundus as branch of vinculum brevum to sublimis (left).

tion of each half of the FDP and to the endotenon connecting these halves (Figs. 5-8 and 5-9). These vascular loops and their connections are present in the FDP from the level of the DIP joint to the midportion of the proximal phalanx (Fig. 5-10). The volar and lateral surfaces of the FDP are virtually avascular. As in the FDS, a cross-over zone exists at the midproximal phalanx between the dorsally based vincular system and the paratenon system.

Sublimis-profundus vascular interrelationships

In the digital sheaths, the segmental vascularization to flexor tendons takes the form of the vinculum longum and vinculum brevum. For the FDS, the VB is a midline dorsal vessel arising from the proximal transverse digital branches of the digital vessels at the level proximal to the PIP joint over the volar plate. Similarly, at the DIP joint, the VB of the profundus tendon arises from a second distal transverse digital branch.[5] The VL to the profundus tendon takes a course intricately associated with the FDS. The VL arises as a branch of the VB of the FDS just proximal to the PIP joint (Figs. 5-10 to 5-13) or as a branch from the VL to the sublimis tendon at the level of the decussation of the FDS.

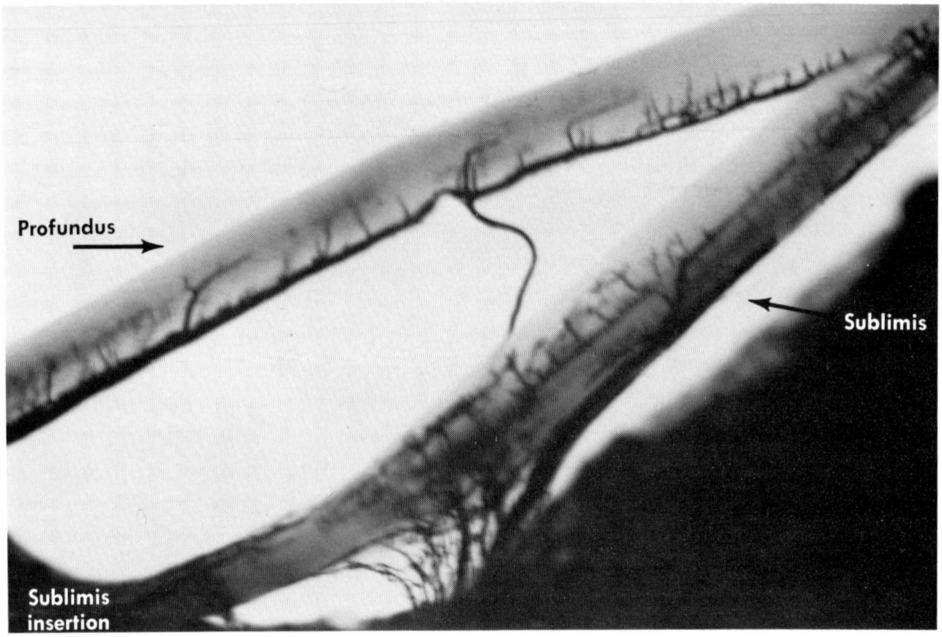

Fig. 5-11. Vinculum longum to the flexor digitorum profundus arising from the vinculum brevum of the flexor digitorum sublimis and passing through Camper's chiasm (insertion of the flexor digitorum profundus on the left; decussation of sublimis on the right). Note the perpendicular vascular connections (vascular loops) on both flexor digitorum sublimis and flexor digitorum profundus.

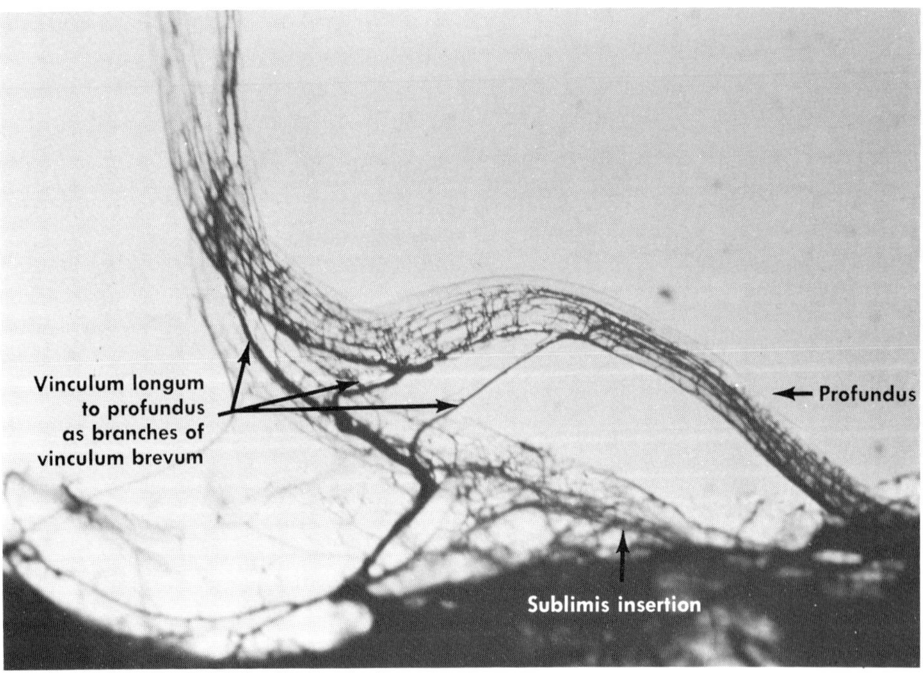

Fig. 5-12. Branches of vinculum brevum of flexor digitorum sublimis reaching flexor digitorum profundus as vinculum longum in two areas. Insertion of flexor digitorum profundus is on the right.

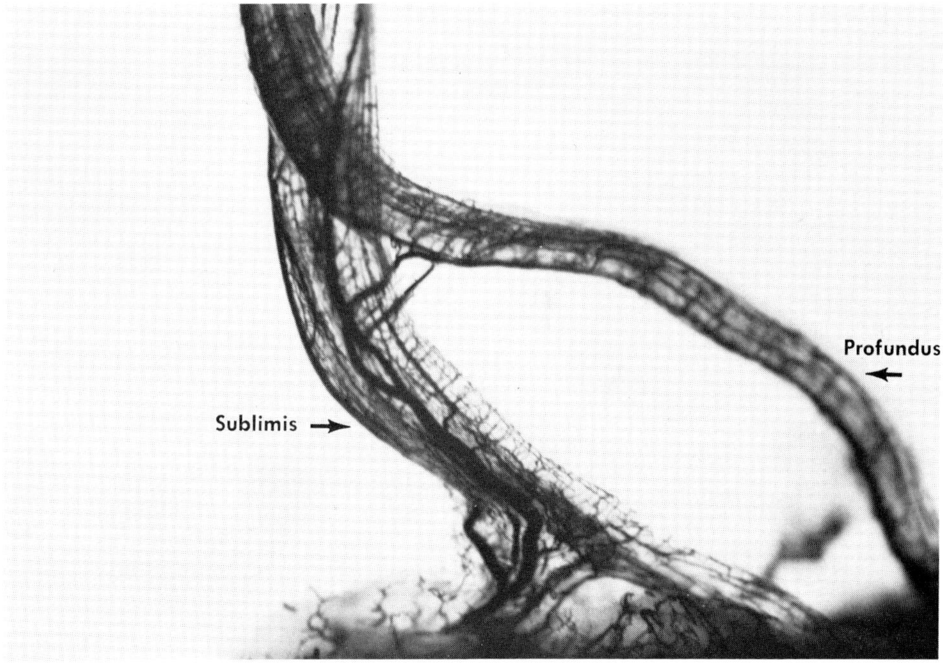

Fig. 5-13. Vascularization of flexor digitorum profundus off vinculum brevum of flexor digitorum sublimis at decussation of flexor digitorum sublimis. Insertion of flexor digitorum profundus is on the right.

DISCUSSION

If one assumes that tendon healing is related to the periadventitial cells of blood vessels, the presence of an intrinsic vascularity as we have demonstrated would support the concept of end-to-end healing of tendons. We have not been able to demonstrate intrinsic vessels in dog FDP in the area where the classic experiments in tendon healing were conducted and this would be a possible explanation of the need for an extrinsic source of fibroblasts for tendon healing. The implication of finding two separate nutritional systems is unclear. Does the more evenly distributed interfascicular paratenon system account for the more predictable good result in the palm? Is the dorsally-based vascular loop vincular system a more delicate diffusional system that, when injured, leads to a more unpredictable surgical result? The interface between the paratenon and vincular systems at the level of the midproximal phalanx probably explains the findings of Peacock[7] and Young and Weeks[10] regarding the inability of the intrinsic vascularization to support isolated tendons over long distances. The presence of two systems also emphasizes the importance of exact localization of level of injuries in relationship to a fixed point—the phalanges with the finger in the fully-extended position. This could possibly help in making clinical correlations in respect to the type of vascularity in the area injured.

The finding of the passage of the VL along the sublimis to the FDP is probably the most significant as to clinical implications. If one resects the sublimis while repairing the FDP at the level of the midproximal phalanx, one could render the distal FDP avascular by destroying its VL. This could explain why Verdan's[9] repair of both FDS and FDP did better than the repair of FDP with excision of the FDS.

The concept of a dorsally-based nutritional system in the digital sheath could affect the choice of suture method. The more volarly placed Kessler stitch (placed parallel to the intrinsic vascular pattern) will interfere with the nutritional system less than the Bunnell suture (crossing vessels tangentially and being placed more dorsally).[1] Interference with the nutritional system, increases the "gap" and thus increases the scar.

Further studies are being carried out on adults as well as various animal models in hopes of correlating results of experiments in one species with clinical dogma in humans.

References

1. Bergljung, L.: Vascular reactions after tendon suture and tendon transplantation, Scand. J. Plast. Reconstr. Surg. Supplementum 4, 1968.
2. Brockis, J. G.: The blood supply of the flexor and extensor tendons of the fingers in man, J. Bone Joint Surg. **35B**:131-138, Feb., 1953.
3. Edwards, D. A. W.: The blood supply and lymphatic drainage of tendons, J. Anat. **80**: 147-152, 1946.
4. Edwards, E. A.: Organization of the small arteries of the hand and digits, Am. J. Surg. **99**:837-846, 1960.
5. Field, P. L.: Tendon fibre arrangement and blood supply, Aust. N. Z. J. Surg. **40**:298-302, Feb., 1971.
6. Mayer, L.: The physiologic method of tendon transplantation, Surg. Gynecol. Obstet. **22**: 298-306, 1916.
7. Peacock, E. E., Jr.: A study of the circulation in normal tendons and healing grafts, Ann. Surg. **149**:415-428, 1959.
8. Smith, J. W.: Blood supply of tendons, Am. J. Surg. **109**:272-276, 1965.
9. Verdan, C. E.: Half a century of flexor tendon surgery: current status and changing philosophies, J. Bone Joint Surg. **54A**:472-491, April, 1972.
10. Young, L., and Weeks, P. M.: Profundus tendon blood supply within the digital sheath, Surg. Forum **21**:504-506, 1971.

6. Tendon sheath reconstruction with artificial implants: a study of ultrastructure

Roger E. Salisbury, M.D.
Norman S. Levine, M.D.
Daniel W. McKeel, Jr., M.D.
Basil A. Pruitt, M.D.
Clarence W. R. Wade, Ph.D.

INTRODUCTION

For many years, flexor tendon injuries in no-man's-land, with attendant destruction of the sheath, pulleys, and surrounding soft tissue consistently defied good operative results regardless of the surgeon's knowledge of the hand, preoperative planning, or technical skill. Far too often the repaired tendon healed with dense adhesions resulting in severely limited range of motion. Experiments with drugs[4] to decrease adhesions, while provocative, have not been practical in humans. Efforts to prevent adhesions from interfering with tendon gliding by surrounding the anastomosis with blocking agents[2] have caused many foreign body reactions and more scar or prevented wound healing, resulting in tendon necrosis.

During the past ten years, however, markedly improved results in previously unsalvageable fingers have been achieved by Hunter[3] using an artificial tendon implant to reconstruct the normal anatomy before performing a tendon graft. The remodeling of undifferentiated connective tissue around an implant to form a new synovial tendon sheath is such a unique example of the clinical surgeon controlling wound healing that further experiments were performed in the laboratory to better understand this process.

METHOD

The chicken was chosen for the experimental studies because the anatomy of its foot is analogous to that of the human hand; each digit has a flexor digitorum profundus and flexor digitorum sublimis tendon surrounded by a synovial sheath. Since the foot is prehensile, function can be easily evaluated as a measure of the success of tendon surgery. The experimental tendon used in this study was made by the U. S. Army Biomechanical Research Laboratory and consisted of medical grade silicone rubber coating a porous dacron tape 3 mm. wide and 1 mm. thick. Because the silicone rubber could be easily peeled back from the tape, implant length could be adjusted for any size digit.

In a series of 35 chickens, each animal was restrained in a towel and the foot was scrubbed with Betadine soap and alcohol. After a digital block was achieved with a 1% Xylocaine injection, an Esmarch bandage was applied to effect a bloodless field and the long toe was explored through a midlateral incision. The digital sheath was carefully excised (except for the pulleys), the flexor digitorum sublimis and flexor digitorum profundus excised and discarded, and the artificial tendon sutured to the distal flexor digitorum profundus stump in a fishmouth anastomosis with two #5-0 nylon simple sutures. An artificial tendon was also inserted into the soft tissue of the chicken's back, either above or below the dorsal muscles, to determine if location or lack of motion of the implant changed the nature of the neosheath. All casts were removed 3 weeks after surgery, and the chickens were allowed to ambulate freely in a grated cage that allowed unlimited flexion of the toes. The toes were reexplored 8 weeks after surgery, and the artificial tendon, with surrounding neosheath and pulley, was dissected out. The implant and neosheath from the back were also removed, as well as a normal flexor synovial sheath from another toe to serve as a control. Neosheath specimens were fixed in formalin or glutaraldehyde and submitted for light scanning and electron microscopy.

RESULTS

In all the animals, undifferentiated connective tissue in the back and foot responded to the presence of an implant by forming a neosheath around it. The sheaths in the back were thinner (Fig. 6-1) than the normal control, translucent, and very vascular. The neosheath in the foot was thicker (Fig. 6-2) than the control. Hematoxylin and eosin preparations of sheaths from all locations revealed marked similarities and a few differences. Although normal tendon sheath and the neosheaths from the foot and back had fibrous and areolar types of synovium, the neosheaths from the foot were predominantly fibrous with the collagenous portion of the sheath being more developed than in the others. The neosheaths formed in the foot most often had an intimal layer consisting of one layer of flattened fibroblasts (Fig. 6-3) whereas the normal tendon sheath and the neosheaths from the back had intima several cells thick consisting of plump cuboidal cells.

Scanning electron microscopy of specimens from all three locations was very similar and revealed two predominant patterns. In some parts of the sheath the surface was very cellular (Fig. 6-4) and resembled rugae interspersed with pores. In other areas the surface showed wavy pleats (Fig. 6-5) of parallel collagen bundles. The pleating of the sheath would effectively increase the surface area, perhaps important during motion. Pores also have been noted by others[1]

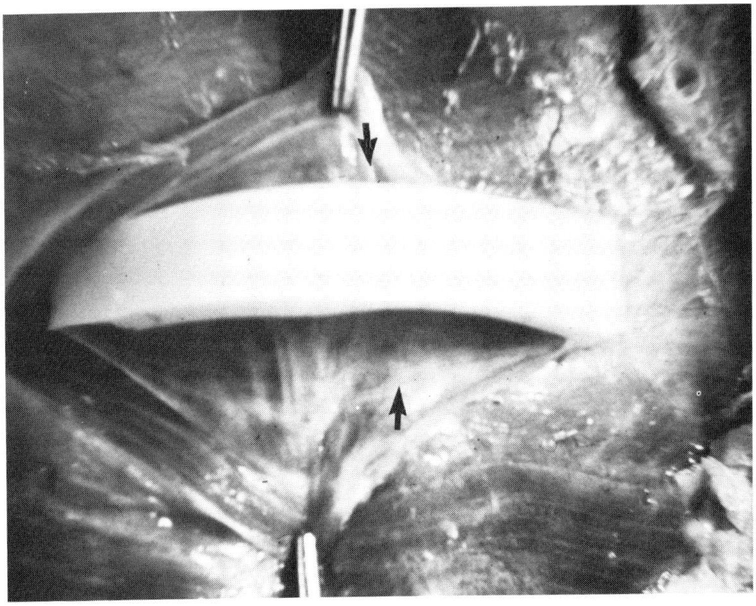

Fig. 6-1. Neosheath from the back of a chicken (8 weeks old) has been slit open longitudinally and retracted to reveal a filmy, translucent wall (arrow).

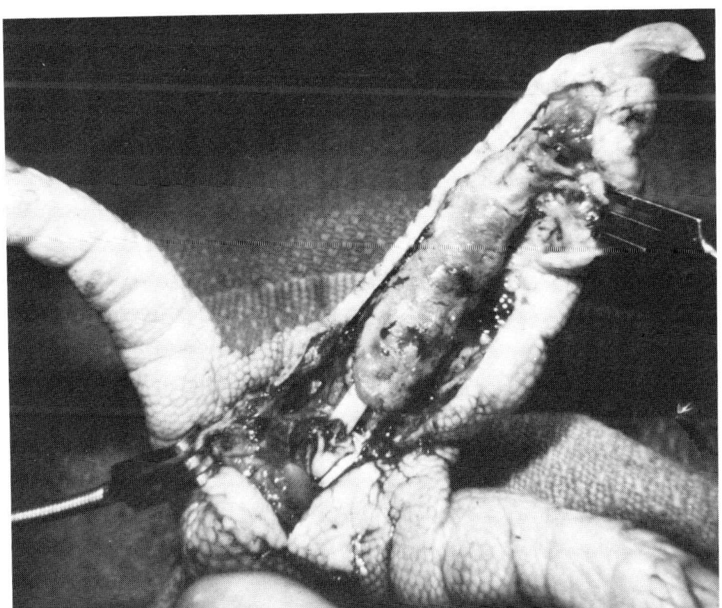

Fig. 6-2. Thick neosheath in the toe of a chicken 8 weeks old.

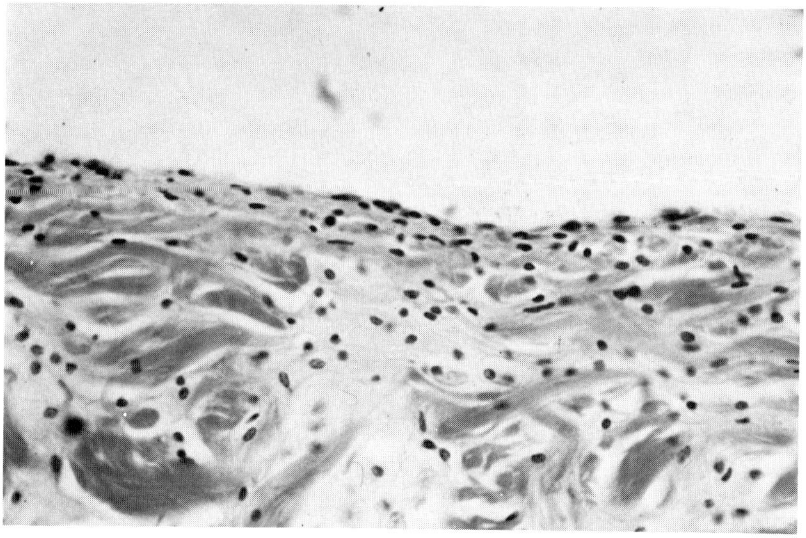

Fig. 6-3. Fibrous neosheath from foot of chicken, revealing intimal layer of fibroblasts over layer of collagen (hematoxylin and eosin ×40).

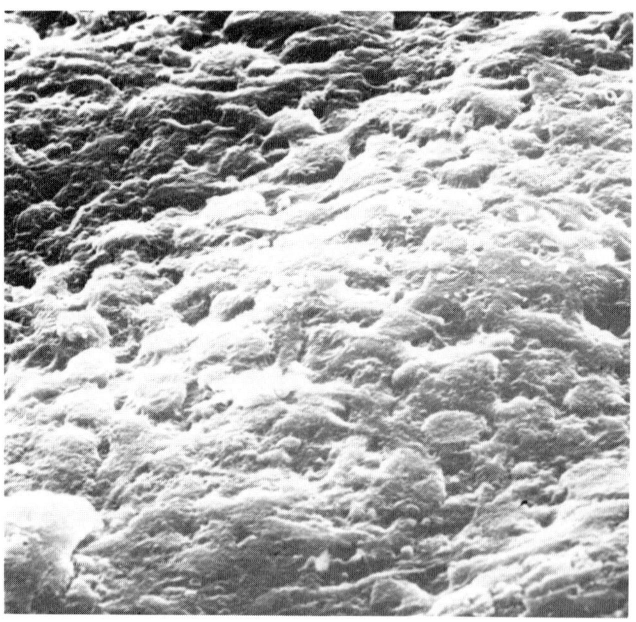

Fig. 6-4. Scanning electron microscopy of cellular portion of neosheath (×800).

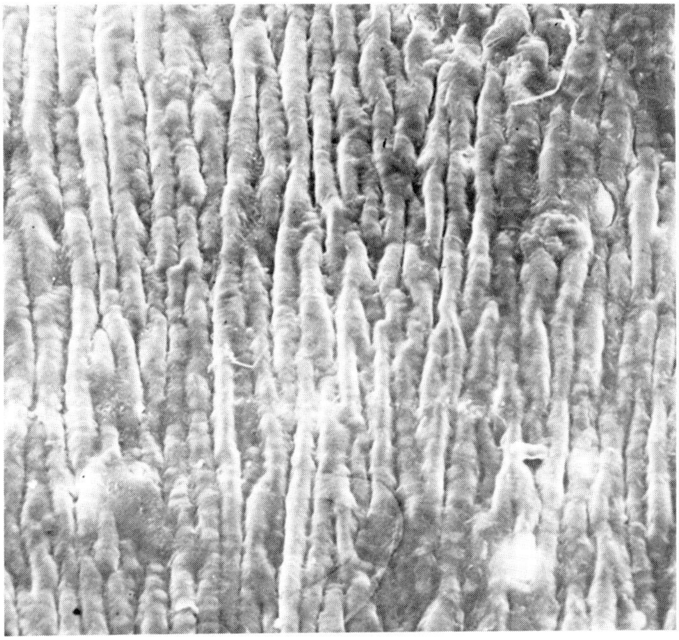

Fig. 6-5. Scanning electron microscopy of neosheath, showing fibrous pleated surface (×200).

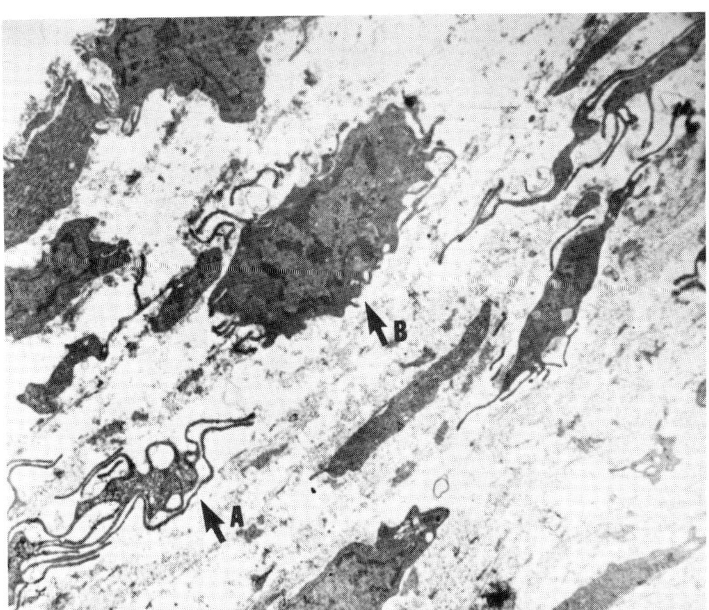

Fig. 6-6. Transmission electron microscopy of neosheath, with cells similar to Type A and Type B (arrows) (×24,000).

in examining synovial tissue and measured to be 1 micron in normal synovium. It may be speculated that they provide passage for nutrients to the intimal surface and that the valleys between the pleats may trap the lubricating synovial fluid essential for tendon gliding.

Transmission electron microscopy further clarified the cellular and fibrous structure of the sheath. All neosheaths from the back and toes, and the controls, contained predominantly fibroblasts, as well as macrophages, intermediate cells, mast cells, and Schwann cells. The intimal cellular layer in contact with the tendon was noncontinuous in all specimens and lacked a basement membrane. These findings confirm that the pores seen by scanning electron microscopy were not artifacts. The intimal cells were rich in cytoplasmic vacuoles and the surface was remarkable for many cytoplasmic processes. In the neosheaths of the back and foot were Type A– and Type B–appearing cells (Fig. 6-6), seen also in the controls and previously identified only in synovial tissue. The Type A–like cells (called phagocytic by Wysocki[5]) characteristically had a surface topography broken by many cytoplasmic processes and an interior rich in cytoplasmic vacuoles, mitochondria, fibrils, and filopodia. Type B–appearing cells were characterized by dilated cysternae of endoplasmic reticulum, but few cytoplasmic processes, vacuoles, or mitochondria. Other intermediate cells showed characteristics of both cell types as well as fibrils and lysosomes, often indicative of a role in collagen synthesis. The underlying fibrous layer was of variable thickness and contained collagen, reticulum, elastic, and unmyelinated nerve fibers.

DISCUSSION

Light scanning and transmission electron microscopy reveal that the neosheath is not just a tube of scar, as some have claimed, but analogous to normal synovial tendon sheath. The neosheath possesses a two-layer structure and cells very similar to those previously described only in synovial tissue. Differences in the character of the sheath from different locations appear to be quantitative rather than qualitative. For instance, the neosheath in the back contained the same cellular and fibrous population as the neosheath in the foot but was not as thick. A possible explanation for this difference is that the implant in the back is static while the one in the foot was subjected to motion. Even though the implant was only anastomosed distally, passive flexion of the toe occurred as the chicken's toe hit the grating. The constant mechanical trauma of motion most likely resulted in a greater collagen response to the implant. The fibrous component of the neosheath is not random but oriented longitudinally along the axis of the implant as the collagen is oriented along the lines of stress in a normal tendon sheath. Although the sheath contained fibroblasts and many immature cell types, Type A– and Type B–appearing cells have been identified. The Type B cell with its abundant ergastoplasm has been shown by others to be very specialized and synthesizes and secretes protein while the Type A cells are phagocytic.

SUMMARY

The management of severe flexor tendon injuries in the hand has been significantly improved by tendon sheath reconstruction with an artificial implant followed by conventional tendon grafting. Studies of the ultrastructure of the neosheath reveal little difference from the normal synovial tendon sheath helping to explain why Hunter's two-stage technique gives superior results to other less physiologic procedures in patients with severe tendon injuries.

References

1. Barland, P., Novikoff, A. B., and Hamerman, D.: Electron microscopy of synovial membrane, J. Cell Biol. **14**:207-220, 1962.
2. Hochstrasser, A. E., Broadbent, T. R., and Woolf, R.: Sheath replacement in tendon repair: experimental study with ivalon, Rocky Mt. Med. J. **57**:30-33, 1960.
3. Hunter, J. M., and Salisbury, R. E.: Flexor tendon reconstruction in severely damaged hands, J. Bone Joint Surg. **53A**:829-858, 1971.
4. Peacock, E. E., Jr., Madden, J. W.: Some studies on the effect of B-aminoproprionitrile in patients with injured flexor tendons. Surgery **66**:215-223, 1969.
5. Wysocki, G. P., and Brinkhous, K. M.: Scanning electron microscopy of synovial membranes, Arch. Pathol. **93**:172-177, 1972.

7. Preliminary observations on the use of chemically stored tendinous allografts in hand surgery

François Iselin, M.D.

Whenever a tendinous graft is necessary, the use of allografts facilitates the surgery of repair by making the operation quicker and simpler and by avoiding the creation of additional lesions caused by taking an autograft.

For nearly 20 years we have been using, in our unit, homogenous tendons stored in a German-made mercurial solution named Cialit.

The utilization is very simple. The tendons are taken from fresh cadavers or from amputated limbs. They are carefully cleaned of the paratenon and sunk in a 1:5,000 solution of Cialit, that is 1 gm. of Cialit powder in 5 liters of sterile water. The container is glass with a glass and rubber top because the Cialit may corrode any metal. The tendons are first stored for 3 weeks in the solution, then thoroughly rinsed in sterile water, sunk again in a new solution at the same dilution, and are then ready for use.

When it is decided to insert a graft, a nurse, using long forceps, simply takes one from the container, puts it into sterile water where the graft is bathed for 15 minutes, and then rinses it before it is put into place. The liquid is completely bactericidal and no bacteria have been found by routine bacteriologic cultures.

The liquid for storage should be changed every 2 months by a simple shift of containers. Tendons may be preserved up to 6 months, but this has never been experienced because there is always a minimal supply.

This type of graft is standard for us. There are no significant differences in results from those with autografts that we are compelled to use whenever no chemically stored tendons are available.

The storage of anatomical pieces in Cialit was initiated in 1947 by Guntz[1] from Frankfurt and was started by Marc Iselin in Nanterre in 1955, essentially with bones. The idea of preserving nerves, skin, and tendons soon arose in our team, and an experiment was made by Karl Seiffert, from Frankfurt, who issued, in 1966,[12, 13] the results of a tremendous work that is the basis of this paper. It is therefore dedicated to the memory of Dr. Seiffert, who died in 1972 at 42 years of age.

The questions were: is there a difference between autografts and allografts, or fresh and preserved grafts, and how does storage in Cialit interfere with revascularization of grafts?

Teneff has shown that revascularization of grafts follows the same process whatever their type, autografts or allografts. The formation of vessel-carrying adhesions during reconstitution of the tendinous tissue is considered by all experimenters as necessary and unavoidable.

Nageotte's[6] theory that grafts should first die before being revitalized is hardly acceptable, because it is most unbelievable that fibroblasts could resume normal relationship of mutation with the denatured tissue of a chemically fixed transplant.

Other authors, such as Lindsay[3-5] and Potenza,[11] think that a graft can survive as long as it is intact. Peacock[9] has demonstrated that a graft survives only weakly and that it must necessarily be revascularized.

The quality of the graft is important. We get rid of the paratenon because Potenza[10] has shown that it is of no use and that it may also be a cause of supplementary adhesions. The graft may be the complete tendinous unit with its intact sheath, described by Peacock[8] as "composite tissue allografts."

The process of graft assimilation and the reactions between grafts and the site of transplantation were studied by Seiffert.[13] He compared autografts, fresh allografts, and preserved allografts on dog gastrocnemius that were cleaned of paratenon. Samples were taken every week from 1 to 9 weeks, then again at 3 months and 6 months.

Seiffert's first finding is that fresh allografts create a significant inflammation, with local infiltration of round cells that causes hypertrophic scarring. Fresh autografts create no inflammation. Allografts preserved in Cialit show no inflammatory reaction and an early disappearance of enzymatic activity.

Second, revitalization of preserved allografts occurs by a conjunctive cellular invasion in the collagen fibers coming from the stumps, starting in the second week. Reconstitution of an oriented tissue is complete in 4 to 8 weeks. Surrounding adhesions may go to the skin but are rather weak, because the conjunctive proliferation coming from the transplantation site is originated by peripheral inflammation.

The gliding spaces remain obliterated until the fourth week and reappear after the sixth week. Secondary freeing is achieved by gaps that appear, not at the border between the transplant and the receiving site, but in a kind of cuff of new conjunctive tissue.

A "creeping substitution" of collagen that gives a close to normal appearance to the graft appears in 6 to 9 months. This is interpreted as a functional metaplasia. Actually as Peacock and Madden[9] call it, it is a pseudotendon, but

Seiffert[13] assumes that the vitality of a conjunctive graft is not important for the functional result.

Third, the oriented revitalization of these grafts supports the theory of the "guiding rail," which states that implanted tissues could exert a determining influence on the process of regeneration, as demonstrated by Dr. Greenley. This directing influence is believed to be mechanical, and the functional tension given to a tendon graft is considered most important. This could explain the complete transformation of the composite tissue allografts by the difference of forces that are applied on the different anatomical structures of this type of graft.

At this point we may state that a graft is accepted without problems by the receiving site and there is no difference between fresh autografts and preserved allografts.

Also, assimilation of these grafts is made through peripheral revitalization that reorients the collagen of the transplant toward the reconstitution of a new tendon, very much like a normal one, under the influence of mechanical factors. The most astonishing observation is the essentially identical transformation of a graft into an effective new tendon.

Finally, we feel that preservation of a graft, especially in Cialit, in skipping the time of devitalization, will diminish the immunologic reactions, and at least avoid inflammatory adhesions. Since we now do most of our graftings in two-stage operations, we also eliminate most surgical adhesions and have an impression of improvement in the quality of our latest results.

CONCLUSIONS

Preserved allografts are well accepted and well revitalized. They are superior to fresh allografts, which have strong immunoinflammatory reactions, the preservation avoiding these reactions by devitalizing the grafts.

Preserved allografts are theoretically superior to fresh autografts because they are already reduced to their collagenic framework, which induces an immediate revitalization without primary resorption, thus avoiding part of the peripheral conjunctive reaction. Therefore, we feel that preserved allografts are the materials that should be the least surrounded by accidental adhesions and the most likely to easily pull free from normal vascular adhesions.

Finally, the type of preservation is not so important, and Seiffert has demonstrated that lyophlized allografts show reactions absolutely similar to the chemically preserved allografts. The study of the behavior of the collagenic molecules under lyophilization and in mercurial solution shows identical findings. The choice between these types of preservation is therefore a question of possibilities and finances. Chemical storage in Cialit is inexpensive but necessitates a devoted staff always in search of donors; lyophilization provides ready-packed tendons that are very simple to handle, but its cost, especially in Europe, is still above the possibilities of public hospitals.

References

1. Guntz, E.: Langenbecks, Arch. Klin Chir. **279**:56, 1954.
2. Lindsay, W. K., and Thomson, H. G.: Digital flexor tendons, an experimental study, part I, Br. J. Plast. Surg. **12**:289-319, 1960.
3. Lindsay, W. K., and Walker, F. G.: Digital flexor tendons, an experimental study, part II, Br. J. Plast. Surg. **13**:1, 1960.
4. Lindsay, W. K., and McDougall, E. P.: Digital flexor tendons, an experimental study, part III, Br. J. Plast. Surg. **13**:293-304, 1961.
5. Lindsay, W. K., and Birch, J. R.: The fibroblast in flexor tendon healing, Plast. Reconstr. Surg. **34**:223, 1964.
6. Nageotte, J.: L'organisation de la matière dans ses rapports avec la vie: Etudes d'anatomie générale et de morphologie expérimentale sur le tissu conjonctif et les nerfs, Paris, 1922, Alcan.
7. Peacock, E. E.: Biological principles in the healing of long tendons, Surg. Clin. North Am. **45**:461, 1965.
8. Peacock, E. E., and Madden, J. W.: Human composite tissue tendon allografts, Ann. Surg. **166**:624, 1967.
9. Peacock, E. E., and Madden, J. W.: Some studies of the effects of B-amino propionitrile in patients with injured flexor tendons, Surgery **66**:215-223, 1969.
10. Potenza, A. D.: Critical evaluation of flexor tendon healing and adhesion formation within artificial digital sheaths. J. Bone Joint Surg. **45A**:1217-1233, 1963.
11. Potenza, A. D.: Prevention of adhesions to healing digital flexor tendons, J. A. M. A. **187**: 187-191, 1964.
12. Seiffert, K., Hartleib, J., and Schmidt, K. P.: Uber den biologishen umbau von frischem und in Cialit conserviertem Schnengewebe in funktionstruchtige gehne, Brun's Beitr. Klin. Chir. **209**:444-463, 1964.
13. Seiffert, K.: Biologische Grundlagen der homologen transplantation konseivreter bundegewebe, Habilations schrift vorgelegt Medizinischen Fakultät JW Goethe Universität, Frankfurt, 1966.
14. Seiffert, K., and Schmidt, K. P.: Preserved tendon grafts. In Hand surgery trans. Fifth Int. Congr. Plast. Surg. London, 1971, Butterworth & Co. (Publishers) Ltd.

8. Tendon suturing methods: analysis of tensile strengths

James R. Urbaniak, M.D.
James D. Cahill, Jr., M.D.
Rod A. Mortenson, M.D.

In the past two decades, a voluminous amount of literature has been concerned with the many problems and questions posed by tendon surgery. Numerous articles have been devoted to discussion of suture materials, tendon suturing,* grafting,[3, 9, 13] healing,[1, 2, 11, 13, 18] rate of healing,[7] nutrition,[16, 17] and related clinical and laboratory endeavors. Thus a discussion of suture materials and various methods of anastomosing tendons is certainly not new. However, since the classic work of Mason and Allen,[7] no experimental work can be found in the English literature comparing the tensile strengths of the various methods of tendon anastomoses now available. Thus it is the purpose of this chapter to review several suturing methods currently in use, to compare their relative tensile strengths initially and during healing, to determine the most satisfactory suture material, and to measure the tensile forces on intact human tendons in vivo for clinical correlation.

MATERIALS AND METHODS

A technique was required in which a stress could be uniformly and quantitatively applied to the suture materials and tendon anastomoses, and could be measured up to the point of failure. Other investigators dealt with this problem by adding standard weights to the repaired tendon until the sutures broke or pulled out of the approximated ends.[15] However, this method is cumbersome and does not permit continuous monitoring of a progressively increasing load. In this study, these problems were avoided through use of an Instron Tensile Tester. This device consists of a pair of pneumatic clamps to hold the specimen, a strain transducer coupled to the upper clamp, a constant speed gear that drives the clamps apart, and an amplifier and graph to provide a continuous record of the load applied and its duration. The unit was calibrated daily with standard metric weights.

*See references 4-6, 8, 10, 12, 14.

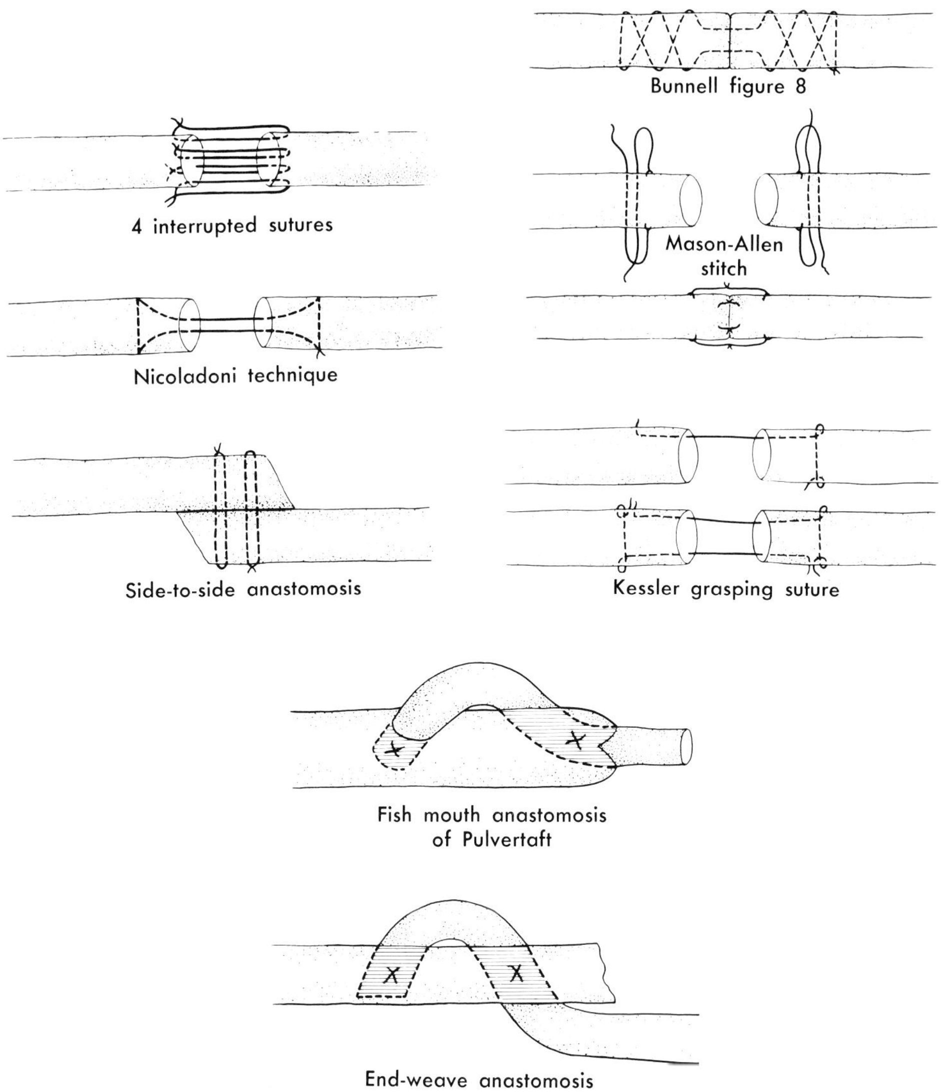

Fig. 8-1. The eight tendon anastomoses tested were classified into three groups based on the strength of their union.

Many suture materials are now available that meet the basic requirements of tendon surgery: high tensile strength, ease of handling, and minimal tissue reaction. Four such materials were chosen for comparison: 4-0 stainless steel, 4-0 Ethilon, 4-0 Tevdek, and 4-0 Mersilene.* A single strand of each material was placed in the Instron and ruptured. This procedure was repeated with a single square knot in a single strand, with two knotted strands, and with two

*Ethilon is nylon, Tevdek is Teflon impregnated braided polyester fiber, Mersilene is braided polyester fiber (Dacron).

unknotted strands of each material. Ten determinations were made for each test.

In order to compare the immediate strength of different methods of anastomosis, fresh digital flexor tendons of approximately equal cross-sectional diameter were taken from adult male mongrel dogs. The tendons were immediately cut, repaired, and tested in the Instron using 4-0 stainless steel and these eight suture methods: four interrupted sutures, the Nicoladoni stitch,[10] the side-to-side stitch, the Mason-Allen stitch,[6] the Bunnell stitch, the fish-mouth anastomosis of Pulvertaft,[14] the end-weave stitch, and the "grasping" suture recently described by Kessler[4, 5] (Fig. 8-1). Twenty examples of each method were tested and the failing strength and mode of failure were recorded for each.

To determine the relative strengths of various methods of anastomosis during healing, the Nicoladoni, the Kessler, the Bunnell, and the end-weave anastomoses were used to repair surgically cut digital flexor tendons in the forepaws of adult mongrel dogs. Care was taken to use tendons of approximately equal cross-sectional diameter. The paws were cast in flexion, and the dogs were sacrificed at 5-day intervals through 20 days. The tendons were removed immediately and tested in the Instron as previously described. Five repairs of each type at each time interval were performed and equal numbers were done with 4-0 stainless steel and 4-0 polyester fiber. For controls, the same anastomoses were also placed in the dog tendons without the tendon being cut.

Measurement of the tension in intact human digital flexor tendons was per-

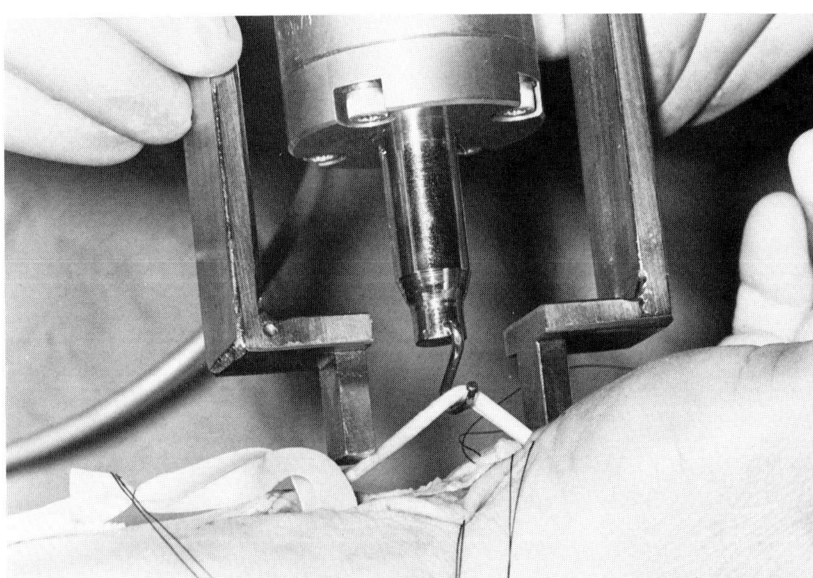

Fig. 8-2. A strain transducer is applied to the flexor digitorum profundus tendon in the wrist of an alert patient to measure the tension of the tendon during active and passive motion.

formed in patients undergoing surgery for relief of median nerve compression. All patients were awake, under local anesthesia, and had a tourniquet in place. The device used to measure this tension incorporates a strain transducer (Fig. 8-2) and recorder, and operates on the principle illustrated in Fig. 8-3. This device was calibrated before each use with standard metric weights. Tension in the tendons was measured under the following conditions: rest, passive flexion-extension, active flexion without resistance, active flexion against slight resistance, and active flexion against moderate resistance.

RESULTS

Analysis of the tensile strengths of the various suture materials revealed some interesting facts. All the materials showed an almost linear increase in

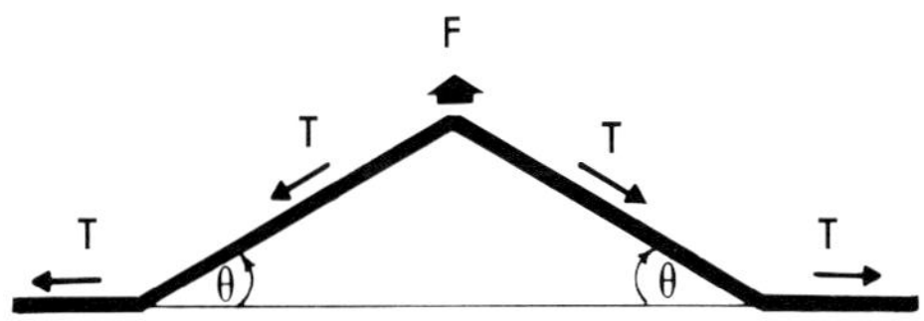

$$F = 2 \times T \sin \theta$$

$$T = \frac{1}{2} \frac{\sin \theta}{F}$$

if $\theta = 30°$

$$T = F$$

Fig. 8-3. The geometric principle of measuring the tension of human flexor tendons at the wrist with the strain transducer (T, tension; F, force).

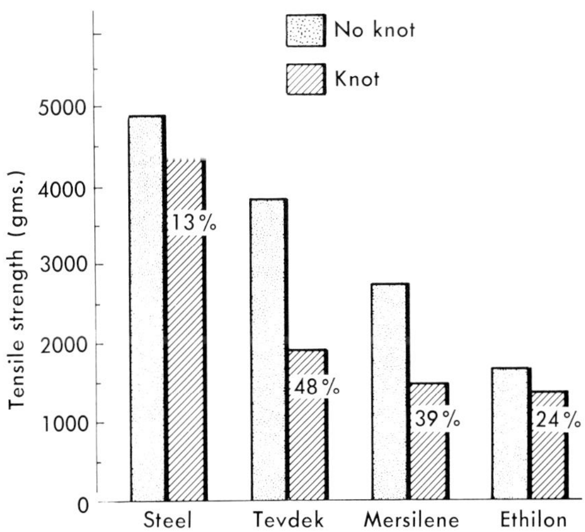

Fig. 8-4. Tensile strength of two strands of the 4-0 suture materials tested. Stainless steel was the least affected by knotting.

strength relative to the number of strands tested. Of the synthetic materials tested, Ethilon had the lowest tensile strength and Tevdek had the strongest (Fig. 8-4). However, tying a knot in the suture markedly altered its tensile strength as well as its ability to withstand an applied load. Ethilon showed approximately a 22% reduction in tensile strength when knotted, Mersilene a 36% reduction, and Tevdek a 46% to 47% reduction, which was the greatest loss of strength. However, in absolute terms, none of the synthetic materials were as strong as 4-0 stainless steel, which was also the least affected by knotting with only a 10% to 13% reduction in original tensile strength.

The inherent strength of a tendon repair is dependent upon the type of anastomosis utilized in the repair. Whether the wire suture pulled out of the tendon substance or whether disruption of the anastomosis occurred by fracture of the wire seemed to be an inherent property of the type of tendon anastomosis that was employed. The eight different methods of tendon anastomosis that were studied break down into three basic groups:

Group I in which the pull of the suture is parallel to the collagen bundles of the tendon and the stress of the anastomosis is transmitted directly to the opposing tendon ends

Group II in which the stress applied is directly transmitted across the anas-

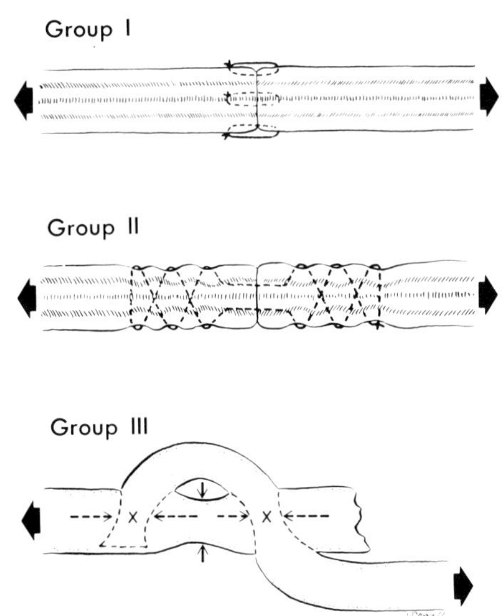

Fig. 8-5. The eight different methods of tendon anastomoses could be placed into three basic groups. In Group I, the suture applied a shearing force to the tendon ends parallel to the collagen bundles and resulted in a very weak repair. In Group II, the longitudinal pull of the suture is converted either to an oblique or transverse compressive force on the tendon, and the strength of the repair approaches the strength of the suture material. In Group III, the strongest union, loading of the tendon applies a compressive force of tendon to tendon at right angles to the longitudinal shearing forces.

tomosis by the suture material and thus dependent upon the strength of the suture itself

Group III in which the sutures are placed perpendicular to both the collagen bundles of the tendon and the stress applied to the repair (Fig. 8-5)

In Group I, the suture applied a shearing force to the tendon ends parallel to the collagen bundles and resulted in a very weak anastomosis. The suture repair methods that can be included under Group I include the following: the interrupted circumferential sutures, the Nicoladoni repair, and the side-to-side anastomosis. In all cases the suture pulled out of the tendon repair without breaking the suture itself. Interrupted sutures placed around the circumference of the tendon provided the weakest anastomosis with failure of the repair at 1683 gm. The Nicoladoni repair was somewhat stronger with failure at 2683 gm. Side-to-side repair is the strongest in this group (Table 1). Thus a weak anastomosis should be expected in any type of tendon repair where the shearing force of the suture is parallel to the longitudinal collagen bundles of the tendon.

In the Group II anastomosis, the longitudinal pull of the suture is converted either to an oblique or transverse compressive force on the tendon and results in a much better purchase of the tendon by the suture. The repairs described by Bunnell, Kessler, and Mason and Allen can be included in Group II. Because of the improved purchase of the tendon by the suture, the suture itself now broke in the majority of cases before it pulled out of the tendon substance. The Bunnell criss-cross stitch withstood a load of 3,930 gm. before exceeding the tensile strength of the suture material, breaking the suture. The Kessler and the Mason-Allen repairs withstood greater loads of 3,970 gm. and 4,030 gm., respectively (Table 1). These methods of anastomosis transmit still more of the longitudinal pull of the suture to a transverse compressive force on the tendon with better purchase of the tendon as reflected by the type of anastomosis failure seen in these repairs. In 80% of the cases, disruption of the anastomosis was a result of the wire suture breaking and only in 20% of the cases did the suture pull out of the tendon substance without breaking. The strength of the repair utilizing

Table 1. The tensile strength of the eight different tendon anastomoses tested

		Suture	
Anastomosis	*Tensile strength*	*Pulled out*	*Broke*
Interrupted	1,683 gm.	20	0
Nicoladoni	2,683 gm.	20	0
Side-to-side	3,230 gm.	20	0
Bunnell	3,930 gm.	12	8
Kessler	3,970 gm.	4	16
Mason-Allen	4,030 gm.	4	16
Fish-mouth	4,055 gm.	20	0
End-weave	6,430 gm.	20	0

these three methods is approaching the tensile strength of the suture material used and thus dependent upon the suture material chosen for the repair. Obviously, if 4-0 Ethilon were used for the anastomosis the strength of the repair would have been much less.

The Group III anastomosis includes the fish-mouth repair described by Pulvertaft and the end-weave anastomosis. In the Group III anastomosis, there is no direct pull on the suture because the suture is placed perpendicular to both the collagen bundles of the tendon and to the stress applied to the tendon. That is, the suture applies a compressive force of tendon to tendon at right angles to the longitudinal shearing forces when the tendon is loaded. Thus a very strong repair was achieved with the end-weave repair, and to a lesser extent by the fish-mouth stitch. The former far exceeded the tensile strength of the suture material and was able to tolerate a load of 6,430 gm. before failing; the latter withstood a shearing force of 4,055 gm. (Table 1). The longitudinal pull did not break the wire suture in any of the cases. Thus the strength of these two repairs, especially the end-weave, is not directly related to the tensile strength of the suture material, but rather, the strength of the repair is related to the redistribution of the shearing forces across the anastomosis, which is an inherent property of these types of repair where tendon grasps tendon.

The strength of the various methods of anastomosis during early healing is much less than those in the corresponding fresh preparations, especially in the first 10 days. However, the degree of weakening of some methods was unexpected. Predictably, the Group I repair, the Nicoladoni, provided the weakest repair at all times tested, as low as 560 gm. at 5 days. It was however, a relatively atraumatic repair to perform, and none of the uncut controls could be broken

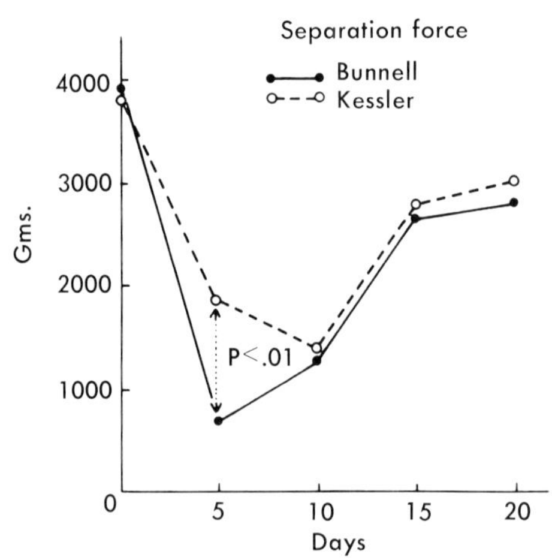

Fig. 8-6. A comparison of the Bunnell and Kessler sutures during early healing in dog flexor tendons. Although nearly equal in strength initially, by the fifth day the Kessler stitch was nearly three times stronger than the Bunnell.

at loads exceeding 13 kg. when the tendon pulled out of the pneumatic clamps of the Instron.

The Bunnell and Kessler sutures of Group II provided the greatest surprise. Although nearly equal in strength initially, there was a threefold difference in strength between the two methods at the fifth day (Fig. 8-6). The strength of the Bunnell was 630 gm. while that of the Kessler was 1,830 gm. From the tenth day onward, there was no significant difference between the strengths of the two methods. The controls ruptured at 10 days at stresses of 10 kg. to 12 kg. The Bunnell double figure-8 suture appeared to have more of a "strangling" effect on the intact tendon than the "grasping" suture of Kessler. In all cases of controlled rupture, the separation occurred within the length of the applied suture.

The end-weave from Group III showed the greatest loss of strength during early healing. However, its weakest point at 5 days of 1,550 gm. makes it one of the strongest repairs in locations where this type of repair is practicable (Fig. 8-7).

Comparison of the results of repairs performed with 4-0 stainless steel and 4-0 Mersilene revealed no significant difference in results during early healing. All anastomosis failures during this time were the result of suture pulling out of tendon, not the result of suture fracture (Fig. 8-8).

The forces measured in intact human digital flexor tendons revealed that active flexion of the digit against mild resistance did not place more than 900 gm. of stress on the tendon. The stress of passive flexion-extension ranged from 200 gm. to 300 gm., but seldom exceeded 200 gm. Flexion against moderate resistance was on the order of 1,500 gm. In one instance, a grip meter placed in the hand registered 2 pounds while tension measured in the ring finger profundis

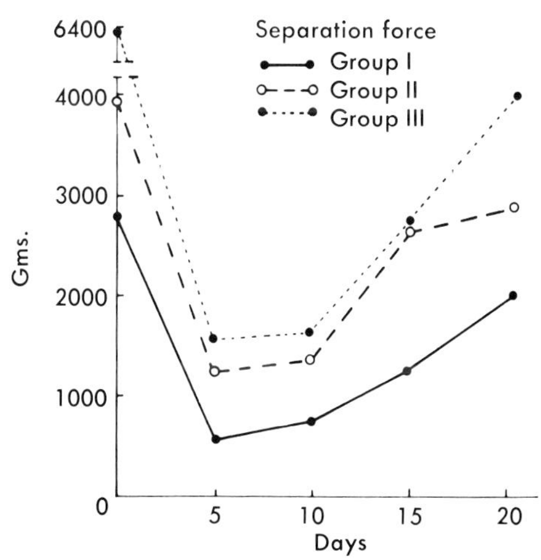

Fig. 8-7. A comparison of the tensile strengths of the three groups of tendon anastomoses during early healing. A sharp drop at 5 days exists in all repairs, but the end-weave suture of Group III withstands 1,550 gm. of tension.

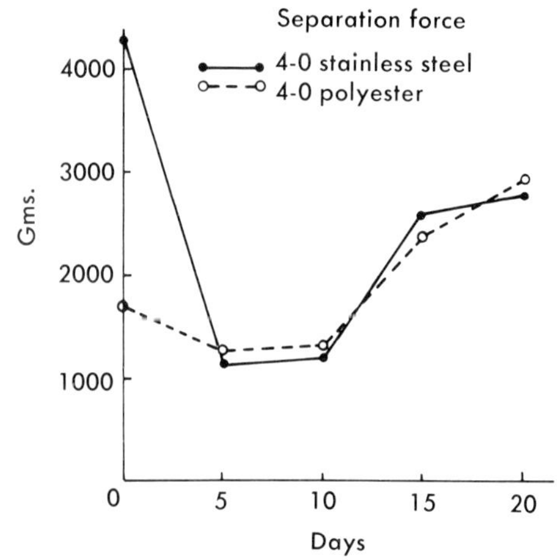

Fig. 8-8. Although 4-0 stainless steel was stronger than 4-0 polyester fiber (Mersilene) in the fresh tendon, there was no significant difference in the separation force during early healing.

tendon was 1,250 gm. The tourniquet reduced the maximum force of contraction, but the subjects were able to produce tensions of approximately 5,000 gm. with maximum effort. These tension studies on intact human flexor tendons are very preliminary. A study is now being conducted on a large group of patients without the use of a tourniquet at the time of testing.

DISCUSSION

The main objective of tendon repair is the restoration of the mechanical union and tensile strength without compromising the gliding function of the tendon. One of the major questions in tendon surgery has been when to begin motion. Immobilization permits fibroblasts to invade the approximated tendon ends to initiate the normal reparative process, but prolonged immobilization often results in dense adhesions of the tendon to surrounding connective tissue and subsequent loss of gliding motion. In older patients, prolonged immobility frequently results in decreased joint mobility. Early motion allows the vascular and collagenous adhesions to the tendon to stretch and thus maintain gliding function.

Before permitting early motion, several factors must be considered: tensile strength of the suture material, holding power of the suture for the tendon, bulkiness of the repair, and the stress that must be withstood. As shown by the work of Mason and Allen,[7] the strength of an anastomosis for the first 2 days is due primarily to the suture alone. If early motion is anticipated, either stainless steel or the polyester sutures provide adequate strength. While the steel is stronger, the polyester, being more flexible, is easier to handle, has adequate strength, and may result in less mechanical trauma to smaller tendons. Later, from approximately the third to the twelfth day, softening of the tendon occurs, greatly diminishing the purchase of tendon by suture. The strength of all repairs reaches a minimum at this time and no stress may be permitted that would

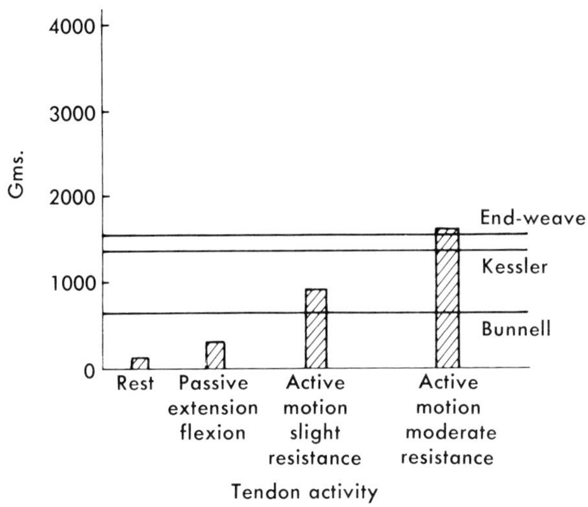

Fig. 8-9. The horizontal lines represent the tensile strength of the end-weave, Kessler, and Bunnell repairs at 5 days of healing in dog flexor tendons. The vertical bars indicate the forces measured in intact human digital flexor tendons. The end-weave and Kessler repairs appear to maintain enough strength to withstand the stress of active early motion against mild resistance.

exceed or closely approach the failure point of the anastomosis. Any type of anastomosis where the pull of the suture is parallel to the collagen bundles would be sure to fail with motion at this time. Only if the longitudinal shearing force is converted to a compressive force either by suture or by tendon itself will the softened repair maintain its integrity. The Kessler and end-weave methods of anastomosis maintain enough strength in this manner to withstand the stress of active early motion against mild resistance (Fig. 8-9). The Nicoladoni and widely-used Bunnell techniques did not meet this criterion in this study. This study still leaves several important questions unanswered: the effect of repeated submaximal stress on the strength of the anastomosis, the resistance to motion as a result of edema, and the increase in anastomosis strength with increase in tendon diameter.

These results indicate that the Group II and the Group III repairs, specifically the Kessler and end-weave anastomoses, provide the greatest strength whether or not early motion is to be attempted. The weave allows tendons of unequal diameter or multiple tendons to be joined. Its major disadvantage is the bulkiness of the repair, requiring careful placement in an area in which the surrounding tissue is not constricting, to permit gliding. Also, adequate tendon length is necessary for this anastomosis. The "grasping" suture of Kessler provides a stronger repair than the Bunnell double figure-8 for joining tendons of equal diameter in a confined space such as the digital flexor sheath.

SUMMARY

Four suture materials were studied. It was found that the tensile strength of all the materials tested was linear to the number of strands used. Knotting and manipulation greatly reduced the tensile strength of all the materials tested except stainless steel. The strongest suture material available and least affected by handling was 4-0 stainless steel. Polyester suture was much easier to handle and provided adequate strength.

The tensile strengths of eight different methods for repairing tendons were compared in fresh preparations. The end-weave and fish-mouth repairs were by far the strongest, but they should be used only in sites surrounded by loose areolar connective tissue. The Mason-Allen, Bunnell, and Kessler technique provided repairs of moderate strength, useful in areas of limited space. The interrupted circumferential sutures, Nicoladoni repair, and side-to-side anastomosis provided weak repairs.

In vivo testing in dogs revealed much weakening of all repairs during early healing. Of the methods tested, the Kessler and end-weave techniques maintained apparent adequate strength to permit early motion against mild resistance as measured in the human flexor tendons.

References

1. Flynn, J. E.: Healing of tendon wounds, Am. J. Surg. **109**:315-324, March, 1965.
2. Flynn, J. E., and Graham, J. H.: Healing following tendon suture and tendon transplants, Surg. Gynecol. Obstet. **115**:467-472, Oct., 1962.
3. Gaisford, J. C.: Tendon grafting: a suggested technique, Plast. Reconstr. Surg. **38**:302-308, 1966.
4. Kessler, I.: The "grasping" technique for tendon repair, The Hand **5**:253-255, 1973.
5. Kessler, I., and Nissim, F.: Primary repair without immobilization of flexor tendon division within the digital sheath, Acta Orthop. Scand. **40**:587-601, 1969.
6. Mason, M. L.: Primary and secondary tendon suture: a discussion of the significance of the technique in tendon surgery, Surg. Gynecol. Obstet. **70**:392-402, 1940.
7. Mason, M. L., and Allen, H. S.: Rate of healing of tendons: an experimental study of tensile strength, Ann. Surg. **113**:429-459, 1941.
8. Mason, M. L., and Shearon, C. G.: Process of tendon repair: an experimental study of tendon suture and tendon graft, Arch. Surg. **25**:4, 616-691, 1932.
9. McFarlane, R. M.: Flexor tendon injuries within the finger: a study of the results of tendon suture and tendon graft, J. Trauma **8**:987-1003, 1968.
10. Nicoladoni, C.: Ein Vorchlag zur Sehnennaht. Wien. Klin. Wochenschr. **52**:1413-1417, 1880.
11. Peacock, E. E., Jr.: Fundamental aspects of wound healing relating to the restoration of gliding function after tendon repair, Surg. Gynecol. Obstet. **119**:241-250, Aug., 1964.
12. Peacock, E. E., Jr.: Some technical aspects and results of flexor tendon repair, Surgery **58**:330-342, Aug., 1965.
13. Potenza, A. D.: The healing of autogenous tendon grafts within the flexor digital sheath in dogs, J. Bone Joint Surg. **46A**:1462-1484, 1964.
14. Pulvertaft, R. G.: Suture materials and tendon junctures, Am. J. Surg. **109**:346-352, 1965.
15. Schink, W., and Gerbach, B.: Experimentelle studie uber die Festigkeit genahter sehnen bei verschiedenen Nahtmethoden. Langenbecks Arch. Chir. **297**:191-235, 1961.
16. Smith, J. W.: Blood supply of tendons, Am. J. Surg. **109**:272-276, March, 1965.
17. Urbaniak, J. R., Bright, D. S., Gill, L. H., and Goldner, J. L.: Vascularization and the gliding mechanism of free flexor-tendon grafts inserted by the silicone-rod method, J. Bone Joint Surg. **56A**:473-482, 1974.
18. Urbaniak, J. R., and Goldner, J. L.: Laceration of the flexor pollicis longus tendon—delayed repair by advancement, free graft, or direct suture—a clinical and experimental study, J. Bone Joint Surg. **53A**:1123-1148, 1973.

9. The finger flexor tendon sheath and pulleys: anatomy and reconstruction

James R. Doyle, M.D.
William Blythe, Ph.D.

Surgeons who perform flexor tendon surgery of the hand recognize the importance of the tendon sheath and associated pulleys.[3, 6-9] It is generally agreed that these pulleys are required for the maintenance and restoration of useful flexor tendon function.[5, 9-11] The purpose of this chapter is to present our understanding of the gross and macroscopic anatomy of the flexor sheath and pulleys, certain practical observations that deal with function, and methods used for reconstruction of pulleys.

TECHNIQUE

The basis for these observations is personal experience gained in a hand surgery practice, anatomical dissection in fresh cadaver specimens using low-power magnification, and study of specially embedded and sectioned whole fingers.[14]

Fresh cadaver specimens were studied by first injecting the sheath in the region of the distal palm with methylene blue solution. This was injected under minimal pressure using a 30-gauge needle. Care was taken to inject only enough dye solution to distend the sheath. Dissection could then be performed with some ease since the more easily distended and stained synovial sheath would be seen in distinct contrast to the annular and cruciform components of the pulley mechanism. A loupe or dissecting microscope aided in identification of these structures. Whole fingers from the midmetacarpal region to the tip of the digit were embedded in nitrocellulose and then serial longitudinal sections were cut and stained with hematoxylin and eosin. These sections were studied under low power magnification and the position and morphology of the pulleys correlated with the gross dissection.

The relative functional value of the respective pulleys was determined by excision of the pulleys in a serial fashion and then measuring the distance the fingertip failed in approximating the midaspect of the palm in flexion. The amount of force required and distance of tendon excursion was determined for

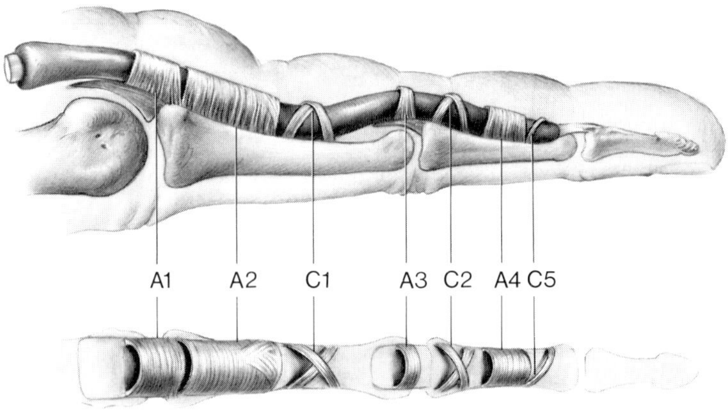

Fig. 9-1. The flexor sheath is a double walled, hollow, synovial-lined connective tissue tube that encloses the flexor tendons. Four annular and three cruciform pulleys are noted in their relative locations. The annular pulleys are thick, rather rigid fibrous tissue structures in contrast to the cruciform bands, which are thin and pliable. The second and fourth annular pulleys are the most important from a functional viewpoint.

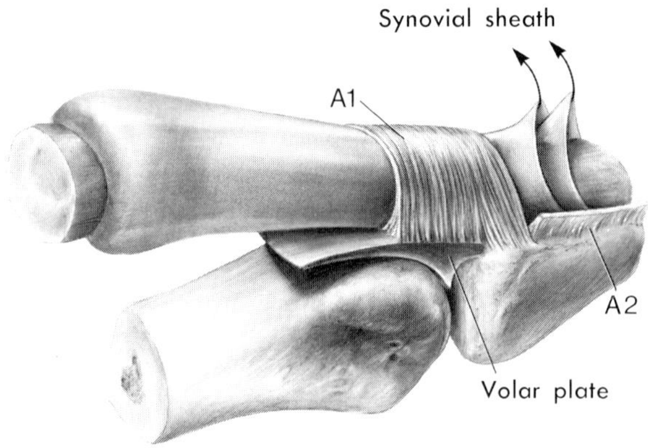

Fig. 9-2. The flexor sheath is a double walled tube with two distinct layers of synovia. One layer is visceral and envelops the tendon, the parietal layer lines the flexor canal. The volar plate at the metacarpophalangeal joint provides attachment for about two-thirds of the first annular band.

the profundus tendon in each of the tested fingers in order for the tip of the digit to touch the palm. Serial resections of pulleys were then performed and the same force and excursion applied to the profundus tendon. The distance in millimeters was measured from the pulp of the terminal phalanx of the digit to the underlying palm.

FINDINGS

The flexor synovial sheath is a double walled hollow tube sealed at both ends. It begins at the distal palmar skin crease and at the level of the neck of the metacarpal. Its distal end is just proximal to the distal interphalangeal joint (Figs. 9-1 and 9-2).

On top of this sheath and closely applied to it are a series of annular and cruciform fibers that vary in length or width from 2 or 3 mm. to 20 mm. and in thickness from less than 0.1 mm. to 0.75 mm.

Four discrete annular bands have been identified along with three cruciform bands. The first of these annular bands begins about 5 mm. proximal to the metacarpophalangeal joint line. This annular band is 0.5 mm. thick and 8 mm. to 10 mm. long. It has been arbitrarily designated annular one and is separated from the next and largest of the annular bands by a 1 mm. to 3 mm. gap through which the synovial sheath bulges with flexion. The first annular band gains about two-thirds of its origin from the underlying volar plate and the remainder from the proximal phalanx (Fig. 9-2). The second annular band originates entirely from the proximal phalanx and begins about 5 mm. to 7 mm. distal to the metacarpophalangeal joint line. The second annular band is 18 mm. to 20 mm. long and varies in thickness from 0.25 mm. to 0.75 mm. Its annular fibers are overlaid with interdigitating layers of cruciform fibers at its distal end. Its greatest thickness is in the distal half.

At the distal end of annular two, oblique fibers arch upwards to meet and interdigitate with fibers from the opposite side to form the first cruciform band. This band is quite thin, relative to the adjacent annular band, and is 3 mm. to 4 mm. wide at the confluence of its fibers.

Table 2. Serial resection determination of the relative functional importance of the various pulleys*

		Pulleys					*Failure to touch palm (mm.)*
A1	A2	C1	A3	C2	A4		0
	A2	C1	A3	C2	A4	C3	0
	A2				A4	C3	0
	A2				A4		0
A1	A2	C1	A3	C2			2-5
A1	A2	C1	A3				5-8
A1	A2	C1					10-12
	A2						12-15
		C1	A3	C2	A4	C3	12-15
					A4		20-25
							25-30

*Annular two and four were required for normal tendon function. If annular four was absent the fingertip failed to touch the palm by 2 mm. to 5 mm. when a predetermined force and excursion was applied to the profundus tendon. Of the two critical pulleys, annular two was noted to be the most important since the fingertip more closely approximated the palm (12 mm. to 15 mm.) when only annular two was intact in contrast to a 20 mm. to 25 mm. loss of flexion when only annular four was present.

The third annular band is located at the level of the middle joint and appears to arise principally from the volar plate of the proximal interphalangeal joint. It is 3 mm. to 4 mm. wide and 0.33 mm. thick. The second cruciform appears at the level of the base of the middle phalanx. It is similar to cruciform one although somewhat thinner and is less likely to have a distinct cruciform configuration. In comparison to the cruciform bands, the fourth annular is a thick and readily identifiable structure that occupies the middle third of the middle phalanx. It is 10 mm. to 12 mm. in length. A third cruciform band begins at the distal margin of annular four. Although sometimes cruciform in shape with interdigitating fibers, it is more often a single oblique band of fibers.

Relative functional importance of the various pulleys was determined by serial resection and demonstrated that annular two and annular four were the two most important or critical pulleys for maintenance of flexion in the digit (Table 2). Annular one was readily expendable without noticeable loss of function. The single most valuable or critical pulley was annular two. This band, although normally 18 mm. to 20 mm. in length was narrowed to 5 mm. without noticeable alteration of its function. Complete motion of the finger occurred only if annular four and two were present. Annular one appeared to be less important than annular two in our studies.

PULLEY RECONSTRUCTION

Pulleys may be reconstructed by insertion of a free tendon graft around or through phalanges or by using portions of the superficialis tendon near its insertion (Fig. 9-3).[2, 4, 13] Both Boyes and Littler agree that a full-length fibrous sheath is not required for good flexor tendon function.[3, 10] Both along with Rank, Wakefield, and Hueston[12] agree that two critical pulleys are required, one at the base of the proximal phalanx and one at the mid portion of the middle phalanx.

A loop of free tendon can be passed around the phalanx and sutured to itself. In the proximal phalanx the loop may be passed beneath or around the extensor mechanism.[2, 4] Riordan has advocated placing the free graft through a drill hole in the base of the proximal phalanx in order to assure adequate anchorage of the pulley. The pully loop is rotated after suturing so that the suture junction is pulled into the bone.[13] The reconstructed pulley should restrain the underlying flexor tendon as close as possible to bone without inhibiting free gliding of the underlying flexor tendon. An attached slip of the superficialis tendon makes an ideal pulley for the middle joint or middle phalanx.[2] The slip may be attached to the contralateral side of the proximal phalanx where it may prevent hyperextension of the proximal interphalangeal joint and also act as a pulley. However, passing it more directly across the base of the middle phalanx is more likely to prevent its distortion and relative lengthening with flexion. If remnants of a pulley remain, they may be used as anchors to which a free tendon graft may be sutured to act as a pulley. In general, reconstructed pulleys should be as

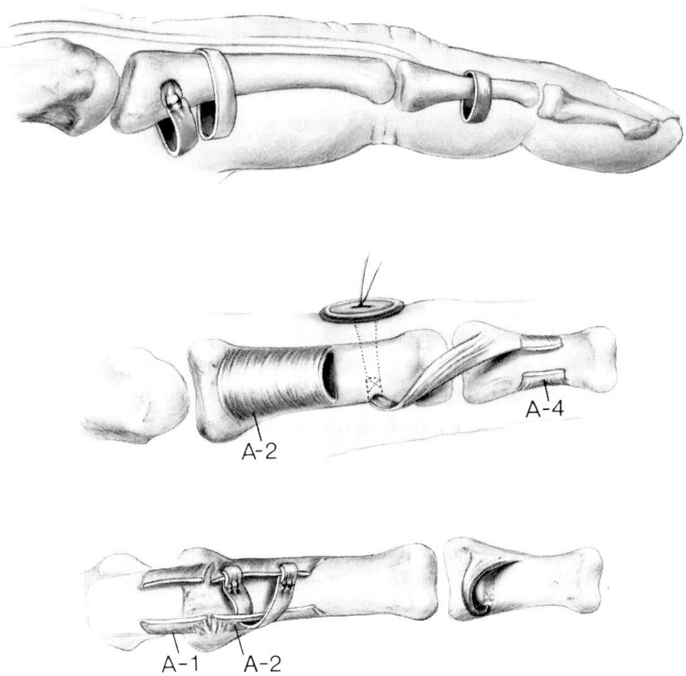

Fig. 9-3. Pulleys may be reconstructed by using free tendon grafts or by using a slip of the superficialis tendon near its insertion. In the proximal phalanx, grafts may be placed through the bone (Riordan), or around or underneath the extensor tendon (Boyes, Bunnell). Remnants of the annular bands may be used as anchors for a free graft that can be woven into and sutured to the band. Attachments of the reconstructed pulleys must be strong and preferably to bone. The reconstructed pulley should hold the flexor tendon as close as possible to the bone without loss of free tendon motion.

broad and as tight fitting as possible. Their attachments must be quite strong in view of the magnitude of forces placed on them in flexion.[1] Soft tissue adjacent to bone (other than substantial portions of one of the annular pulleys) is usually not strong enough to provide a good attachment for the reconstructed pulley.

DISCUSSION AND CONCLUSIONS

The gliding mechanism of a tendon varies according to the functional demands placed upon it and upon the arc of motion of the joints that it serves. Tendons that pull straight and have very little arc of motion or bending usually travel through a special type of connective tissue called paratenon. Paratenon is a pliable, filmy, and loose tissue that acts as an accommodating interface between the tendon, its underlying bed and overlying fascial compartments. In the finger, special adaptations are required because of the relatively confined space and also because the flexor tendon must work or bend around corners.[4] It moves around an arc riding on a film of synovial fluid between two synovial-lined surfaces. This double-walled hollow tube that encloses the digital flexor tendons consists of a visceral layer and a parietal layer that join each other at both ends to make a self-enclosed, self-lubricating system. The inner layer of this sheath (visceral layer) is closely applied to the tendon and is called epitenon.[4]

Pulleys are condensations of fibrous tissue that occur at strategic locations along the flexor sheath. These pulleys are located on top of the parietal layer of the sheath and are always lined with synovium. Plicae or pouches in the parietal sheath may be noted at either end of these pulleys to accommodate for movement or stretching between the tendon and sheath interface. The annular configuration is seen at areas of greatest stress or pull of the flexors. The annular bands, however, being somewhat like rigid tubes are divided or separated from one another to allow flexion of the digit without buckling or deforming of the pulleys. In complete flexion the rigid annular bands are noted to nearly approximate each others' margins. This point is especially easily recognized in the 1 mm. to 3 mm. gap that exists between the first and second annular bands at the metacarpophalangeal joint. If this gap were not present, then this long rigid tube would no doubt interfere with flexion of the joint and gliding of the underlying flexor tendon (Fig. 9-1). The widest annular bands (two and four) appear between joints. The more narrow annular bands (one and three) arise either partially or completely from the volar plates. The relative narrowness (3 mm. to 4 mm.) of annular three no doubt allows it to accommodate quite well to the great amount of flexion that occurs at the proximal interphalangeal joint. In contrast to the annular bands, the cruciform pulleys are narrower, thinner, and more pliable. These cruciform bands appear to provide a supporting system for the stronger and more important annular pulleys.

The fact that the first annular is readily expendable if the second annular band is intact is easily understood by all surgeons who perform trigger finger releases. Little or no functional loss occurs after such surgery.

In summary, four annular and three cruciform pulleys have been identified in the flexor mechanism of the finger. The second annular band, located in the proximal phalanx, and the fourth annular band, located in the middle phalanx, appear to be the most important. They should be preserved or reconstructed if normal tendon function is to result. The relative significance of these two pulleys has been described by Littler and Boyes, and by Rank, Wakefield, and Hueston.[2, 10, 12] Reconstructed pulleys must be firmly anchored to bone, as broad as possible and should restrain the tendon as close as possible to the underlying bone.

References

1. Blythe, W.: Unpublished data, 1974.
2. Boyes, J. H.: Bunnell's Surgery of the hand, ed. 5, Philadelphia, 1970, J. B. Lippincott, pp. 403-404.
3. Boyes, J. H., and Stark, H. H.: Flexor tendon grafts in the fingers and thumb, J. Bone Joint Surg. **53A**:1332-1342, 1971.
4. Bunnell, S.: Surgery of the hand, ed. 3, Philadelphia, 1956. J. B. Lippincott, pp. 431 (Fig. 433), 434-435.

5. Doyle, J. R., and Blythe, W.: Macroscopic and functional anatomy of the flexor tendon sheath, J. Bone Joint Surg. **56A**:1094, 1974.
6. Flatt, A. E.: The care of minor hand injuries, ed. 3, St. Louis, 1972, The C. V. Mosby Co., pp. 9-11.
7. Green, W. L. and Niebauer, J. J.: Results of primary and secondary flexor tendon repairs in no-man's-land, J. Bone Joint Surg. **56A**:1216-22, 1974.
8. Kleinert, H. E., Kutz, J. E., Atasoy, E., and Stormo, A.: Primary repair of flexor tendons, Orthop. Clin. North Am. **4**:865-876, 1973.
9. Littler, J. W.: Discussion of paper by Verdan, C. E.: Primary repair of flexor tendons, J. Bone Joint Surg. **42A**:647-657, 1960.
10. Littler, J. W.: Free tendon grafts in secondary flexor tendon repair, Am. J. Surg. **74**:315-321, 1947.
11. Milford, L.: The hand, St. Louis, 1971, The C. V. Mosby Co., p. 107.
12. Rank, B. K., Wakefield, A. R., and Hueston, J. T.: Surgery of repair as applied to hand injuries, ed. 4, Baltimore, 1973, The Williams & Wilkins Co., pp. 34-35, 248-249.
13. Riordan, D. C.: Personal communication, 1973.
14. Sakovich, L., and Burn, H. F.: Vacuum embedding of tissues in nitrocellulose, Am. J. Clin. Pathol. **43**:396-398, 1965.

10. Early management of fresh hand wounds with specific reference to delayed repair

François Iselin, M.D.

Any hand wound may cause severe functional impairment. Restoration of function as close to the normal as possible may necessitate complex surgical procedures and the result may be compromised by infection.

Avoiding infection is not so much a matter of antibiotics but of surgery performed on a thoroughly decontaminated wound and surrounding skin. This is to emphasize the necessity of a complete excision of the bruised tissues that otherwise would turn to necrosis and the necessity of covering with good, clean, and adequately placed skin the underlying repairs of tendon, nerves, and bones.

We believe that it is difficult to meet these requirements in the usual conditions of emergency and surgery and we therefore advocate the method of delayed complete repair after early preparation.

This procedure has been routine in our unit since 1960 when it was originated by Dr. Marc Iselin, who stated that there is nothing adverse in thoroughly preparing a patient for early reparative surgery at a time convenient to all concerned and when conditions are optimal for success. The surgical team must be ready to perform an operation that repairs in one stage all the lesions, whether they are of bone, tendon, or nerves, and to meet the conditions of adequate skin cover even if this requires skin autoplasties or grafts. If there are no local possibilities for this total reparative surgery, the patient should be referred to a more specialized center without inconvenience as long as the immediate care of the wound has been correctly performed.

DELAYED REPAIR MUST BE COMPLETE REPAIR

More than 7,500 cases have been treated this way without inconvenience and for the sake of simplicity we have studied the method on 100 consecutive cases treated in our outpatient department. This study therefore refers only to light cases but many of them are compound fractures of the distal phalanx and the results appeared as significant.

The delay between injury and surgery may vary between a few hours and 10 days. The more bruised and dirty a wound is, the longer the delay for surgery will need to be. Of these 100 cases, five were treated after 2 days, 90 after 4 days, four after 5 days, and one after 10 days.

It must be stressed that there should not be any delay for some superficial (no nerves or tendons lacerated), neat, and clean wounds, and that emergency action is compulsory for hemorrhages, dislocations, and severely displaced fractures that may endanger the vitality of a hand or a finger. In these cases emergency reduction and fixation without immediate skin closure is advocated as a first step to secondary early repair.

All 100 cases of this study have sustained preoperative bacteriologic swabs before operating room cleaning. Seventy-nine cases were free from germs and 21 were contaminated, 15 of which were nonpathogen and six were pathogen. Of the 94 wounds without preoperative pathogens, 85 healed aseptically and nine had postoperative infections.

We believe that the six wounds with preoperative pathogens had aseptic evolution because the excision of bruised tissues was complete and skin closure was of good quality.

More important is the finding that only 29 out of 100 were neat linear wounds while 71 were bruised wounds. Nevertheless, after preparation we were able to close simply in 85 cases. This means that on delayed closure, the skin was fit for suturing in 56 cases of crush injuries. We wonder what these figures would have been in immediate repair and how many skin grafts would have been used. We therefore think that *delaying the excision seems to be as economical as possible in this matter.*

Out of these 100 cases, 91 recovered with no sequelae. Sixty-seven returned to work before 30 days, 21 between 30 and 60 days 30 of which were compound fractures of the distal phalanges.

These results emphasize that we did not get into any trouble in treating these cases with delayed repair.

PRACTICAL MANAGEMENT

Only the surgeon on duty at the emergency room is entitled to decide to delay the repair of a wound. It is his responsibility to determine how long the preparation delay will be depending on the importance of the wound, its complexity and cleanliness.

Emergency care has two facets, local and general.

Local management

The hand is cleaned by soaking it in a diluted ammonium solution. Any foreign body is removed and necessary hemostasis is performed.

Dressing is made with grease gauze and fluffy cotton pads, with splinting in the natural position, the splint being placed on the opposite side of the wound.

General management

Antitetanous precautions are checked and given as needed, general examination, including physical and biologic, is performed just the way it would be for a secondary repair. Any disturbance such as dysproteinemia, diabetes, or uremia should be detected and checked.

More important is the psychologic preparation. The reasons for the delay and the necessity of fitting the hand and the patient for surgery must be emphasized and clearly explained to the patient, to the family, and especially to the referring doctor, if there is one.

Tranquilizers are given routinely to help the patient through the delay and also to prevent postoperative dystrophy, which we have constantly found to be related to psychologic disturbances.

We do not use antibiotics as a routine treatment, unless the patient is referred to us with infection. In this case we take bacteriologic samples and wait till we have a chart of the germ and its sensitivity to antibiotics before prescribing the correct drug.

The procedure is the same in the postoperative period in which we do not use systemic antibiotic therapy. This delay is the same whether done in the hospital for serious cases or in the outpatient department for ambulatory patients.

The management during the waiting period must be repeated *daily* under the personal control of the surgeon who puts the patient on the operative schedule, because as soon as the patient is ready, surgery must be performed. The concept of emergency is still valid as long as the optimal conditions are obtained.

The surgery of repair must, in these conditions, be as complete as possible and we firmly believe that it must be a thorough repair of whatever has to be repaired. Adequate, complete surgery is always long and tedious. It may perhaps have to associate bone fixation, tendon repair, nerve repair, skin coverage with flaps. It may have to be completed by secondary operations, especially tenolysis, but in our experience the number of secondary operations is minimal if the primary repair has been performed in optimal conditions. It is our conviction that these optimal conditions can only be met after adequate preparation, which must be an emergency gesture that will lead to the best possible early surgery.

11. Primary repair of zone 2 flexor tendon lacerations

Harold E. Kleinert, M.D.
Joseph E. Kutz, M.D.
Myles J. Cohen, M.D.

The successful treatment of flexor tendon lacerations between the distal palmar crease and middle phalanx has been one of the most difficult problems in hand surgery. In 1918 Sterling Bunnell wrote "my first attempts at repair of tendons in the fingers resulted in immediate success, but as the succeeding days went by, motion became less and less until at the end of a few weeks it became nil. The tendons had become firmly embedded in scar tissue and had united to the surrounding finger in a solid mass."[7] Faced with consistently unsatisfactory results the term no-man's-land was coined to describe this region that Verdan later termed zone 2 (Fig. 11-1). Anatomically it consists of that portion of the fibro-osseous canal between the first annular pulley and the flexor digitorum superficialis insertion.

ANATOMY

Within this region the unique anatomy presents special obstacles to the restoration of smooth tendon gliding. The flexor digitorum superficialis and flexor digitorum profundus lie juxtaposed as they pass through the fibro-osseous canal. They are separated from each other and the surrounding canal by only a film of synovial fluid (Fig. 11-2).

The fibro-osseous canal is a closely applied, semirigid tunnel through which the tendons pass. The fibrous portion of the canal is comprised of three annular pulleys, which are dense condensations of transversely oriented fibrous bands. The first is at the level of the metacarpophalangeal joint. It attaches to the junction of the volar plate and the deep transverse intermetacarpal ligament. The second and third pulleys are at the mid portions of the proximal and middle phalanges, respectively. They attach firmly to the volar lateral ridges of the phalanges. Between each annular pulley is a cruciform portion that is filmier, flexible, and overlies each joint. The most important elements of this system are the second and third annular pulleys. Destruction of either of these will result

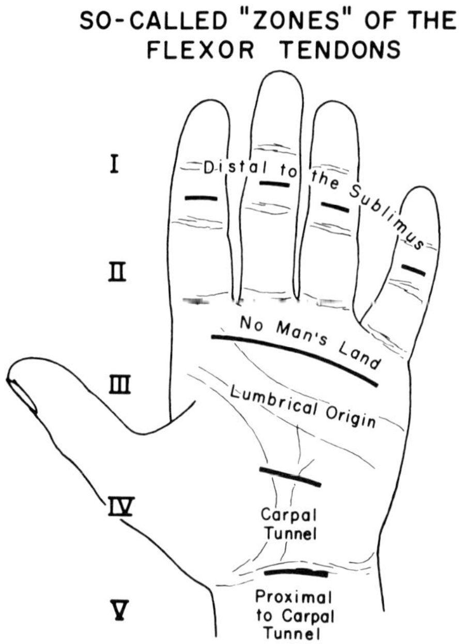

Fig. 11-1. The surface anatomy of zone 2. Zone 2 extends from the distal palmar crease to the mid middle phalanx. (From Kleinert, H. E., et al.: Primary repair of flexor tendons, Orthop. Clin. North Am. 4(4): 866, October, 1973. Courtesy W. B. Saunders Co., Publisher.)

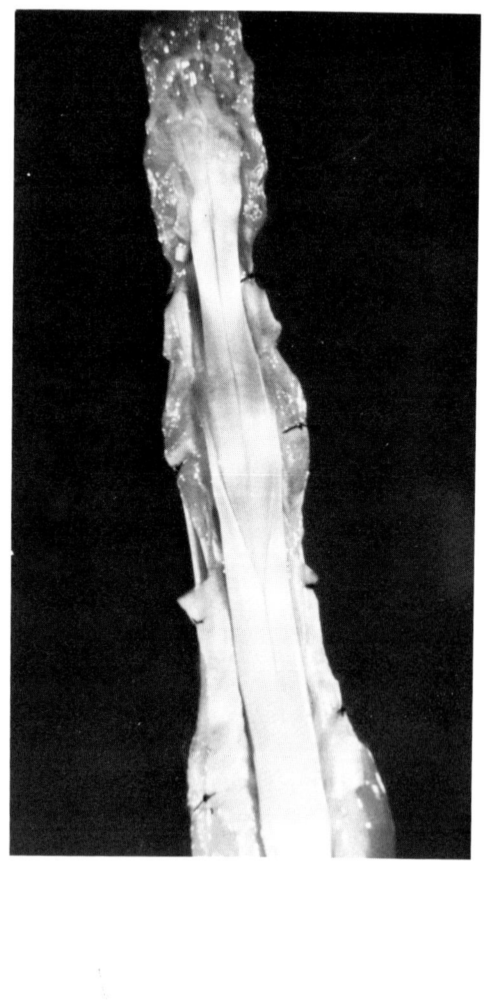

Fig. 11-2. The flexor digitorum superficialis and flexor digitorum profundus pass through zone 2 without interposed loose areolar tissue. Any scarring here will bind the tendons together and eliminate the normal differential gliding. (From Johnson, M. K., and Cohen, M. J.: The hand atlas, 1975. Courtesy Charles C Thomas, Publisher, Springfield, Illinois.)

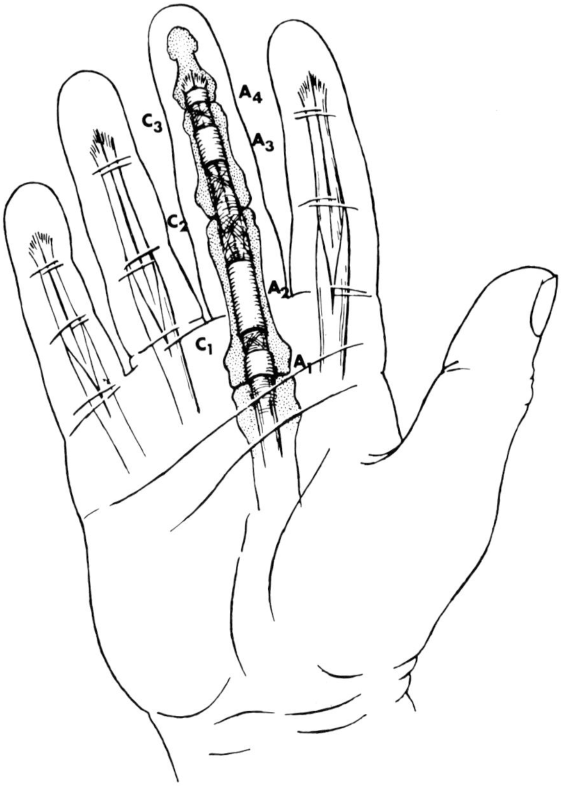

Fig. 11-3. The fibro-osseous canal in zone 2 is comprised of three annular and two cruciform pulleys. The annular pulleys are thick and rigid preventing tendon bowstringing on flexion. The third cruciform and fourth annular pulleys lie beyond zone 2.

in bowstringing of the flexors (Fig. 11-3). The floor of the fibro-osseous canal is the volar aspect of the phalanges and volar plates of the metacarpophalangeal and proximal interphalangeal joints. Fractures and volar plate lacerations thus abut directly on the gliding tendons.

The flexor digitorum superficialis enters the fibro-osseous canal volar to the profundus. Just beyond the first pulley it splits. Each half rolls outward 180° as it passes lateral and then dorsal to the profundus. Once dorsal to the profundus these two bands rejoin and decussate forming Camper's chiasm before passing distally to insert at the mid middle phalanx. This creates a sloping ring aperture through which the profundus passes to become superficial to the decussation (Fig. 11-4). Kaplan has demonstrated a differential excursion of these tendons at the level of the metacarpophalangeal joint. The flexor digitorum profundus moves between 2.7 cm. and 3 cm., the flexor digitorum superficialis moves 0.5 cm. to 0.75 cm. less.[14] The capacity for synchronous full range of motion thus requires smooth gliding not only of the tendons against the fibro-osseous canal but also of each tendon upon its mate. The close approximation of the tendons

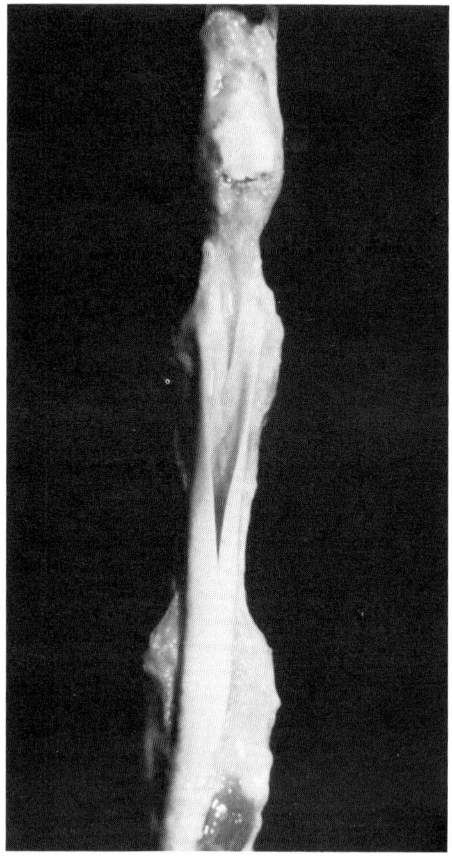

Fig. 11-4. The flexor digitorum sublimus splits. Each leaf rolls laterally and dorsally prior to Camper's chiasm. An oblique tunnel is thus formed for passage of the flexor digitorum profundus. (From Johnson, M. K., and Cohen, M. J.: The hand atlas, 1975. Courtesy Charles C Thomas, Publisher, Springfield, Illinois.)

to each other and to the surrounding sheath and the lack of surrounding loose areolar tissue provides little leeway for scar formation. The smallest cicatrix tends to be rigid and limits motion.

The tendon blood supply is limited. Arteries pass through four folds of mesotenon called vincula (Fig. 11-5). The short vinculum of the profundus arises at the neck of the middle phalanx. It attaches to the profundus as a short flat sheet just proximal to its insertion. The short vinculum of the superficialis arises at the level of the neck of the proximal phalanx. It enters the superficialis decussation either in the center of the chiasm or as two branches entering each slip of the decussation separately. The arterial supply to these vincula comes through transverse branches of the digital arteries. These branches will be interrupted in a midlateral approach to this zone. The profundus at this level is volar to the superficialis. Its long vincula arises from this decussation to enter the

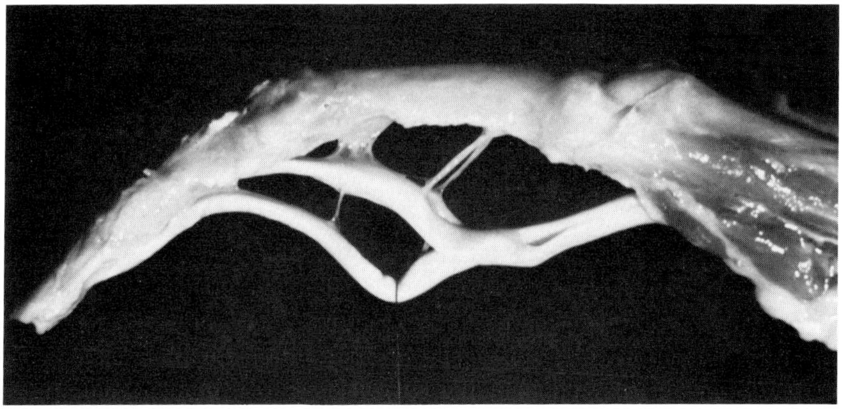

Fig. 11-5. The vinculae of the flexor tendons carry the major blood supply within the sheath. The long vincula of the profundus relies upon the integrity of the decussation and the short vincula, the superficialis. (From Johnson, M. K., and Cohen, M. J.: The hand atlas, 1975. Courtesy Charles C Thomas, Publisher, Springfield, Illinois.)

profundus more proximally. The viability of the midportion of the profundus is thus dependent on the integrity of its own long vincula, the superficialis decussation, and short vincula to the decussation. Interference with any of these structures places the profundus at increased risk of necrosis.[18] The intratendinous blood supply has been recently shown to be primarily dorsal. It may be assumed that sutures in the dorsal portion of the tendon would lead to increased vascular compromise.[9]

TREATMENT

Two approaches have evolved in the management of zone 2 lacerations. The reader is referred to the excellent work of Boyes,[1] Boyes and Stark,[2] and Pulvertaft[23, 24] for a comprehensive analysis of the use of tendon grafting in these injuries. Primary repair has advantages over delayed tendon grafting. In certain cases function can be restored as well or better with primary repair. Both profundus and superficialis function may be restored. Patient rehabilitation is shortened. Hospitalization and attendant cost is lessened. These advantages have stimulated continued interest in primary repair and spurred the development of this technique.

Despite its potential advantages, primary repair may have catastrophic results if careful case selection is waived. This is not a procedure for the surgeon who occasionally performs hand surgery, nor for one not specially trained in this technique.

> The specific procedure decided upon in any case is rarely as important as the manner in which it is carried out.
>
> *Harrison McLaughlin*

The absence of adequate personnel and facilities to perform this surgery is an absolute contraindication to primary repair. Other contraindications include: (1) the inability to convert the laceration to a clean tidy wound such as in human bites and severe crushing injuries, (2) the inability to obtain adequate skin cover, and (3) the presence of inadequate pulleys.

Preoperative evaluation includes details of the mechanism of injury and posture of the hand at the time of injury. A general history and physical examination should be done. X-ray films are taken. The patient is given tetanus prophylaxis. The wound is cleansed, dressed, and prophylactic antibiotics are begun in the emergency room. The patient is then taken to the operating room.

OPERATIVE TECHNIQUE

An axillary block using 1% Carbocaine* will provide 3 hours to 4 hours of anesthesia. If a longer block is required, 0.5% Marcaine* is effective for 12 hours to 18 hours. The hand is prepped, fingernails cleaned and trimmed, and the injured part is washed for 10 minutes. The arm is draped and irrigation of the wound is performed with 500 cc. of Ringer's lactate and 100 cc. of 0.5% Neomycin solution. If the wound is contaminated, several liters of Ringer's lactate may be delivered using a surgical jet lavage. The arm is exsanguinated and the pneumatic tourniquet inflated. Loupe magnification of between 2× and 3.5× is used routinely. A determination of whether and how to extend the wound depends upon wound inspection and the history of finger position. The tendon laceration is rarely at the level of the skin laceration (Fig. 11-6). The wound is extended only as much as necessary to gain exposure, usually proceeding either proximally or distally, rarely both. The method of Bruner is preferred (Fig. 11-7).[3, 4] The

*Winthrop Laboratories.

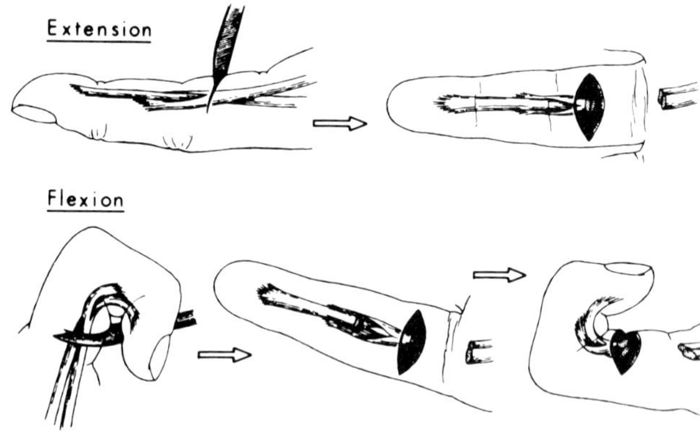

Fig. 11-6. The position of the finger at the time of injury determines the level of the tendon laceration. It may or may not coincide with the skin wound.

dissection proceeds carefully to avoid further damage to the fibro-osseous tunnel and neurovascular bundle. All questionably viable tissue and foreign material are debrided. The laceration in the fibro-osseous tunnel is utilized to create a laterally based flap for exposure of the underlying tendons, which is usually 2 cm. or less in length. It is designed to preserve all or at least 1 cm. of each major pulley. The proximal tendon is often tethered by the vincula and prevented from withdrawal into the palm. Wrist and finger flexion coupled with milking the forearm and hand will bring the proximal tendon stump into the wound (Fig. 11-8). Occasionally if the tendon has retracted into the palm, a palmar incision

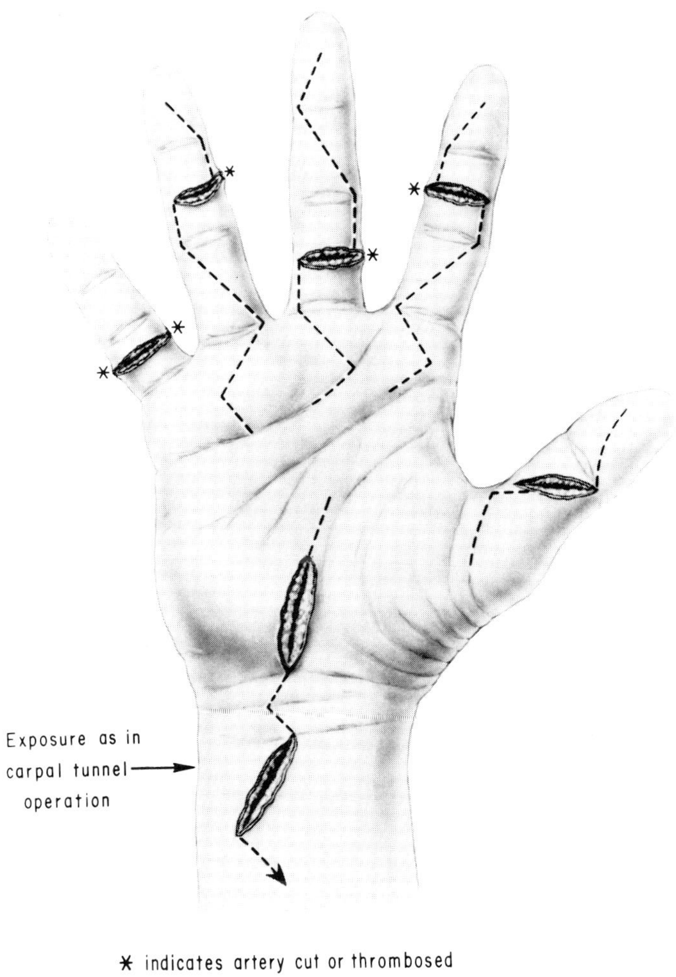

Fig. 11-7. The skin wound is lengthened either distally or proximally, rarely both. The technique of Bruner is preferred for both improved exposure and limited injury to the tendon blood supply. (From Bruner, J.: Surgical exposure of flexor tendons in the hand, Ann. R. Coll. Surg. Engl., 53:84, August, 1973.)

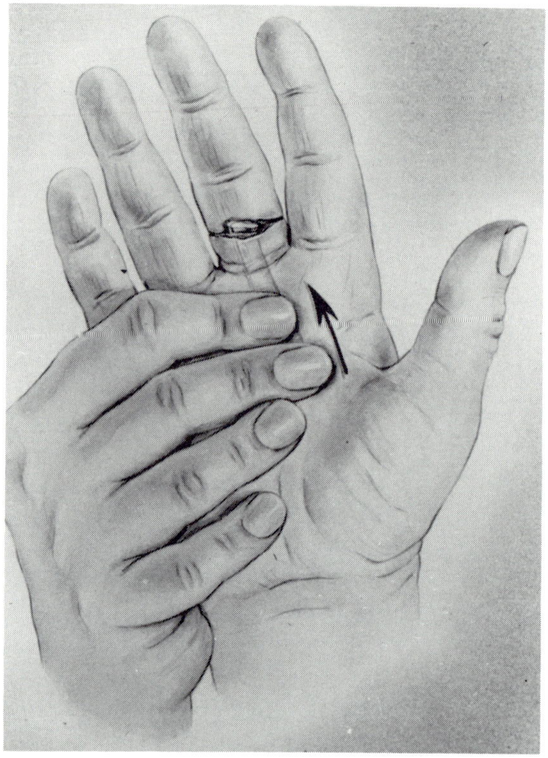

Fig. 11-8. The proximal tendon may be advanced into the wound by flexing the wrist and fingers while milking the forearm and palm.

may be required to pass the tendon into the canal (Fig. 11-9). The tendons are handled only by their cut end. They are held advanced by a Keith needle inserted through the digital sheath and tendon to allow repair without tension. Fractures, if present, are fixed with Kirschner wires. The periosteum is repaired over the fracture site. Lacerations of volar plate and collateral ligaments are repaired with 5-0 Mersilene.*

In a clean, sharply incised laceration no tendon debridement is required. If the tendon cut surface is ragged it may be recut with a straight razor blade. A criss-cross 4-0 or 5-0 Mersilene stay suture is placed (Fig. 11-10). The cross limbs are placed at least 1 cm. from the cut end of the tendon. This suture is placed in the volar half of the tendon to prevent additional vascular compromise. The suture is tied so there is no puckering and no concertina effect. The tendon ends should be comfortably coapted. During suture of the profundus the volar longitudinal groove may be used for alignment. A running 6-0 Mersilene suture is placed coapting only the epitenon in 1 mm. bites. The tendon fascicles are not sutured. Using the tails of the knotted suture, control of the tendon is effected.

*Ethicon, Inc.

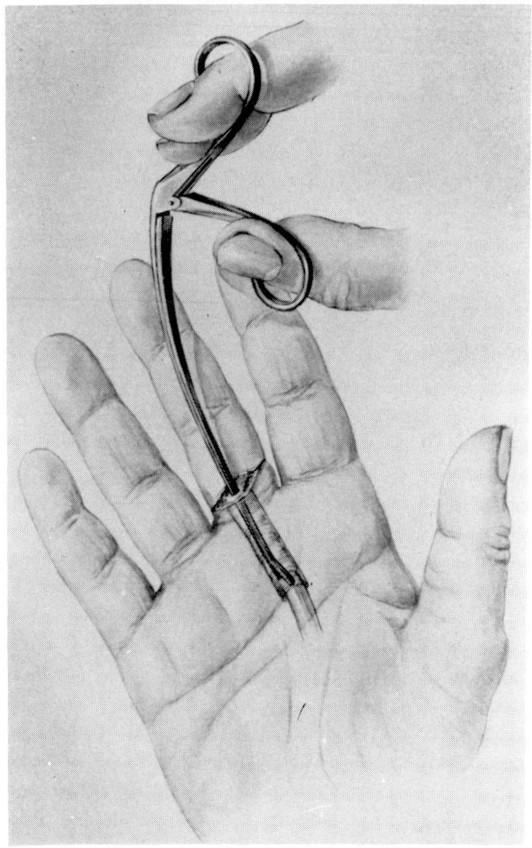

Fig. 11-9. A tendon retriever may be of help to grasp the end of the retracted tendon.

After the volar running suture is completed the tendon is reversed in a fashion similar to vessel repair and the dorsal epitenon is approximated. All loose ends are satisfied leaving a smooth suture line. If both superficialis and profundus have been lacerated both are repaired when possible. If the superficialis is lacerated distal to its division both slips are repaired. On completing the tendon repair the temporary fixation needle is removed. Nerves and vessels are repaired next.

The flap or window in the fibro-osseous sheath, necessary to gain exposure, is usually excised. More recently it has been replaced and tacked with interrupted 5-0 Mersilene to reconstruct an intact sheath. Adequate intact pulleys must be maintained.

The tourniquet is released, pressure is held until the arterial flush has passed, and complete hemostasis is obtained with either ligatures of 6-0 Dexon* or bipolar bovie to prevent hematoma formation.

The skin is closed with multiple fine interrupted 6-0 nylon sutures. A double

*Davis and Geck.

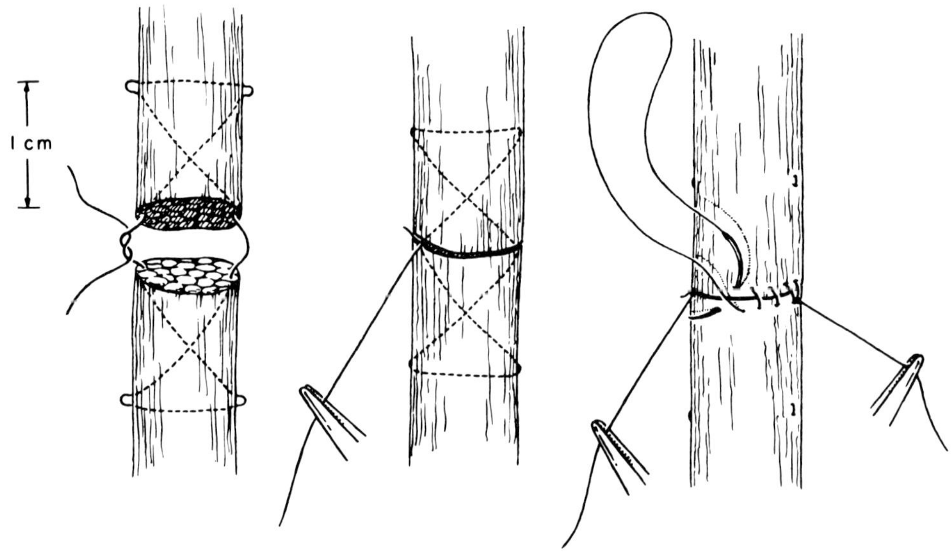

Fig. 11-10. The cross limb of the criss-cross suture is placed at least 1 cm. from the site of laceration. When tied, the tendon should not pucker nor should there be any concertina effect. The 6-0 running suture is in the epitenon only. Suture tails are left long to provide control of the tendon.

loop of 5-0 nylon suture is passed through the nail and knotted. A rubber band is attached.

A thin, nonconstrictive dressing of 1 inch Kling* is used for the wound.

A plaster dorsal and dorsolateral splint is constructed with the wrist 45° angle of flexion and the metacarpophalangeal and proximal interphalangeal joints flexed from 10° to 20° (Fig. 11-11). This position is obtained by holding the arm pronated with the elbow extended and supported under the lower humerus. The splint extends from beyond the involved fingertips to the high forearm and has bilateral side supports for strength. Aside from the Kling, no further dressing is placed beyond the distal palmar crease.

A loosely applied reverse spiral ace wrap is used for an overwrap. The rubber band is placed on traction and attached to a safety pin fastened proximal to the wrist and taped to hold position.

The patient is continued on prophylactic antibiotics for approximately 5 days. Outpatients are seen in the office within 2 to 3 days. At that time, instructions in active finger extension are given. The fingernails should touch the distal portion of the splint. The patient is advised to avoid strong active finger flexion and passive extension. The patient is rechecked once a week to ensure proper function and use of the dynamic splint.

After 21 days the splint is removed and active exercises are begun. Assistive

*Johnson and Johnson.

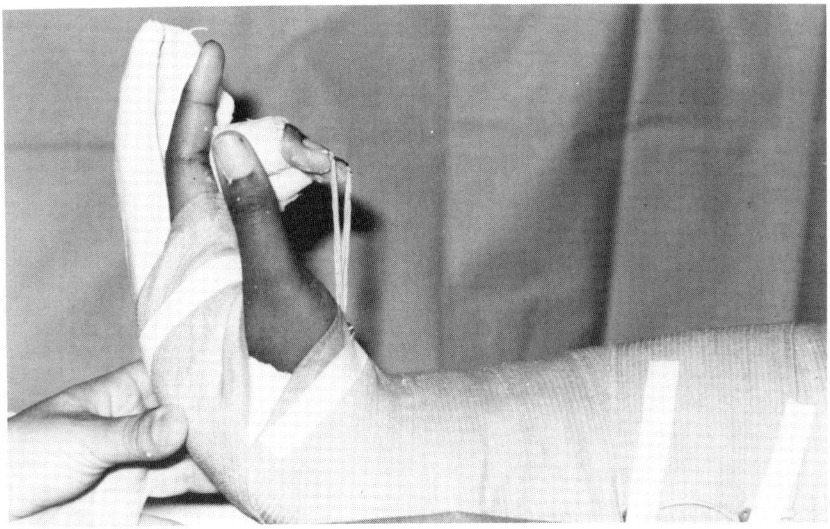

Fig. 11-11. The plaster dorsal splint is constructed to hold the wrist at 20° to 30° less than full flexion. It allows finger joint motion to within 10° to 20° of full extension. Side supports are used for added strength.

finger joint flexion may be started but the patient is not allowed to use the hand for any power function nor passive extension. At 6 to 8 weeks postoperatively, assistive extension and dynamic and static splinting may be begun to increase the range of motion. The patient is followed closely during the interval. Tendolysis (when indicated) is not performed until 6 months following injury.

RESULTS

This technique has resulted in 80% of our patients achieving good or excellent results. Criteria for these classifications are the ability to actively bring the distal pulp to within 1.5 cm. of the distal palmar crease and flexion contracture of the proximal interphalangeal joint of less than 30°. In cases of both superficialis and profundus lacerations the best results were obtained when both tendons were repaired. Of our patients, 18% required tendolysis or secondary grafting for tendon rupture. These ruptures all occurred within the 2 weeks following dynamic splint removal. Younger patients tended to achieve better results. The end results did not correlate with either associated structural damage or preoperative wound "tidiness."[26]

DISCUSSION

The anatomical and functional peculiarities of zone 2 have presented a formidable challenge to the hand surgeon. Primary repair has been performed in carefully selected cases by many surgeons. Bunnell reported his technique in 1947.[6] Later reports of Hauge,[11] Kelly,[15] and Lindsay[19] revealed limited motion following repair. This was particularly discouraging in view of the results of tendon grafting reported by Boyes[1] and Pulvertaft.[23] Tendon grafting has not met with uniform success in all hands. Alex Kelly wrote in 1957: "The widespread adoption of secondary tendon grafting by surgeons not intimately familiar with the problems of hand surgery who hope they will have results comparable to those published by Boyes or Pulvertaft is not realistic. It is akin to the sandlot ballplayer who thinks that he will be able to bat like Ted Williams by eating the right brand of breakfast food."[15] In 1951 Dr. Claude Verdan became dissatisfied with results from tendon grafting as the principle treatment for these injuries and developed his own technique of primary repair. To protect his suture line, he used a temporary proximal transtendon pin to eliminate tension on his repair. The results he felt were much improved over his experience with grafting. We agree with Dr. Verdan[27, 28] that in appropriate cases, primary repair of both tendons yields results superior to grafting in our hands. The senior author has used the techniques presented here since 1954. Case selection remains important. Where contraindications exist, primary wound closure and delayed tendon grafting is the treatment of choice.

We feel that early controlled mobilization in a dynamic splint contributes significantly to the management of these injuries. The electromyographic studies

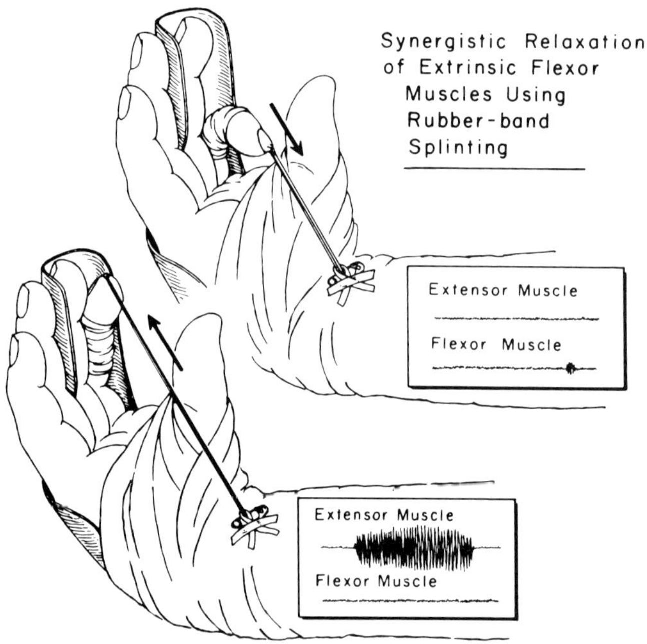

Fig. 11-12. Electromyography confirms reciprocal relaxation of the extrinsic flexors during finger extension in the splint. On relaxation of the extensors, finger flexion is achieved by the rubber band.

of Dr. Graham Lister (Fig. 11-12) have demonstrated that in dynamic (flexor) traction the extrinsic flexors are quiescent. During active extension they reciprocally relax. During flexion the rubber band carries the finger into flexion as soon as the extensors relax with only a short terminal burst of flexor electrical activity.[17] It is felt that this early motion combined with meticulous technique limits the formation of rigid adhesions between the tendons and surrounding sheath.

References

1. Boyes, J. H.: Evaluation of results of digital flexor tendon grafts, Am. J. Surg. **89**:1116, 1955.
2. Boyes, J. H., Stark, H. H.: Flexor tendon grafts in the fingers and thumb, a study of factors influencing results in 1,000 cases, J. Bone Joint Surg. **53A**:1332, 1971.
3. Bruner, J. M.: Surgical exposure of flexor tendons in the hand, Ann. R. Coll. Surg. Engl. **53**:84, Aug., 1973.
4. Bruner, J. M.: The zigzag volar digital incision for flexor tendon surgery, Plast. Reconstr. Surg. **40**:571, Dec., 1967.
5. Bunnell, S.: The early treatment of hand injuries, J. Bone Joint Surg. **33A**:807, July, 1951.
6. Bunnell, S.: Primary repair of severed tendons, the use of stainless steel wire, Am. J. Surg. **47**:502, 1947.
7. Bunnell, S.: Repair of tendons in the fingers and description of two new instruments, Surg. Gynecol. Obstet. **26**:103, 1918.
8. Burnham, P. J.: Repair of tendon injuries in the hand, Arch. Surg. **78**:316, Feb., 1959.
9. Caplan, H. S., Hunter, J. M., Merklin, R. J.: Intrinsic vascularization of flexor tendons in the human, Presented at Am. Soc. Surg. of the Hand, San Francisco, Feb., 1975.
10. Green, W. L., Niebauer, J. J.: Results of primary and secondary flexor tendon repair in no-man's-land, J. Bone Joint Surg. **56A**:1216, Sept., 1974.
11. Hauge, M. F.: The results of tendon suture of the hand, a review of 500 patients, Acta Orthop. Scand. **24**:258, 1955.
12. Holm, C., and Embrick, R.: Anatomical conduction in the primary treatment of tendon injuries in the hand, J. Bone Joint Surg. **41A**:509, June, 1959.
13. Johnson, M. K., Cohen, M. J.: The hand atlas, Springfield, Ill., In press, Charles C Thomas Publisher.
14. Kaplan, E.: The structural and functional anatomy of the hand, ed. 2, Philadelphia, 1959, J. B. Lippincott Co.
15. Kelly, A. D.: A study of 789 consecutive tendon severances, J. Bone Joint Surg. **41A**:581, April, 1959.
16. Kleinert, H. E., Kutz, J. E., Ashbell, T., and Martinez, E.: Primary repair of flexor tendons in no-man's-land, J. Bone Joint Surg. **49A**:577, 1967.
17. Kleinert, H. E., Kutz, M. E., Lister, G. D.: Immediate controlled mobilization following primary flexor tendon repair, In press.
18. Leffert, R. D., Weiss, C., and Athanasoulis, D.: The vincula with particular reference to their vessels and nerves, J. Bone Joint Surg. **56A**:1191, Sept., 1974.
19. Lindsay, W. K., McDougall, E. P.: Direct digital flexor tendon repair, Plast. Reconstr. Surg. **26**:613, 1960.
20. Mason, M.: Primary tendon repair, J. Bone Joint Surg. **41A**:575, June, 1959.
21. McLaughlin, H. L., Baab, O. D.: Symposium on orthopaedic surgery: Carpectomy, Surg. Clin. North Am., **31**:451-461, April, 1951.
22. Posch, J. L.: Primary tenorrhaphies and tendon grafting procedures in hand injuries, Arch. Surg. **73**:609, 1956.
23. Pulvertaft, G.: Problems of flexor tendon surgery of the hand, J. Bone Joint Surg. **47A**:123, January, 1965.

24. Pulvertaft, G.: Repair of tendon injuries in the hand with special reference to flexor tendons, Postgrad. Med. **8**:81, 1950.
25. Rank, B. K., and Wakefield, A. R.: The repair of flexor tendons in the hand, Br. J. Plast. Surg. **4**:244-253, 1952.
26. Rank, B. K., Wakefield, A. R.: Surgery of repair as applied to hand injuries, ed. 2, Baltimore, 1960, The Williams and Wilkins Co.
27. Verdan, C. E.: Half a century of flexor tendon surgery, J. Bone Joint Surg. **54A**:472, 1972.
28. Verdan, C. E., and Crawford, G. P.: Flexor tendon suture in the digital canal, Fifth World Congress of Plastic and Reconstructive Surgery, London, 1971, Butterworth & Co. (Publishers) Ltd., p. 485.
29. White, W. L.: Secondary restoration of finger flexion by digital tendon grafts: an evaluation of seventy-six cases, Am. J. Surg. **91**:662, 1956.

12. Controlled passive motion following flexor tendon repair in zones 2 and 3

Robert J. Duran, M.D.
Robert G. Houser, M.D.

INTRODUCTION

The purpose of this chapter is to review a method of controlled passive motion used immediately after flexor tendon repair in zones 2 and 3.[13] A preliminary report, the study has been expanded and more cases are being added for further evaluation of the method.

HISTORY

Early motion following tendon repair is not new. However, all the methods that are used appear to be different. Our review of the literature indicates that early motion has been used and reported by a number of surgeons extending over a period of almost 70 years.

Our interest in this concept was based on the work and subsequent report by Young and Harmon.[15] Young states that he has used a technique of passive motion without splinting since 1942.[14] He also introduced the nail suture and elastic traction. We were further encouraged to continue our study and use of this method by the excellent results reported by Kleinert and associates[10] in 1967.

Other important studies, experimental and clinical, have been reported by Lahey,[11] Murray,[12] Kessler and Nissim,[9] Hernandez and associates,[8] Furlow,[2] and others. We were greatly impressed by the reports of Torr Wagner Harmer[3-7] who developed a special suture technique allowing early active motion. His clinical experience with the technique began in 1909 and continued for approximately 30 years.

BASIC CONSIDERATIONS

It would appear from experimental and clinical observation that 3 mm. to 5 mm. of extension motion of the tendon anastomosis in a passive exercise program is sufficient to prevent firm adherence of a repaired flexor tendon in zones 2 and 3 of the hand. It is important to state further that we have used this procedure in tidy wounds only.

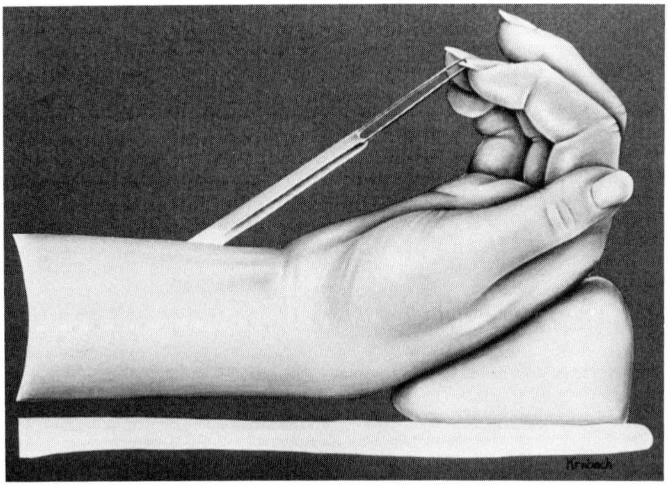

Fig. 12-1. Removable inclined wedge sponge to be used in tendon lacerations of index and thumb. Note nail suture and rubber band traction.

SURGICAL TECHNIQUES AND POSTOPERATIVE MANAGEMENT

It is important to repair the flexor digitorum superficialis as well as the flexor digitorum profundus. If joint capsule, nerves, and arteries are severed, they are also repaired.

Tenorrhaphy is achieved by a modified 5-0 Bunnell suture of synthetic material supported by peripheral mattress sutures of 6-0. If the flexor digitorum superficialis has become thin as it nears its insertion, then mattress sutures alone are used.

Considerable attention is given to the annuli or pulley system. It is frequently necessary to release the annulus laterally for a few millimeters in order to move the repair distally or in extension for 5 mm., otherwise the repair site may not clear the area.

After repairs are complete the wrist is placed in 20° to 30° of flexion (Fig. 12-1) and the metacarpophalangeal (MCP) joint of the finger is held steady in its normal balanced position. Under direct vision, the distal phalanx is moved enough in extension to see the anastomosis glide 3 mm. to 5 mm. (Fig. 12-2). This must be a motion of extension to be certain of a moving anastomosis. This has assured us that the anastomosis of the flexor digitorum profundus has been moved, not only away from fixed structures that may have been damaged in the area (sheath, capsule), but also away from the repair of the flexor digitorum superficialis.

Next, the middle phalanx is grasped and extended until both anastomoses glide distally 3 mm. to 5 mm. This motion is essential for the flexor digitorum superficialis anastomosis. Actually measuring the DIP and PIP joint range may be helpful as a guide later in the passive motion exercises (Fig. 12-3).

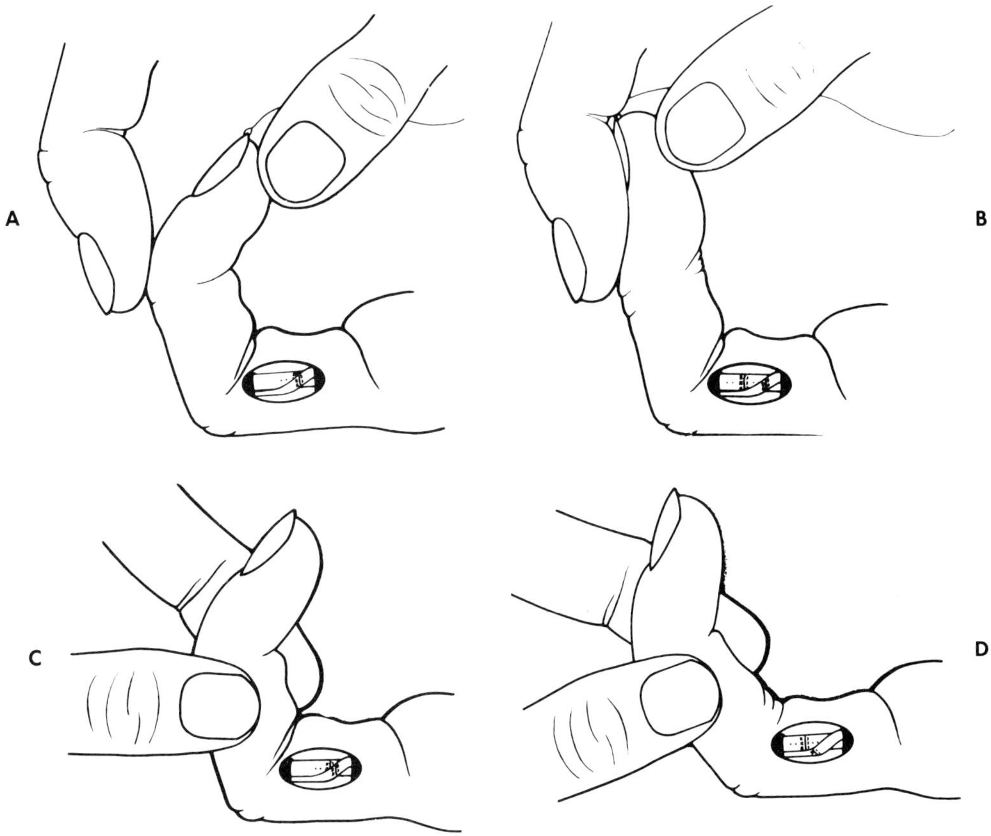

Fig. 12-2. Diagrammatic representation of controlled passive motion exercises. The metacarpophalangeal joint should be in normal balanced position. **A,** Extension of the distal interphalangeal joint sufficient to move anastomosis 3 mm. to 5 mm. This would have been previously determined at surgery under direct vision. **B,** Note distal migration of anastomosis of the flexor digitorum profundus tendon away from that of the flexor digitorum superficialis tendon. **C,** Grasping middle phalanx, both anastomoses glide distally. **D,** Anastomoses thus moved away from fixed structures that may have been injured.

A removable inclined sponge wedge beneath the hand may be helpful in managing the thumb and index fingers because the flexed wrist places them in considerable extension at the terminal joint creating difficulty with the extension exercises (Fig. 12-1). During exercises, the wedge can be removed and the wrist allowed to be in a neutral position. The wedge is replaced after passive exercises are complete. This has not been a problem in the long, ring, and little fingers, and the wrist may remain in 20° to 30° of flexion during the exercises.

At the end of the procedure, a hole is placed in the free border of the nail and a nylon suture is placed through it, tied, and connected to a rubber band. The latter is secured to the volar aspect of the forearm dressing under light tension.

Our routine is to carry out the exercises in the morning and evening with

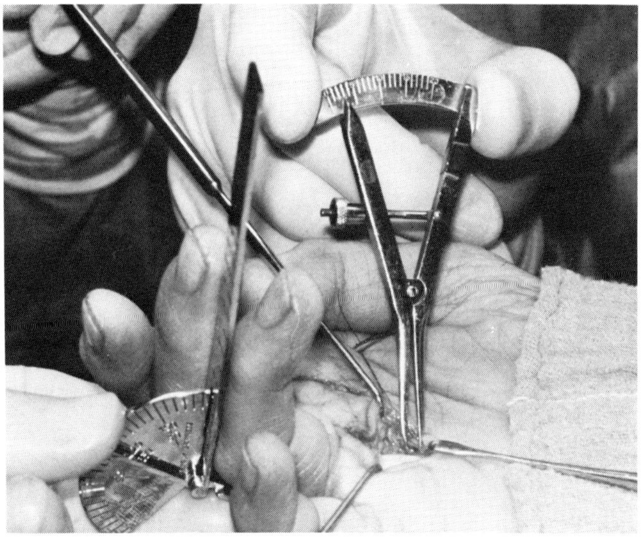

Fig. 12-3. Evaluating degrees of extension of proximal interphalangeal and distal interphalangeal joints necessary to have 3 mm. to 5 mm. of extension motion of the anastomoses. A helpful aid in precise postoperative passive exercises.

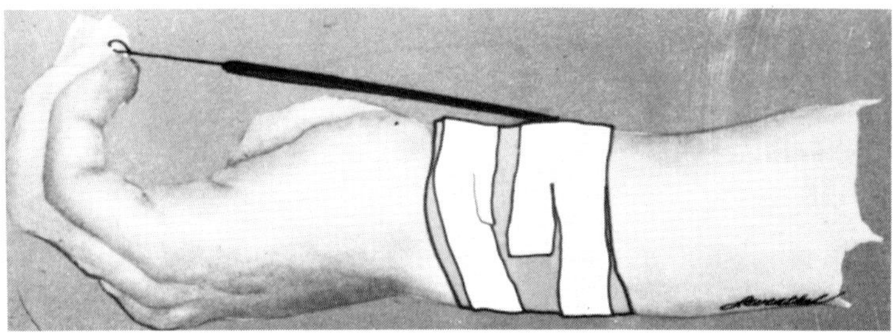

Fig. 12-4. Dorsal splint removed and wrist band applied at 4½ weeks with nail suture and rubber band traction. Passive motion exercises continued an additional week along with gentle active extension exercises.

six to eight motions for each tendon, per session. Between exercises the fingers are covered securely with stockinette. Uninvolved fingers are gently, passively exercised at each session. Training of the patients (or parents) is essential to success of the procedure. This is begun immediately with the patients observing during the first few exercise sessions and then carrying out the exercises themselves when both surgeons and patients are confident.

Controlled passive motion alone is continued for 4 ½ weeks. The dorsal splint is then removed and rubber band traction is attached to a wrist band (Fig. 12-4). Passive motion exercises are continued along with gentle active extension exercises and very limited active flexion. One week later wrist band and the nail suture are removed, and active flexion and extension motion are increased. The anastomosis is protected for two additional weeks as active exercises con-

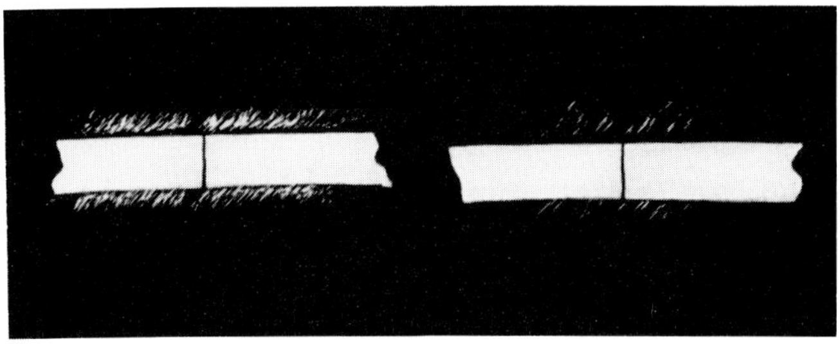

Fig. 12-5. An immobilized anastomosis strengthened by wound adhesion as compared with the anastomosis in a tendon mobilized early that does not have such firm support. This has encouraged protection of the anastomosis from active motion (flexion) for 5½ weeks.

tinue. It is our contention that the anastomosis is more vulnerable to rupture in the tendon that is mobilized early as opposed to the immobilized tendon with its firmer wound adhesion. Therefore, the mobilized tendon requires a longer period of time before active exercises are started (Fig. 12-5). Occasionally it is necessary to use a dynamic splint to correct a PIP contracture whether it is related to primary joint injury or secondary contracture.

RESULTS

Our method of postoperative controlled passive motion in zones 2 and 3 has been performed on 34 patients. Twenty-seven patients, between the ages of 7 and 59 years with an average age of 22 years, were studied for this report.

In an effort to be as critical as possible, a method of evaluation has been used that has been helpful to us (Fig. 12-6). Measurement in degrees of flexion at each joint of the finger (DIP, PIP, and MCP) are made and a second measurement of the PIP joint (flexor digitorum superficialis function alone) is made. These are added together. Loss of extension in the same joints is now subtracted from the total. The measurements are now repeated in the same finger of the opposite uninjured hand and the degrees of motion are totaled. By dividing the total of the normal hand into the total of the injured hand (less the extension defect) and multiplying by 100, a percentage of the normal range of motion of the injured finger is determined (Fig. 12-7). In the thumb, only the IP and MCP joints are measured, but these are measured in full palmar flexion and complete extension.

We have found the subdivision of zones 2 and 3 as established by Boyes and Stark[1] very helpful (Fig. 12-8). By placing each case in its subdivision a single percentage figure (average) could be calculated for that subdivision (Fig. 12-9). For example, in the distal subdivision of zone 2 there were eight cases whose average range of motion was 89% (of the normal). Results in zone

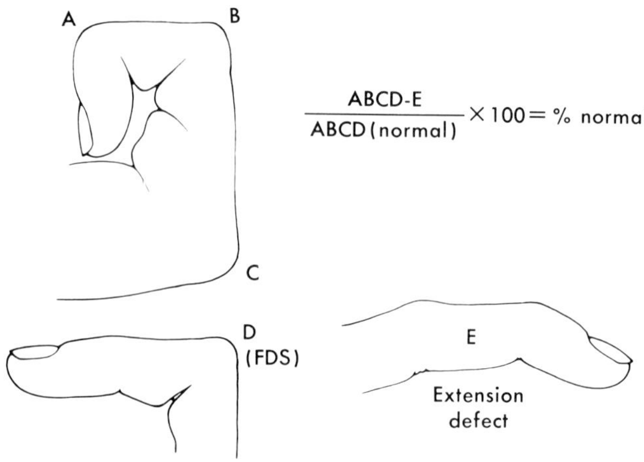

$$\frac{\text{ABCD-E}}{\text{ABCD (normal)}} \times 100 = \%\ \text{normal}$$

Fig. 12-6. Method of calculating percentage of normal range of motion (see text).

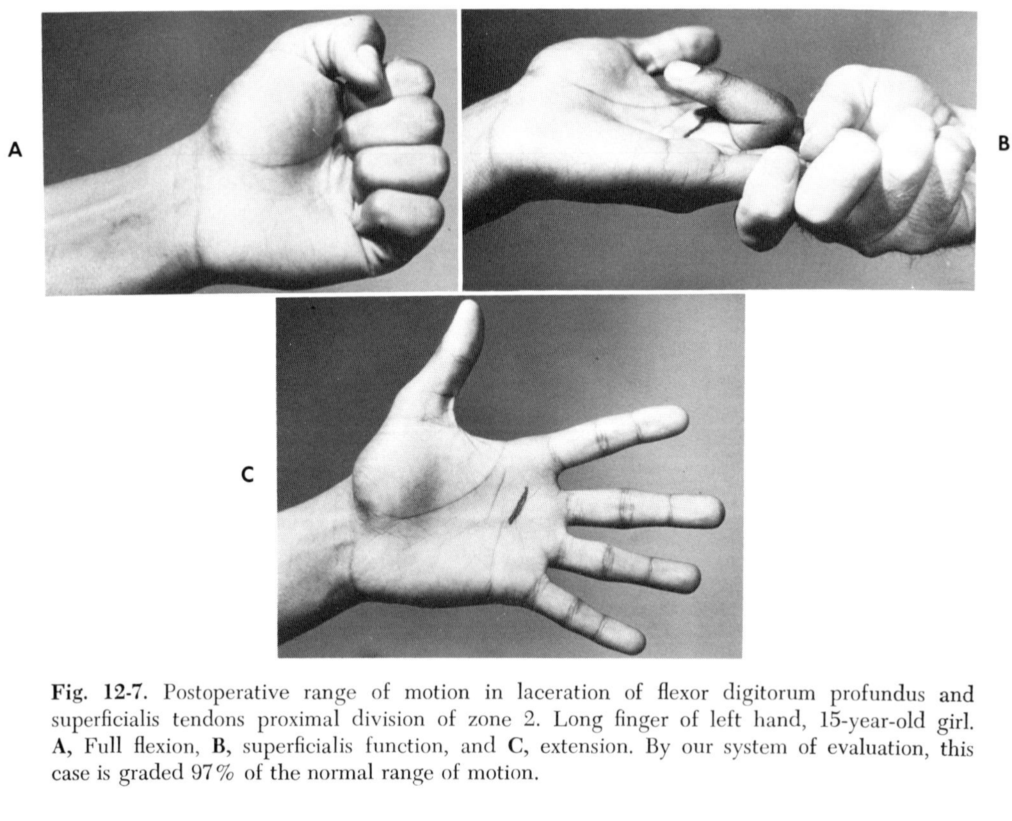

Fig. 12-7. Postoperative range of motion in laceration of flexor digitorum profundus and superficialis tendons proximal division of zone 2. Long finger of left hand, 15-year-old girl. **A,** Full flexion, **B,** superficialis function, and **C,** extension. By our system of evaluation, this case is graded 97% of the normal range of motion.

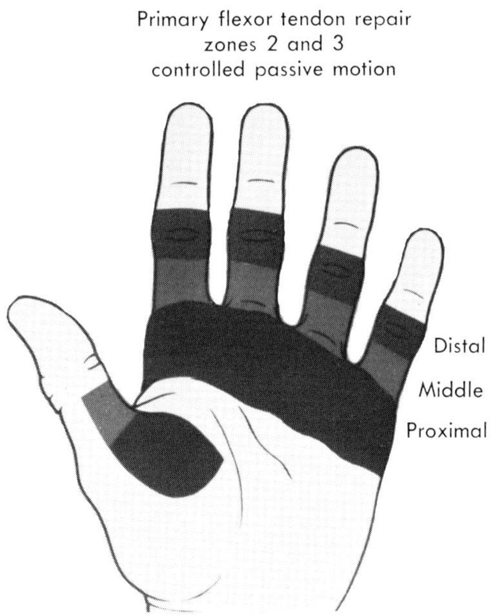

Fig. 12-8. Subdivision of zones 2 and 3 as proposed by Boyes and Stark.

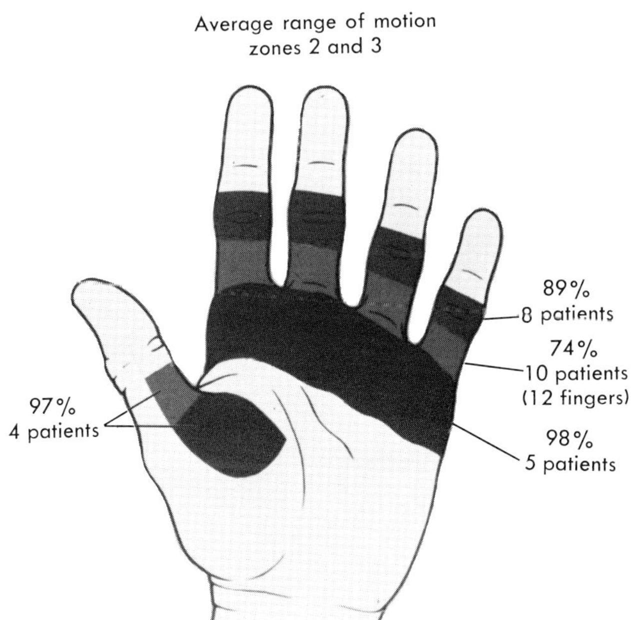

Fig. 12-9. Patients analyzed for this study by divisions. Average percentage of normal range of motion of all cases in each division is calculated.

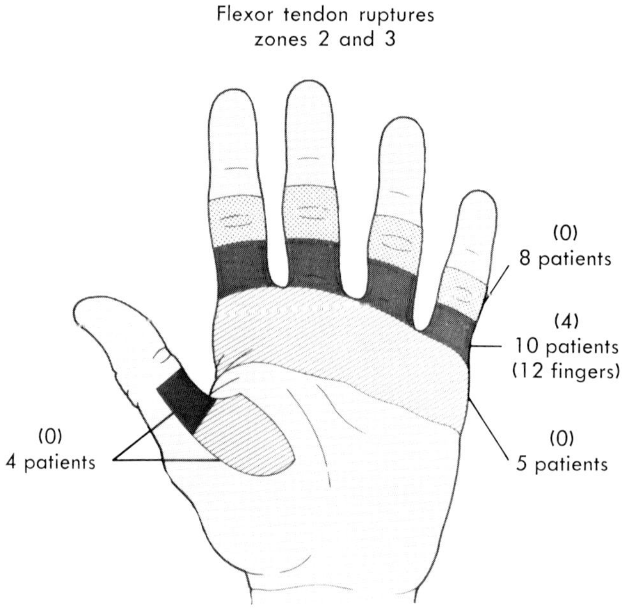

Fig. 12-10. Subdivision of zone 2 and zone 3 as proposed by Boyes and Stark showing all four tendon ruptures occurring in middle division of zone 2.

A

B

C

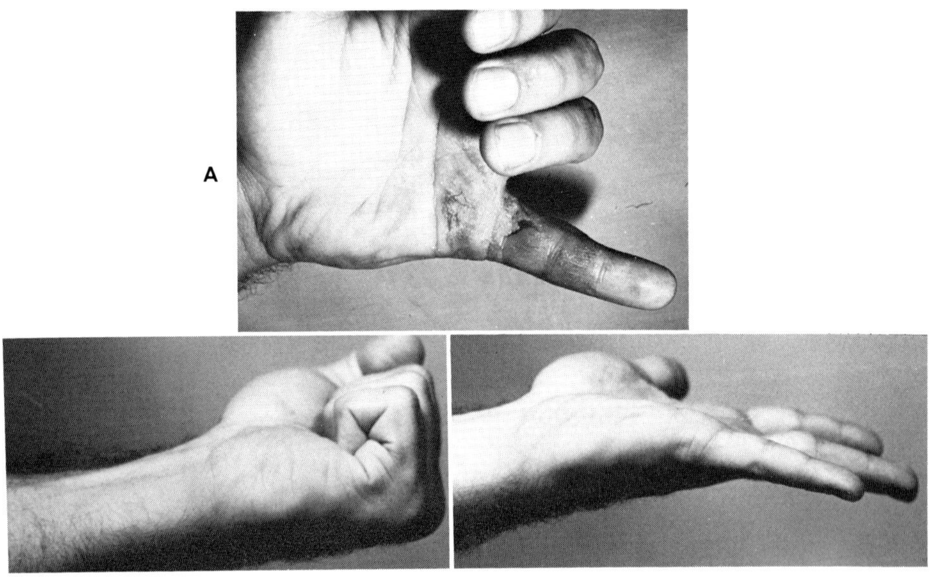

Fig. 12-11. A, Laceration of little finger left hand in middle division, zone 2 in 21-year-old male. Flexor digitorum profundus and superficialis tendons repaired (along with volar digital nerve and artery). **B,** Range of flexion, **C,** extension 3 months postoperatively. By our system of evaluation, this case was graded as normal range of motion.

3 as well as in the proximal subdivision of zone 2 have been encouraging. The disappointing area, middle division zone 2 was the result of four tendon ruptures offsetting some excellent results and thus reducing the overall percentage to 74%.

COMPLICATIONS

Four patients in this group sustained a ruptured tendon and all were located in the middle division of zone 2 (Fig. 12-10). The first two patients in this series resulted in a tendon rupture and should be classified as the surgeon's error. They were the result of too often and too extensive passive motion, and too early active motion. They were not under any precise control. The remaining two ruptures should be classified as patient errors. In one case an excellent result was apparent at 6 weeks when the patient lifted many bales of hay, rupturing a tendon. The final case was a 7-year-old child who mixed uncontrollable active motion with other exercises and ruptured a tendon.

Several of the cases in middivision, however, had near normal range of motion to counterbalance the ruptures (Fig. 12-11). All the patients who had a ruptured tendon were repaired in conventional manner without difficulty. It is interesting to note that as we have developed safeguards, ruptured tendons with this technique should be eliminated.

Distal zone 2 injuries frequently involved the joint and some restriction in extension was not unusual.

CONCLUSIONS

A method of controlled passive motion following tendon repair in zones 2 and 3 has been presented. The method has evolved from a combination of laboratory and clinical experience. We have been encouraged by the results obtained thus far. The tendon ruptures that occurred have been thoroughly studied and, by our present techniques and safeguards, should be preventable. The study has been expanded to accumulate more cases for further analysis.

References

1. Boyes, J., and Stark, H.: Flexor tendon grafts in the fingers and thumb, J. Bone Joint Surg. **53A**:1332, 1971.
2. Furlow, L. T., Jr.: Early active motion in flexor tendon healing, J. Bone Joint Surg. **54A**: 911, 1972.
3. Harmer, T. W.: Cases of tendon and nerve repair, Boston Med. Surg. J. **194**:739, 1926.
4. Harmer, T. W.: Certain aspects of hand surgery, N. Eng. J. Med. **214**:613, 1936.
5. Harmer, T. W.: Injuries to the hand, Am. J. Surg. **42**:638, 1938.
6. Harmer, T. W.: Tendon surgery, Surg. Clin. North Am. **1**(3):809-822, June, 1921.
7. Harmer, T. W.: Tendon suture, Boston Med. Surg. J. **167**:808, 1917.
8. Hernandez, A., Velasco, F., Rivas, A., and Preciado, A.: Preliminary report on early mobilization for the rehabilitation of flexor tendons, Plast. Reconstr. Surg. **40**:354, 1967.
9. Kessler, I., and Nissim, F.: Primary repair without immobilization of flexor tendon division within the digital sheath, Acta Orthop. Scand. **40**:587, 1969.

10. Kleinert, H., Kutz, J., Ashbell, S., and Martinez, E.: Primary repair of lacerated flexor tendons in no-man's-land, J. Bone Joint Surg. **49A**:577, 1967.
11. Lahey, F. H.: A tendon suture which permits immediate motion, Boston Med. Surg. J. **188**:851, 1923.
12. Murray, G.: A method of tendon repair, Am. J. Surg. **90**:334, 1960.
13. Verdan, C.: Primary and secondary repair of flexor and extensor tendon injuries. In Flynn, J. E., editor: Hand surgery, Baltimore, 1966, The Williams and Wilkins Company, p. 220.
14. Young, R. E. S.: Personal communication.
15. Young, R. E. S., and Harmon, J. M.: Repair of tendon injuries of the hand, Ann. Surg. **151**:562, 1960.

13. Repair of zone 1 flexor tendon injuries

Harold E. Kleinert, M.D.
Frank C. Forshew, M.D.
Myles J. Cohen, M.D.

The outlook for the injured hand as to whether it is doomed to disability or returned to useful function depends primarily on the first aid and early definitive treatment rather than upon the care during convalescence.

Sterling Bunnell

Zone 1 of the finger flexion mechanism extends from the terminal portion of the flexor digitorum superficialis insertion to the flexor digitorum profundus insertion (Fig. 13-1). Injuries within this zone involve the terminal portion of the profundus, the third and fourth annular and third cruciform pulleys (Fig. 13-2). Two types of injuries are common within this zone. Lacerations frequently involve not only the tendon and pulley system but also the volar plate of the distal interphalangeal joints. Closed sudden hyperextension injuries at the distal interphalangeal joint cause avulsion of the flexor digitorum profundus from its insertion. This may be associated with an avulsion fracture of the distal phalanx.

Some surgeons have abandoned zone 1 tenorrhaphy. They point to the small contribution of the distal interphalangeal joint to finger flexion, and the fact that a poorly performed repair in the proximal portion of zone 1 may affect an otherwise intact flexor digitorum superficialis. However, failure to restore a functional tendon obviates active distal interphalangeal joint flexion and decreases grip strength. In the little finger, a coexistent weak or absent flexor digitorum superficialis may result in complete loss of active flexion at the proximal as well as the distal interphalangeal joints. Failure to restore the stabilizing function of the profundus leads to muscular imbalance at the distal interphalangeal joint with hyperextension and impaired pinch. The retracted proximal stump of the profundus may act as a mechanical block to the superficialis tendon thus preventing active proximal interphalangeal joint flexion beyond 90°. This may become more pronounced if cicatrix involves the remaining structures of the fibro-osseous canal. Profundus retraction will cause proximal migration of the lumbrical origin. Lumbrical tension is thereby increased and may result in a lumbrical plus finger.[8]

Successful restoration of the flexor digitorum profundus is thus the ideal form of treatment in these injuries.

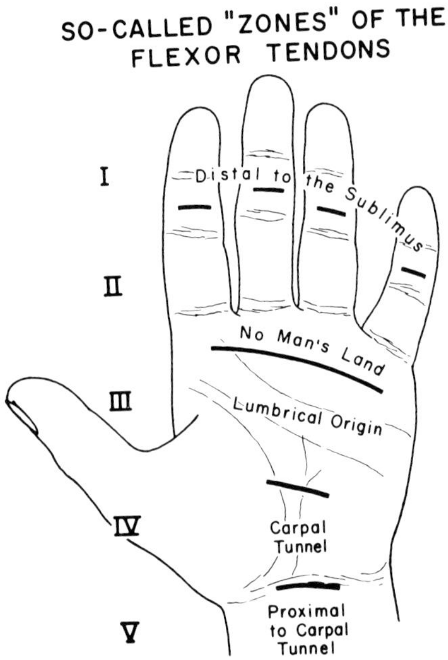

Fig. 13-1

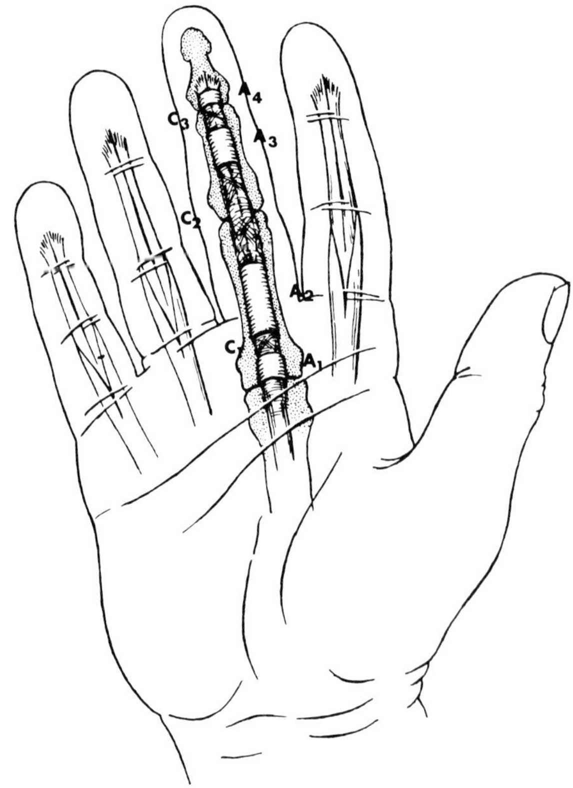

Fig. 13-2

Fig. 13-1. The palmar side of the hand may be divided into five zones on the basis of unique aspects of tendon repair. Zone 1 extends from the termination of the flexor digitorum superficialis to the insertion of the flexor digitorum profundus. (From Kleinert, H. E., et al.: Primary repair of flexor tendons, Orthop. Clin. North Am. **4**(4):866, October, 1973. Courtesy W. B. Saunders Co., Publisher.)

Fig. 13-2. Zone 1 involves the profundus tendon as it passes through the third and fourth annular (A_3, A_4) and third cruciform (C_3) pulleys.

PRIMARY TENORRHAPHY

In clean, fresh, sharply incised wounds more than 1.5 cm. from the profundus insertion, primary tenorrhaphy is employed. Surgical techniques, contraindications, and postoperative management are similar to those used in zone 2 flexor tendon lacerations and are outlined in detail in Chapter 11. In this zone, the third cruciform and fourth annular pulleys may be excised without functional loss. A flap from the third annular pulley may be raised, but we attempt to preserve its proximal portion. If the entire third pulley is resected, distal interphalangeal joint motion of from 40° to 50° may still be possible but some bowstringing will occur.

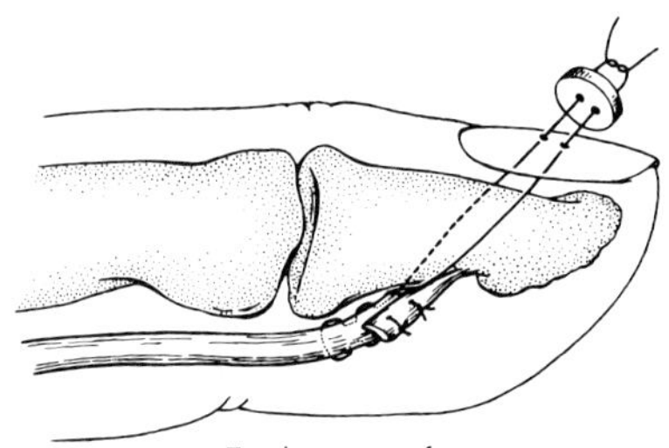

Fig. 13-3. Tendon advancement may be employed in lacerations less than 1.5 cm. from the profundus insertion.

ADVANCEMENT AND REINSERTION

In lacerations within 1.5 cm. of its insertion, the proximal stump of profundus may be advanced and inserted directly into the distal phalanx (Fig. 13-3). This technique eliminates the suture line from the fibro-osseous canal. When estimating the amount of advancement required it should be remembered that the insertion is at the middistal phalanx. Tendon advancement of more than 1.5 cm. will result in a flexion deformity of the finger joints, which is of particular importance in the long, ring, and little fingers where an imbalance may be more pronounced. At the time of advancement, a portion of the distal profundus stump should be resected to prevent mechanical blocking of the repair in the third annular pulley. In this event, active flexion will be limited. Gliding should be checked following tenorrhaphy and before wound closure to ensure that this does not occur.

Avulsion of the flexor digitorum profundus from its insertion usually occurs as a closed injury. Inability to flex the distal interphalangeal joint, volar swelling, ecchymosis, and tenderness are usually present (Fig. 13-4). A fragment of the volar lip of the distal phalanx is often avulsed with the tendon and will be visualized in a lateral x-ray film (Fig. 13-5). This injury may be treated by reinsertion of the tendon into the distal phalanx.

The operative techniques for advancement and reinsertion are similar. The wound is enlarged according to the same principles employed in primary repairs. The tendon is retrieved, drawn distally, and held in position with a Keith needle. A 4-0 monofilament stainless steel wire suture is placed transversely through the tendon 1 cm. proximal to its cut end. It is then woven along each side of the tendon to the cut end. Kinking should be avoided as this weakens the wire and may impair withdrawal. A proximal pull out loop is not used. A distally based osteoperiosteal flap is raised from the volar surface of the distal phalanx. The wire is passed subperiosteally under the flap, around the distal phalanx, and out through the nail where it is tied over a button. The periosteal flap and the distal tendon stump are secured over the repair with 6-0 Mersilene sutures. Dynamic rubber band splinting is employed here as in primary repairs. The dynamic

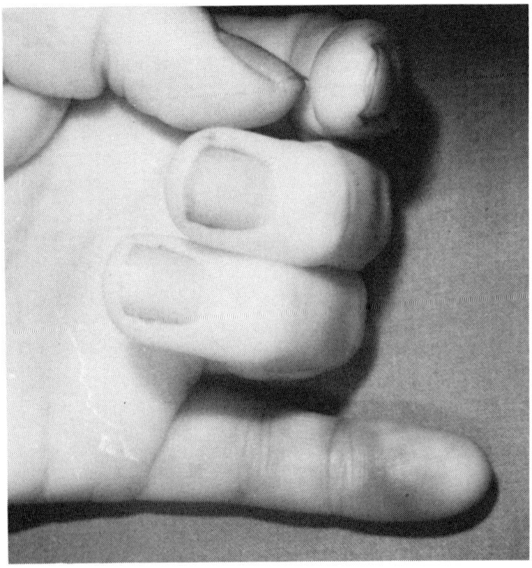

Fig. 13-4. Avulsion is usually seen in closed injuries. Loss of active flexion, ecchymosis, swelling, and tenderness are seen.

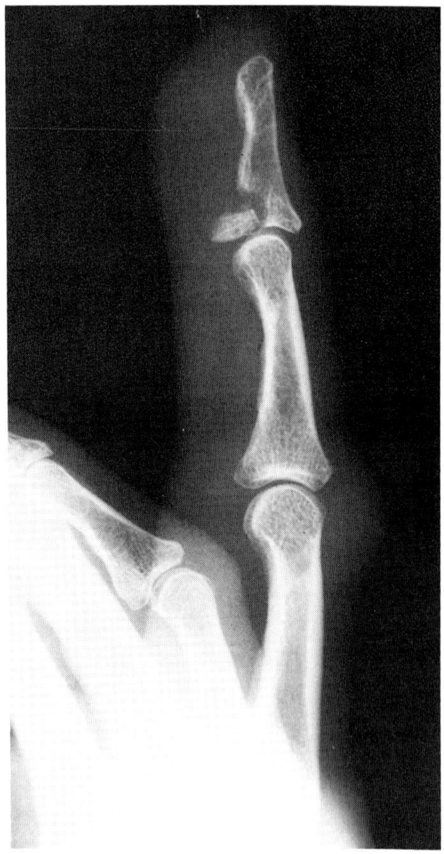

Fig. 13-5. In avulsion of the profundus a small volar fracture of the distal phalanx may be seen on the lateral x-ray film.

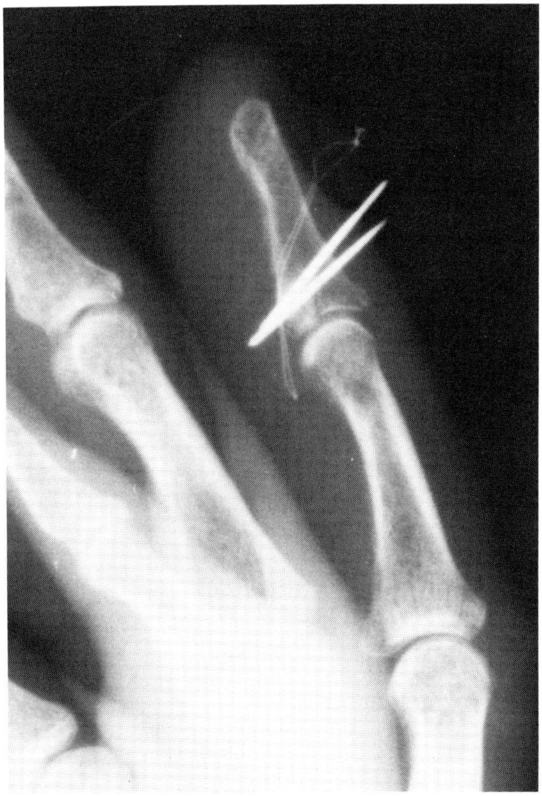

Fig. 13-6. The tendon may be reinserted with a pull-out wire and supplemental internal fixation of the fracture accomplished with a Kirschner wire.

splint is discontinued 21 days after repair. At 5 weeks postoperative the wire is cut and removed by pulling distally on one end of the suture. This technique avoids tension across the repair site. The postoperative exercise and splinting program is otherwise the same as that outlined for zone 2. Any associated fracture may be treated with supplemental internal fixation using a 0.035 Kirschner wire (Fig. 13-6). This is advanced through to the dorsum of the finger and is not allowed to abut on the profundus.

DELAYED AND SECONDARY TENORRHAPHY

Delayed repair may be indicated for patients seen several hours after injury and those who present with impaired circulation, signs of inflammation, or a severely contaminated wound. In the latter case the wound is debrided and left open. Soaks, frequent dressing changes, and systemic antibiotics are begun. If the wound responds favorably to this treatment repair may be accomplished at 3 to 4 days.

Secondary tenorrhaphy, reinsertion, or advancement may be possible as late as 3 to 5 weeks following injury provided the scarring is minimal and proximal retraction has been limited by an intact vincula. In these cases synovitis is frequently found around the severed end of the tendon. The proliferative synovium as well as all scar and granulation tissue must be removed from the sheath prior to tenorrhaphy.

TENDON GRAFTING

Tendon grafting can restore active distal interphalangeal joint flexion in those cases where tenorrhaphy, reinsertion, and advancement are contraindicated. The problem of grafting through an intact superficialis has been well publicized.[9, 10] If this technique is selected, a small caliber tendon graft should be used. We prefer one half of the extensor digiti minimi, which is threaded carefully through the superficialis decussation to avoid damaging it. This can be staged with a silicone rod if scarring or synovitis is a problem or if the third annular pulley must be reconstructed; if the bed is unsatisfactory a graft should be avoided in most instances. Because of the risk of impaired superficialis function, this procedure has been reserved for the well-motivated, younger patient with an otherwise normal finger.

STABILIZATION PROCEDURES

Stabilization procedures such as tenodesis, capsulodesis, and arthrodesis prevent hyperextension and improve pinch. They do not restore either active motion or grip strength. In each of these procedures the joint should be placed in an average of 15° of flexion. Tenodesis provides stability with preservation of passive

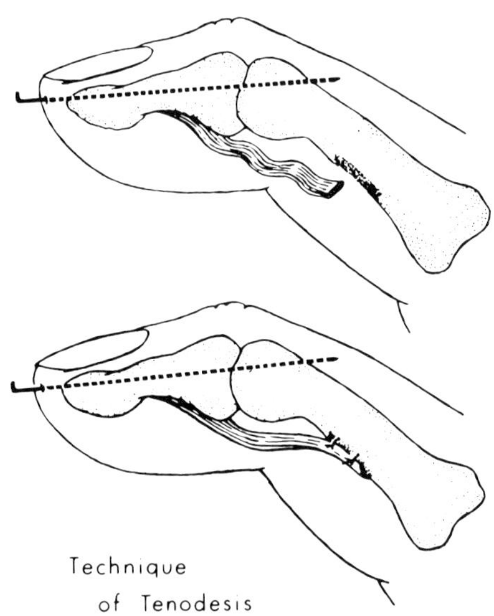

Fig. 13-7. Tenodesis provides distal interphalangeal joint stability in pinch with free passive flexion. The tendon must be secured into bone.

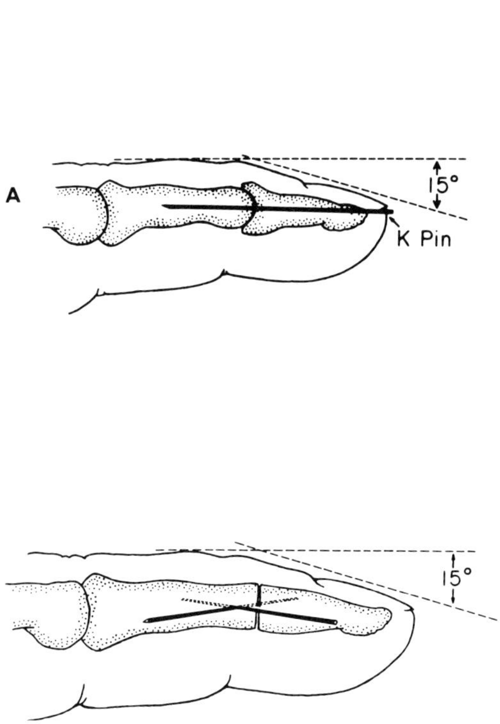

Fig. 13-8. Arthrodesis may be accomplished either by the ball and socket technique, **A,** or by juxtaposition of beveled surfaces using crossed pins, **B.**

flexion (Fig. 13-7). It is indicated when sufficient distal profundus tendon is available to reach the neck of the middle phalanx. When insufficient tendon is available capsulodesis is performed. In both of these cases a 4-0 monofilament stainless steel pull-out wire is used to fix the soft tissue securely into bone.

Arthrodesis provides the greatest stability, but has the concomitant disadvantage of eliminating passive flexion. The ball and socket technique of Carroll[5] may be employed, or the juxtaposed decorticated surfaces may be flattened and beveled. Internal Kirschner pin fixation is used until x-ray films show evidence of union (Fig. 13-8). This may be supplemented with a loop of 4-0 monofilament wire passed through transverse holes drilled in the middle and distal phalanges and then twisted to provide compression and increased stability to the arthrodesis as more recently advocated by Anderson and Bendich.[1]

DISCUSSION

The successful treatment of zone 1 flexor tendon injuries requires restoration of both the active power of the flexor digitorum profundus, and the stability of the distal interphalangeal joint. These are provided by tenorrhaphy, advancement, or reinsertion of the tendon. Meticulous surgical technique and rubber band dynamic splinting have enabled us to use these techniques in the majority of our patients.

Tendon grafting through an intact superficialis may be indicated where profundus repair cannot be effected. It should be reserved for young, well-motivated patients, and performed only by those surgeons who are well versed in the techniques and problems of the procedure.

Tenodesis, capsulodesis, and arthrodesis are useful salvage procedures where the flexor digitorum profundus cannot be repaired. Where grafting is contraindicated, and in the presence of a strong superficialis, these procedures can give a satisfactory result.

References

1. Anderson, G., and Bendich, G.: Fusion of the distal interphalangeal joint, Personal communication.
2. Brown, Paul W.: Laceration of flexor tendons of the hand, Surg. Clin. North Am. **49**:1255-1268, 1969.
3. Bruner, J. M.: The zigzag volar digital incision for flexor tendon surgery, Plast. Reconstr. Surg. **40**:571, 1967.
4. Bunnell, S.: Early treatment of hand injuries, J. Bone Joint Surg. **33A**:807, July, 1951.
5. Carroll, R., and Hill, N.: Small joint arthrodesis in hand reconstruction, J. Bone Joint Surg. **51A**:1219, 1969.
6. Johnson, M. K., and Cohen, M. J.: The hand atlas, Springfield, Ill., In press, Charles C Thomas Publisher.
7. Kleinert, H. E., Kutz, J. E., Atasoy, E., and Stormo, A.: Primary repair of flexor tendons, Orth. Clin. North Am. **4**:865-876, 1973.
8. Parkes, A:. The "lumbrical plus" finger, The hand **2**:164-165, 1970.
9. Pulvertaft, G.: Experience in flexor tendon grafting in the hand, J. Bone Joint Surg. **41B**: 629, 1959.
10. Pulvertaft, G.: Tendon grafts for flexor tendon injuries in the fingers and thumb, J. Bone Joint Surg. **38B**:175-194, 1956.
11. Verdan, C.: Practical considerations for primary and secondary repair in flexor tendon injuries, Surg. Clin. North Am. **44**:951-970, 1964.
12. Verdan, C.: Primary repair of flexor tendons, J. Bone Joint Surg. **42A**:647-657, 1960.
13. Wakefield, A.: The management of flexor tendon repair, Surg. Clin. North Am. **40**:267-273, 1960.

14. Indications for tendon grafting

R. Guy Pulvertaft, C.B.E., M.D.(Hon.), M.Chir., F.R.C.S.

A tendon divided by injury, destroyed by disease or infection, or absent through congenital fault may, under favorable circumstances, be replaced successfully by a tendon taken from elsewhere in the body. A tendon transferred to serve another purpose may, if necessary, be extended by a graft to reach its new attachment. These grafts are taken from the patient and there is no reason in normal practice to use other than autogenous material. Suitable tendons to use are palmaris longus and plantaris and extensor digitorum longus. Flexor digitorum superficialis is chosen for a bridge graft to restore profundus in the palm and wrist.

INJURY

The use of tendon grafts and our knowledge of their behavior stems from the work of Bunnell, whose first published papers on the subject appeared in 1918[5] and 1922.[4] During the half century since then we have learned a great deal concerning the revascularization and survival of grafts, the formation of adhesions, the indications for their use, the operative technique, and the results. During the past decade important advances have been made in the treatment of complicated cases unsuitable for single stage operations. A preformed sheath is developed by the implantation of a flexible silicone rod; later the rod is removed and a graft is inserted into the sheath.[7]

Successful results from the standard grafting method are obtained only when certain rules are followed:

1. The hand is in good overall condition. There is no extensive scarring. Passive movements are full or nearly full. The circulation is satisfactory. At least one digital nerve in the affected digit is intact.
2. A precise and gentle surgical technique is used.
3. The patient is cooperative. A child under 3 years of age is unlikely to assist in the aftercare and it is wise to postpone the operation until the child is older.

Profundus division

Division of flexor digitorum profundus distal to the superficialis insertion may be treated successfully by primary suture. When the division has occurred

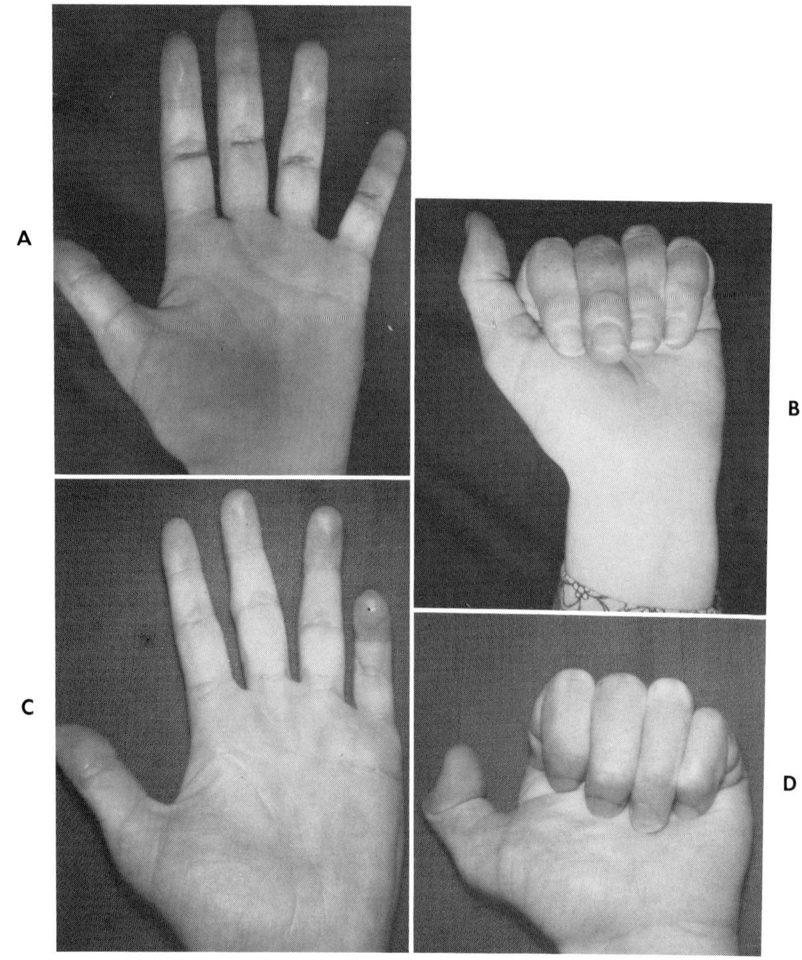

Fig. 14-1. Profundus divisions in all fingers at proximal interphalangeal joints, treated by toe extensor grafts. **A** and **B**, Preoperative state. **C** and **D**, Result. (From Pulvertaft, R. G.: Twenty-five years of hand surgery, J. Bone Joint Surg. **55B**:44, 1973.)

more proximally but the superficialis has escaped injury, it has been my practice to do no more than close the skin wound and to ignore the tendon injury at that time.[9] Whether the profundus division was not observed or ignored deliberately, the choice of later treatment depends upon several factors. Secondary suture may be possible in the distal part of the finger but if this is not practicable, and in all proximal divisions, the ideal treatment is the replacement of profundus by a graft, leaving the intact superficialis undisturbed (Fig. 14-1). It must be emphasized that the operation of tendon grafting is one of some magnitude and should not be undertaken lightly for a comparatively slight disability. It should not be advised unless the patient is determined to seek perfection and the surgeon is confident of his ability to offer a reasonable expecta-

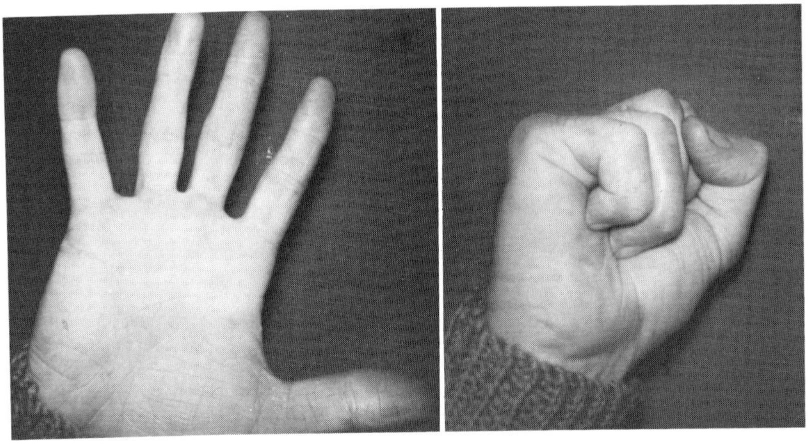

Fig. 14-2. Superficialis and profundus divisions in ring and little fingers, treated by palmaris grafts.

tion of success without undue risk of doing harm. For those who prefer a less involved procedure and will be satisfied with a less perfect result, I advise an arthrodesis or tenodesis of the terminal joint.

Profundus and superficialis divisions

The case for primary suture versus secondary grafting when both tendons are divided within the digital theca remains open. Seeing many failed examples of primary repair and thereby an increased difficulty of subsequent reconstruction has strengthened my view that secondary grafting is the best way to treat this injury. There are others who have consistently practiced immediate suture, or suture after a few days delay, with results comparable or even better than those achieved by grafting.[11] As the general standard of emergency surgery improves, primary suture may become the method of choice; but it must be said that good results can only be obtained by those who are masters of craftsmanship. When skills of this order are not available, I believe that it is wiser to limit the emergency care to wound closure and perform a grafting operation after a suitable delay. Secondary grafting under favorable conditions has a success rate of 70% to 80% (Fig. 14-2).[*] [1, 8]

Flexor pollicis longus division

Division of flexor pollicis longus distal to the metacarpophalangeal joint should be treated by primary suture. Division of the tendon deep to the thenar muscles may also be repaired primarily, but the exposure has dangers owing to the proximity of the digital nerves and the motor branch to the thenar muscles.

---

*Success is defined as flexion to within 2.5 cm. or less of the distal palmar crease and extension restricted by less than a sum total of 40° at the interphalangeal joints.

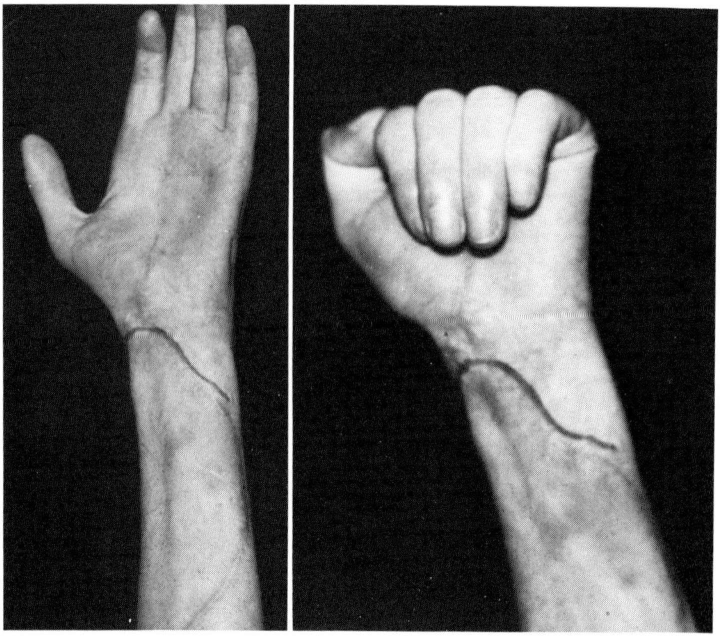

Fig. 14-3. Division of all tendons, nerves, and vessels at wrist, treated initially in error by skin suture only. Result after superficialis bridge grafts for flexor pollicis longus and all profundus tendons; followed by nerve repair and later tenolysis. (From Pulvertaft, R. G.: Problems of flexor tendon surgery of the hand, J. Bone Joint Surg. **47A**:131, 1965.)

My advice to the inexperienced surgeon is to leave this injury for secondary grafting, unless the hand is laid open by the injury. Under these circumstances, repair of all the divided structures is required. Secondary suture of flexor pollicis longus distal to the metacarpophalangeal joint is satisfactory when it is possible to bring the ends together without difficulty. I am not in favor of elongation above the wrist in order to secure extra length. It is better to use a graft. Replacement of the tendon by a graft reaching from above the wrist to the terminal phalanx is a reliable procedure, yielding a success rate of 80% to 90%.*

Divisions in the palm and wrist

The best results come from primary suture. For failed or neglected cases a short bridge graft taken from superficialis is of value in filling the gap in profundus resulting from retraction of the proximal end. Good function can be restored provided the scarring is not severe (Fig. 14-3).

Extensor tendon division

Tendon grafting is indicated in some cases, but, when possible, attachment to an adjacent active tendon or transference of a muscle that can be spared is preferable.

---

*Success is defined as an active range at the interphalangeal joint of 40° or more.

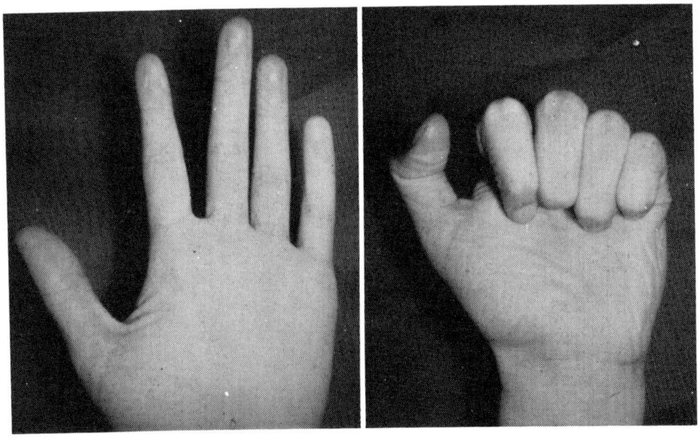

Fig. 14-4. Superficialis and profundus divisions in index finger. Injury at 9 years of age. Result after plantaris graft attached to profundus of same finger at 13½ years of age. (From Tubiana, R., editor: The hand, Philadelphia, W. B. Saunders Co.)

Tendon grafting after long delay

A patient is sometimes first seen several years after a tendon injury has occurred. Previous surgery has failed or the patient has been told that there is no successful treatment for the complaint. This is particularly true for divisions within the digital theca. Function can be restored to many of these hands, provided there is good passive range and sensibility (Fig. 14-4). Surprisingly, the results in my own series have been slightly better than in those for whom operation was performed within 3 to 4 months of injury.[10] The average interval between injury and surgery in the delay series of combined superficialis and profundus loss was 5 years. In all cases one of the muscles of the affected digit was used, although on reflection, it would have been wiser on occasions to have transferred a superficialis tendon, prolonged with a graft, from an adjacent finger.

The better results may be explained to some extent by a stricter selection for operative suitability and because the average age (15 years) was lower than in the general series (24 years). The lessons to be learned from these observations are that delay does not worsen the prognosis and that it is probably advantageous to allow a lapse of 4 to 6 months before operating to permit the tissues to recover completely from the initial trauma. This is of significance when dealing with young children, for the very young cannot cooperate in the aftercare and it is advisable to postpone a grafting operation until they reach 3 or 4 years of age.

RHEUMATOID DISEASE

Tendon rupture is a common feature of rheumatoid disease. Extensor tendon loss can usually be made good by linkage to an intact tendon or by transference of a suitable muscle. It may be necessary to lengthen the transferred tendon

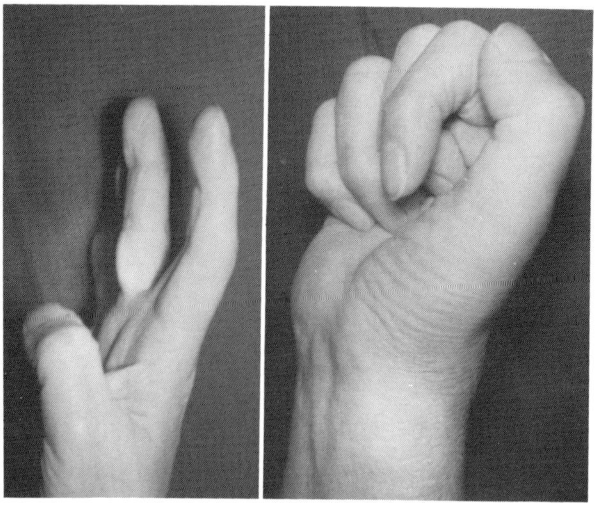

Fig. 14-5. Rupture of superficialis and profundus of index finger, resulting from rheumatoid erosion of carpus; result after palmaris graft.

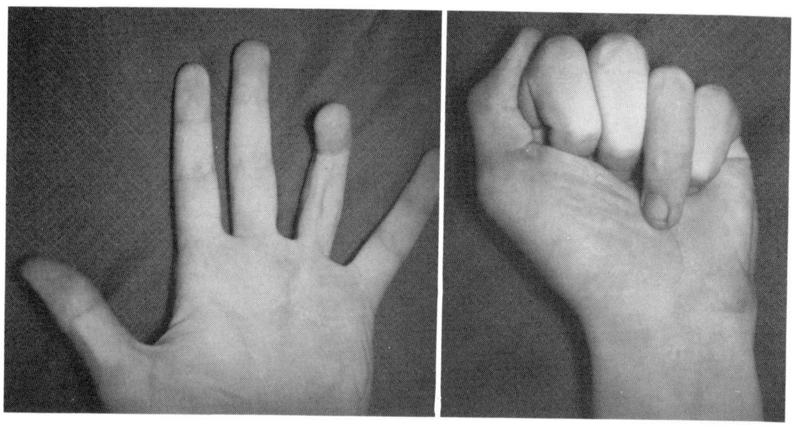

Fig. 14-6. Septic tenosynovitis of flexor tendons in ring finger; result after toe extensor graft.

with a graft. Flexor tendon loss is less frequently seen but is more difficult to treat successfully. I have seen few cases in which the conditions were suitable for tendon grafting (Fig. 14-5).

INFECTION

I have had little experience of tendon replacement after septic teno-synovitis. Very occasionally, a patient is seen in whom the flexor tendons have been destroyed but the finger has retained good passive mobility. Grafting operations were performed upon two such patients. One failed owing to adhesions and the other made a worthwhile, though not brilliant, recovery (Fig. 14-6).

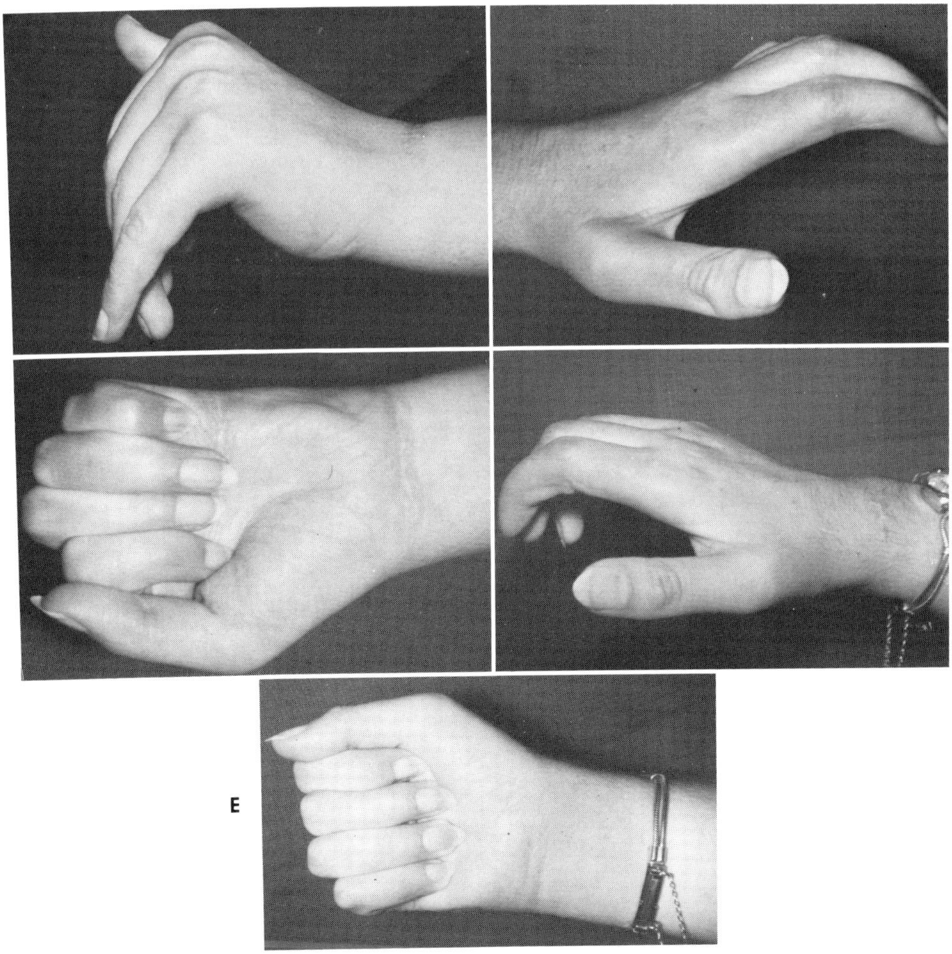

Fig. 14-7. Congenital absence of extensor tendons of all fingers on dorsum of hand. Result after release of palmar structures followed by plantaris grafts reaching from extensor carpi radialis brevis to extensor tendons at metacarpophalangeal joints. Tenolysis was performed later. **A**, Maximum preoperative extension, left hand. **B** and **C**, Result left hand. **D** and **E**, Result right hand.

CONGENITAL ABNORMALITIES

Indications vary and it is not practicable to attempt a classification of congenital abnormalities. In general, it can be said that when a digit lacks adequate control due to absence of muscle, tendon, or both, consideration should be given to providing this control by tendon transference or by a graft to bridge a tendon deficiency (Fig. 14-7).

PARALYSIS

Loss of function caused by irreparable lesions of the spinal cord and peripheral nerves can be overcome in many instances by transference of expendable

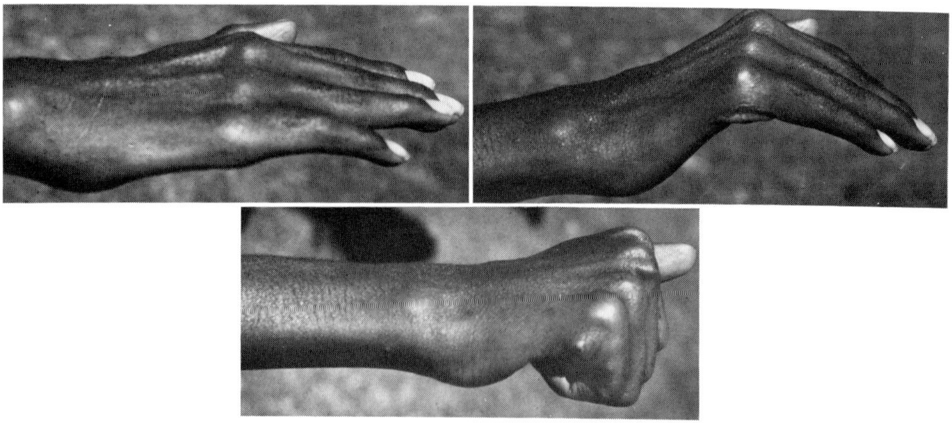

Fig. 14-8. Leprosy involving ulnar and median nerve paralysis. Result after extensor carpi radialis longus transfer, lengthened with plantaris grafts, to lateral bands of extensor tendons of all fingers. Operation by Brand.

active muscles. The tendons of these muscles may need to be lengthened by grafts.

Leprosy is responsible for the majority of peripheral nerve lesions today; consequently it is in this field that the most significant advances in the treatment of permanent ulnar and median nerve palsies have been made. Given suitable conditions and the facilities for effective aftercare, consistently good results can be obtained from operations for the clawed fingers of the intrinsic minus hand using some adaptation of the Stiles-Bunnell technique, which gives an active or a tenodesis control. The muscle chosen for active control is usually a single superficialis divided into four tendon slips to reach each finger without an intervening graft, or extensor carpi radialis longus prolonged by grafts taken from plantaris[2, 3] or from fascia lata (Fig. 14-8).[6]

CONCLUSIONS

Autogenous tendon grafting is a well-proved procedure for the restoration of tendon defects in the hand. The results are not entirely predictable, but when used with precision under suitable circumstances, it offers a good expectation of a successful outcome.

Acknowledgment

It is my pleasure to thank Mr. Barry Wilks and his student, Stephen Watson, of the Photographic Department of the Derbyshire Royal Infirmary for their assistance.

References

1. Boyes, J. H., and Stark, H. H.: Flexor-tendon grafts in the fingers and thumb, J. Bone Joint Surg. **53A**:1332, 1971.
2. Brand, P. W.: The hand in leprosy. In Clinical surgery, Vol. 7, London, 1966, Butterworth and Co. (Publishers) Ltd., p. 279.

3. Brand, P. W.: Paralysis of the intrinsic muscles of the hand. In Operative surgery, ed. 2, Vol. 11, London, 1970, Butterworth and Co. (Publishers) Ltd., p. 129.
4. Bunnell, S.: Repair of tendons in the fingers, Surg. Gynecol. Obstet. **35**:88, 1922.
5. Bunnell, S:. Repair of tendons in the fingers and description of two new instruments, Surg. Gynecol. Obstet. **26**:103, 1918.
6. Fritschi, E. P.: Reconstructive surgery in leprosy, Bristol, 1971, John Wright and Sons Ltd., p. 42.
7. Hunter, J. M., and Salisbury, R. E.: Flexor-tendon reconstruction in severely damaged hands, J. Bone Joint Surg. **53A**:829, 1971.
8. Pulvertaft, R. G.: Tendon grafts for flexor tendon injuries in the fingers and thumb, J. Bone Joint Surg. **38B**:175, 1956.
9. Pulvertaft, R. G:. The treatment of profundus division by free tendon graft, J. Bone Joint Surg. **41A**:1363, 1960.
10. Pulvertaft, R. G.: Twenty-five years of hand surgery, J. Bone Joint Surg. **55B**:32, 1973.
11. Verdan, C. E.: Half a century of flexor-tendon surgery, J. Bone Joint Surg. **54A**:472, 1972.

15. Flexor tendon surgery in children

Martin A. Entin, M.D., C.M., M.Sc., F.R.C.S.(C), F.A.C.S.

Misconceptions that have prevailed in relation to surgical management of injuries in infants and children are that the very young form less scar than adults, that they heal more quickly, that reeducation in attainment of lost function is not necessary, and that one "cannot do wrong in infants." In reality, surgical management of very young patients is a more arduous and demanding task than that of older patients. In fact, considerably greater attention is required for handling of tissues, placing of incisions, providing immobilization, and other details that often spell the difference between success and failure in attainment of function of injured tendons.

REASONS FOR DIFFICULTIES IN CHILDREN

There are several reasons why tendon surgery in infants and children constitutes a more difficult and demanding task than in adults. The diagnosis of severed tendon and of associated nerve injury is most difficult in young children, and it becomes more difficult when time elapses after initial injury and adaptation of function occurs. Observing the child in spontaneous play often provides a clue as to what tendon is not working (Fig. 15-1). The presence and distribution of defects in sensibility that accompany tendon injury are also difficult to establish; exploration of the wound is the final arbiter.

One must also take greater care in placing incisions more accurately, since there is greater likelihood of interfering with growing parts. Problems may arise in children due to formation of hypertrophic scarring. Special care in handling is necessary because the tissues are much more delicate and magnification is helpful.

Since it is almost impossible to appeal to the child to keep the injured part at rest, it is mandatory to provide secure immobilization of the repaired structures; because the various parts of the upper limb are small, the task of providing secure immobilization often taxes all the ingenuity of the surgeon. Finally, reeducation of the infant is often frustrating. Many surgeons prefer to defer repair and reconstruction of the injured tendons until the child is 3 to 4 years of age, when some control is possible.[7, 33]

A

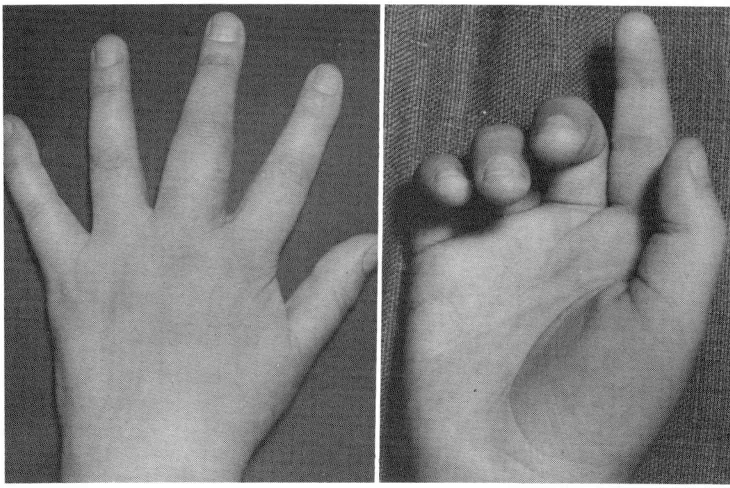

B

Fig. 15-1. A, Hand of a 6-year-old female child. Note the relatively large size of the hand in relation to the fingers that is typical of children's hands. **B,** Diagnosis of severed tendons is difficult in infants. In this 3-year-old girl the position at rest indicates that both flexors were severed through injury with a sharp object at the level of proximal crease of the right index finger. The ulnar digital nerve was also cut.

TENDON HEALING

The key to tendon healing is the understanding of the intrinsic blood supply to the tendons, as well as the understanding of the process of tissue repair.

In the palm and forearm the vessels enter the tendons from all sides. This abundance of blood supply permits fairly rapid healing. In the fibrous sheath, because of the need to keep the tendons close to the bones, the blood vessels reach the tendons through the mesentery-like structures (vinculi) that permit gliding within this complex structure (Fig. 15-2). There are secondary subdivisions into longitudinal vessels within the substance of the tendons.[9, 28]

In children the distances between vinculi are shorter so that segmental blood supply is more abundant. The adhesions that form are consequently more pliable and greater adaptability for tendon gliding can occur (Fig. 15-2).

The process of tendon healing is the result of fibrous tissue formation by the invading fibroblasts.[6] The maturation of the collagenous fibers leads to reorientation of these fibers under the influence of tension forces.[21] It has not been established that the process of tendon healing is qualitatively different in children, although a long-term result with meticulous surgical technique appears to yield more satisfactory function in children than in adults.[9] Investigative work on the influence of early age on healing of tendons would help our understanding of this process.

It is the greater potential of attainment of good functional results in young patients that permits carrying out primary repair of severed structures within the

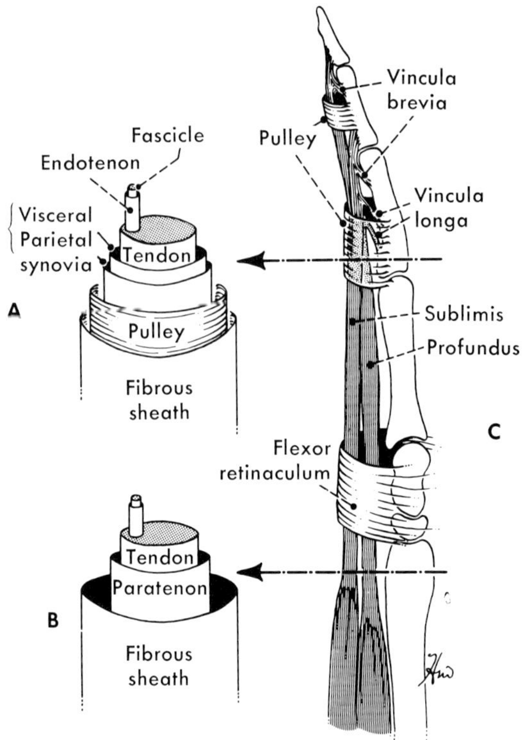

Fig. 15-2. Diagram of the flexor tendons showing the vascular pathways and the various investing layers around the tendons. **A** schematically shows the arrangement of the coverings of the flexor tendons within the fibrous sheath at the level of the proximal pulley, **C.** Special structures permit the entrance of the blood vessels and nerves to the tendon via vinculi from the dorsal aspect (top arrow in **C**). Visceral and parietal synovial lining facilitate gliding within the fibrous sheath. In the palm of the hand and in the forearm the tendons pull in a straight line and are covered by paratenon **B.** (After Entin, M. In Moseley, H. F., editor: Accident surgery, vol. 2, p. 356, New York, 1964, Appleton-Century-Crofts).

fibrous tendon sheath in children. In fact, if the opportunity to carry out either primary or delayed primary repair in flexor tendons in infants is not available, it is wiser to delay reconstruction until the infant is 3 years of age or older. Tendon grafting is extremely difficult to carry out technically because of the small size of the structures involved. Reeducation of specific digit in infants is very difficult.[7]

METHODS OF TENDON REPAIR

The repair of tendons is technically more difficult in infants because the structures are tinier and tissues are more delicate. Magnification and the use of small instruments and sutures are mandatory. Because of the great delicacy of the tendon tissues, great reliance has to be placed upon the stabilization of the joints, and the use of a tethering suture from nail to palm or of small Kirschner wires obliquely across the joint is helpful.

In the past, Sterling Bunnell's admonition about the difficulties of repairing flexor tendons within the fibrous sheath and the choice of secondary elective tendon grafting in this area has dominated the approach in the adult.* In recent years, well documented reports of primary flexor tendon repair by highly skilled surgeons demonstrated that in properly selected cases primary repair can achieve comparable results in children.†

The reason for the success of primary repair is due to the fact that this procedure was carried out by hand surgeons with great experience and skills, utilizing meticulous techniques, using magnification aids, and careful selection of patients. Consequently, these two approaches to flexor tendon repair, instead of being antagonistic, have become accepted as appropriate methods of management for different situations.[8]

In children the primary tendon repair always appeared to have produced better function than in adults. While the reasons are not entirely clear, it is possible that the comparatively better results obtained in the very young patient are due to greater adaptability of tissues and less likelihood of joints to become stiffened. Nevertheless, the surgeon who is lacking the necessary skills or has no access to fine instruments and to magnifying equipment should not "try his luck," banking mainly on this propensity.

SITES OF INJURY AND AGE OF WOUND

As in adults, the site of injury of flexor tendon is important because it demands selection of appropriate management. The hand is arbitrarily divided into various zones[32]:

1. Distal to insertion of superficialis
2. Within fibrous sheath
3. Mid-palm
4. Carpal tunnel
5. Forearm

In addition, the important considerations in the choice of procedure are whether one or both tendons are severed, if there are associated injuries of other tissues, the integrity of bony framework, whether there is loss of skin, and whether the injury is recent.

If the wound is tidy, the elapsed time after injury is short, and the wound can be closed, primary repair is indicated. If the wound is "old," more than 12 hours, a period of observation with the aid of antibiotics is instituted and delayed primary repair can be done within a week or 10 days. While my personal experience with this method is rather limited, a number of surgeons have reported satisfactory results.‡

---

*See references 3, 5, 17, 23-26.

†See references 15, 16, 19, 22, 30-32.

‡See references 1, 11, 14, 18, 22, 27.

A

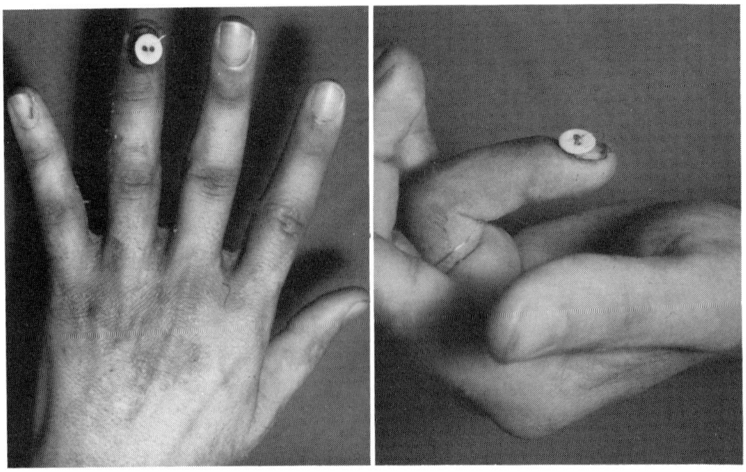

B

Fig. 15-3. Bunnell pull-out stainless steel suture of the terminal tendon to the medulla of the distal phalanx provides accurate and strong approximation. **A,** Appearance of the finger 3 weeks after tendon grafting. **B,** Same as **A,** with patient actively flexing his ring finger. Note the pull-out portion of the wire suture draped over the proximal phalanx.

MANAGEMENT OF UNCOMPLICATED TENDON INJURIES

Profundus tendon only

If the profundus tendon alone is severed just distal to the superficialis insertion, primary repair should be done using coapting 5-0 nonabsorbable sutures, and a 6-0 suture for continuous approximation of the periphery of tendon. If the distal stump is short or if the tendon has been avulsed, Bunnell pull-out stainless steel wire sutures give the strongest apposition against the bone (Fig. 15-3).

Should the profundus tendon not be found or be destroyed, it is probably better to carry out definitive tendon grafting when the infant is older. Tenodesis of distal joint does not give good results in children because it causes a permanent flexion contracture of the distal joint that becomes more pronounced with growth. Arthrodesis of the distal joint is contraindicated in young children for the same reason; moreover, it may interfere with growth of bone.

In the area of fibrous tendon sheath, Pulvertaft attained excellent function in the adult utilizing tendon graft of the flexor profundus in the presence of intact superficialis.[25] Such results cannot be obtained in infants because of the great technical difficulties. However, delay of definitive treatment until the child is older permits carrying out tendon grafting and retaining the intact superficialis. The adaptability of children may aid in the attainment of comparable function.

Both flexors are severed

In young children both tendons should be repaired, unless the two suture lines are in the same position, in which case cross adhesions are more likely to occur. Discarding the superficialis should be done with caution since hyper-

A

B

C

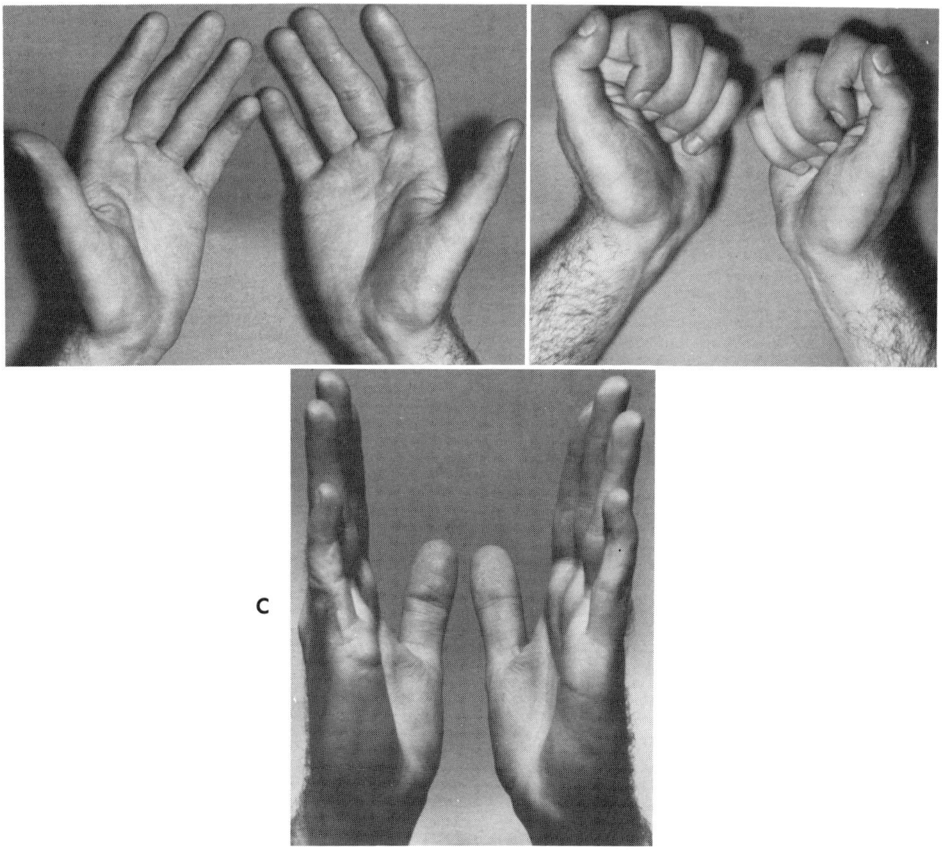

Fig. 15-4. Delayed primary sutures compared to tendon grafting in similar injury of flexor tendons. Both tendons were injured in right and left little fingers of 4-year-old boy through the cut at the level of the proximal interphalangeal joint. In the left hand, delayed primary suture of profundus only was done 2 months after injury. In the right hand, a tendon graft was done. Flexor superficialis was discarded in both hands. **A,** Appearance of both hands 14 years after tendon repair. Sites of injury at the proximal interphalangeal joints of little fingers are imperceptible. **B,** Normal range of flexion was attained in both little fingers. **C,** In extension, the right little finger (tendon graft) shows a slightly greater flexion contracture at the distal joint. Photographed 14 years after repair.

extension deformity may result if the volar plate and capsule are exposed. Only a small portion of the fibrous sheath is excised to permit the suture of the tendons (Fig. 15-4, left hand).

In children, especially the very young, it is preferable to use the original motor for tendon repair, so that reeducation is less taxing. While adaptation is greater in children, it is much more difficult to impart information about substitution of parts for different function. The elapsed time between injury and reconstruction does not necessarily prejudice the final result, provided the finger joints are kept supple, which can be attained by moving the affected finger along with the

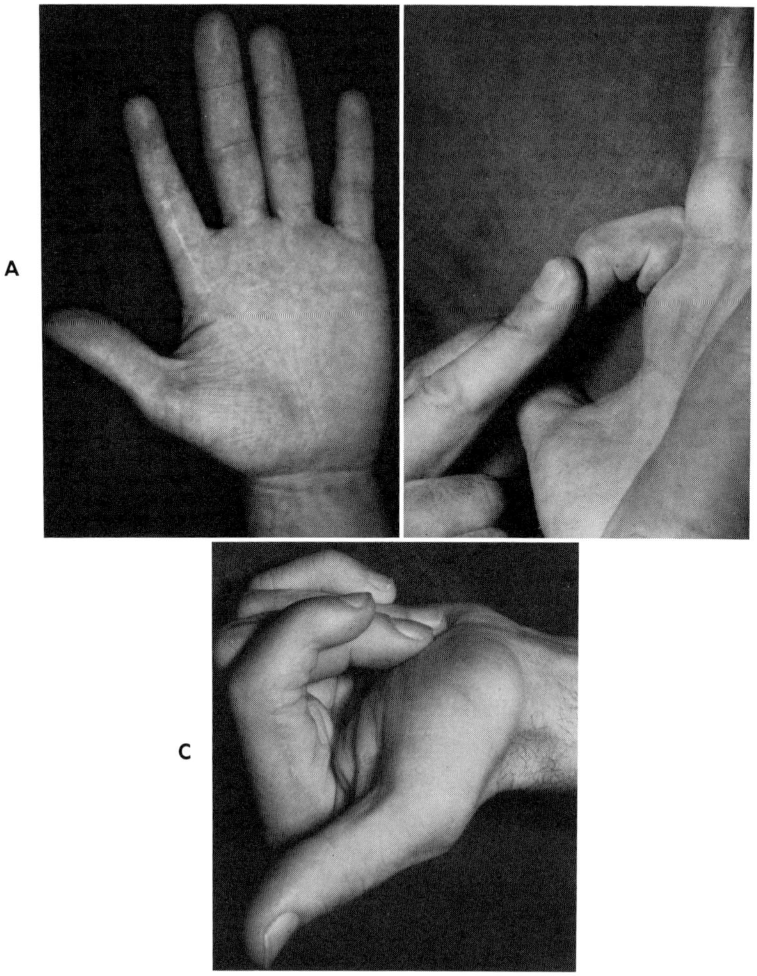

Fig. 15-5. Reconstruction of flexor tendon 14 years after injury. **A,** Photograph of left hand of 22-year-old male who severed both flexor tendons of his left index finger at 8 years of age. The surgeon carried out immediate repair through a midline incision. The tendons attenuated and active flexion was lacking. **B,** Presence of normal sensibility and of good passive range of motion in the index finger as well as relative freedom from scar in the incision influenced the decision to carry out tendon grafting 14 years after injury to provide normal function. **C,** Range of active motion of the index finger 4 months after tendon grafting. Note that a midlateral incision was used. Full function was attained in 1 year.

adjacent finger. Tendon grafting can be carried out years after injury.[2, 7] It may be necessary to use superficialis muscle from an adjacent digit as a motor, if the original profundus is not available (Fig. 15-5).

In the palm both tendons are usually severed and often nerves are also involved. This region is considered less hazardous than the fibrous sheath of the fingers in the adult. In children, however, especially if several digits are involved, cross adhesions may follow the suture of both tendons, especially if the site of injury is near the distal crease of the palm. The most common complication is

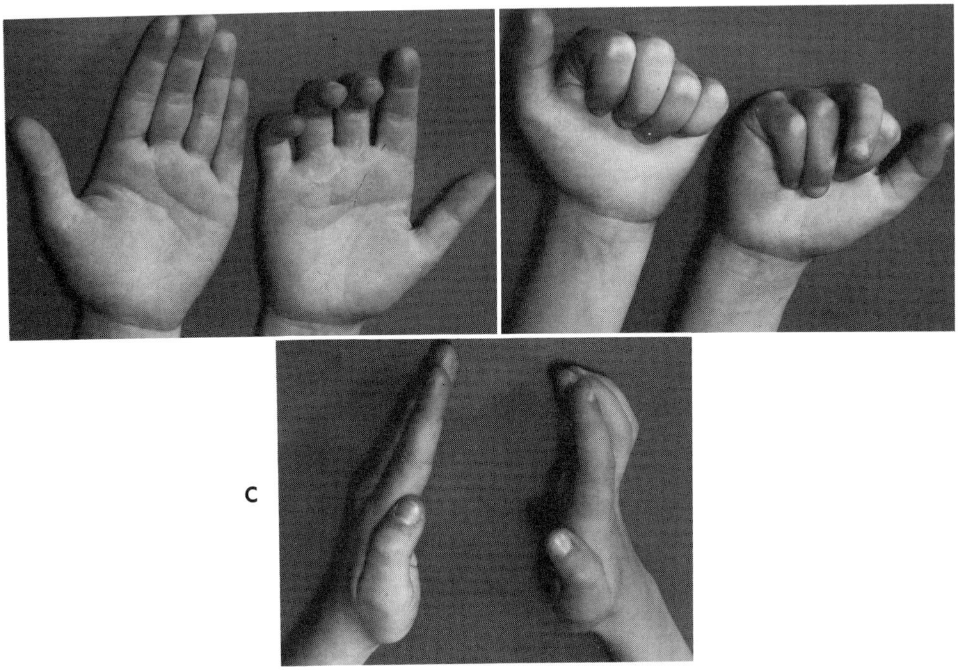

Fig. 15-6. Multiple injuries including digital nerves and tendons. **A,** Volar aspect of both hands of 9-year-old girl. Right hand was cut 3 years previously, severing all flexor tendons and all digital nerves to three ulnar fingers. Immediate repair of nerves and tendons was done at another hospital. Note the position of the scar. **B,** Flexion of fingers demonstrates that the little and ring fingers lack 1.5 cm. and the long finger lacks 3 cm. from distal palmar crease. The severance of tendons was within the proximal pulley of the long finger. **C,** Lateral view shows the limitation of extension of long, ring, and little fingers.

the limitation of extension of the fingers, while finger flexion can be normal or satisfactory (Fig. 15-6).

If the limitation of motion is primarily in the range of extension, I prefer to wait until the child is older for possible gradual adjustment. Tenolysis offers a means of improving restriction of the range of flexion due to adhesions, provided it is done with care and produces the release of the entire flexor system.[31] It is necessary to obtain free gliding of the involved flexors throughout the entire course of their action and this should be evident by producing passive flexion of the involved digit at the time of operation.

Should it become apparent at the time of tenolysis that the tendons are too short or the adhesions are so overwhelming that the likelihood of attaining improvement is very small, alternative management is indicated. For the former, short bridge grafts, as suggested by Bunnell and Pulvertaft[23] are useful in the correction of shortening. These apply primarily to the palm of the hand and to the area of carpal tunnel in the wrist. The bridge grafts are less formidable than the replacement of the entire tendons. Overwhelming adhesions are not likely to yield to a tenolysis and should be handled by a two-stage reconstruction utilizing the silastic implant that was popularized by Hunter[12] and that gives gratifying results even in children.[13]

The sources of tendon grafts are somewhat more limited in children than in adults. The flexor superficialis is usually adequate in length; it cannot be used if it is too short or too bulky (Fig. 15-4, right hand). The superficialis of the little finger is often too delicate for grafting. Similarly, the palmaris longus is not satisfactory in young children. In older children palmaris longus muscle and plantaris muscle may provide satisfactory graft. The long extensors of the toe are usually satisfactory and can be removed through several small transverse incisions.

POSTOPERATIVE MANAGEMENT

Because it is almost impossible to appeal for cooperation from infants or young children, special precautions must be taken to assure complete immobilization to avoid tearing of the repaired tendons. We have alluded to the tethering of the finger tip to the palmar skin by a stout suture preventing excessive pull. Because control of individual digits is not possible, reliance is placed on the control of the limb of moderate flexion of the wrist and right angle flexion of the elbow. The entire limb is held in a cast, extending from fingertips to axilla. In infants it is advisable to have a few layers of soft cling worn like a Sam Brown belt on the opposite shoulder and incorporated into the cast at the elbow; early loss of cast is disastrous. It is wise to place the entire limb with the cast within the shirt or outer garment to restrict vigorous use for ambulatory children during play.

If nonabsorbable sutures are used or when the Bunnell pull-out wires have to be removed, light general anesthesia avoids struggle and excessive pull on the freshly repaired tendon. When supervised exercises are needed, the parents should be instructed regarding such procedures. Formal physiotherapy is difficult and rarely necessary for very young patients.

FLEXOR TENDONS IN THE THUMB

Thumb flexor tendons are relatively less frequently injured in children than in adults. The anatomical configurations are less restrictive, and consequently, primary repair is less difficult in the thumb, but should be carried out with the same delicacy as for finger tendons. Secondary repair of the flexor pollicis longus can be performed for severance distal to the metacarpophalangeal joint in long-standing injuries. Tendon graft is indicated when the tendon is either too short or if the proximal portion of the flexor pollicis longus cannot be identified. The proximal suture should be done in the wrist.

MANAGEMENT OF COMPLICATED INJURIES (LESS THAN OPTIMAL)

Excellent results are difficult to attain consistently even in relatively simple tendon injuries in the hand. In complicated injuries the expectations are reduced,

A B C D

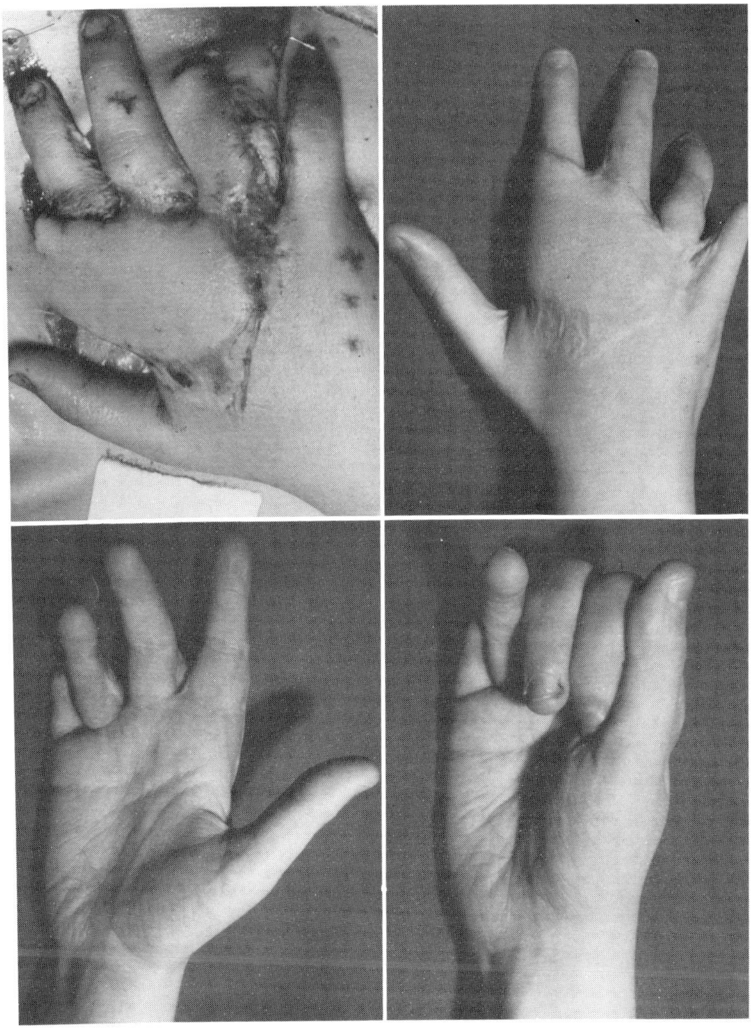

Fig. 15-7. Less than optimal type of injury. Severe injury of the right hand of 11-year-old boy, caused by the moving stairs of an escalator, involving extensor and flexor tendons, compound fracture of bones of ring and little fingers, and extensive loss of dorsal skin. **A**, Initial treatment required stabilization of bone by K-wires and application of two infraclavicular flaps. **B** and **C**, Appearance of hands after primary coverage. **D**, Flexion is lacking in the right ring finger, but impaired function of the proximal interphalangeal joint restricts reconstruction of flexor tendon function.

because conditions for success are less than optimal.[20] These conditions include multiple tendon injuries in several digits, extensive loss of skin, associated nerve injuries, damage to the bony framework, injuries affecting the joints, and severe crushing injuries involving all tissues. Based on the severity of the injuries involved, a useful classification has been determined that gives some indication of the likelihood of attaining good results after tendon repair.[3, 4, 13] We also have a universally acceptable, standardized manner of assessing the final results for comparison between different methods and series of cases.[3, 29, 34]

Primary tendon repair or even tendon grafting does not give satisfactory results in these less than optimal cases, and often preliminary surgical procedures have to be used before definitive flexor tendon reconstruction can be undertaken (Fig. 15-7). Usually the presence of a scar, limitation of joint function, and other clinical features make it obvious that good function is not likely to be achieved by simple tendon repair or conventional tendon graft. Frequently this becomes apparent only at the time of operation when the extensive cicatrization and ubiquitous adhesions are exposed.

The introduction of a two-stage procedure by the initial use of silastic tendon implant to produce a new tendon sheath, followed later by the use of tendon graft, permits salvaging useful function in these complicated injuries.[12] Prior to the availability of this method, simple tendon graft did not attain good function, and occasionally resulted in loss of function.[13] While this method of management was used primarily in adults, it may be utilized for salvaging the function in older children (Fig. 15-8). It is contraindicated in the very young, since it demands some cooperation from the patient.

We have observed that occasionally a discrepancy exists between the size of

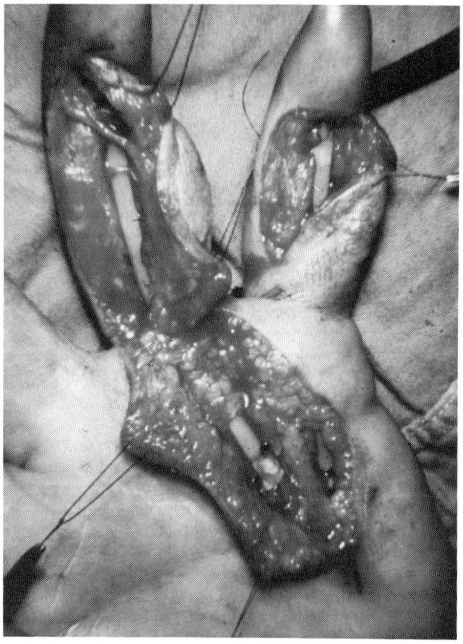

Fig. 15-8. Less than optimal injury. Injury to both flexor tendons of ring and little fingers in the area of fibrous sheath some years previously was complicated by persistent wound, and resulted in extensive fibrosis of all structures on the volar aspect and absence of active flexion when this young man first presented himself for treatment. Surgical exploration revealed complete adhesion of all structures within the fibrous sheath of both fingers. It was not possible to salvage the distal pulleys. Silastic tendon spacers were inserted and distal pulleys were made from portion of removed tendons. Definitive tendon grafting was carried out after passive range of motion was attained.

the finger whose tendon had been injured and its homonymous finger when the two are compared years after injury (Fig. 15-5). Similar observations were made by other authors.[10] The intriguing question was raised whether this is due to the lesser growth of autogenous tendon grafts placed in the young children. However, there is also lesser girth of the involved digit. Although the smaller size of the injured finger is not always found, when it occurs it may result from several factors: interference with the blood supply to the involved digit caused by the initial trauma, additional insult caused by the extension of the wound to expose the tendon, or further dissection inherent in the repair.

Concomitant nerve injury apparently does not contribute to retardation of growth, provided full recovery takes place.[10] We have noted less frequent use of repaired finger in some children, notwithstanding apparent full range of movement of the grafted tendon and clinically satisfactory recovery of sensibility.

SUMMARY

1. Surgical management of flexor tendon injuries in very young children is an arduous and demanding task.
2. The use of fine instruments and magnification aids, and the avoidance of incision in areas of potential growth are necessary.
3. Primary sutures of flexor tendons are indicated in uncomplicated injuries. Absorbable sutures for skin are helpful.
4. Padded casts from fingertips to axilla with tethering soft webbing around the opposite shoulder prevents undesirable distal displacement. Placing the limb with the cast inside outer garments avoids problems in vigorous use in the very young.
5. In complicating injuries with less than optimal conditions for restoration of normal function, useful range of tendon function can be attained through secondary one or two-stage tendon grafting.
6. If sensibility is satisfactory and joints are kept supple, definitive tendon reconstruction can give useful function even after a protracted period of time.
7. Light general anesthesia is suggested for removal of pull-out or nonabsorbable sutures in very young children.
8. It is helpful to involve parents in the postoperative reeducation.

References

1. Arons, M. S.: Purposeful delay on the primary repair of cut flexor tendons in some-man's-land in children, Plast. Reconstr. Surg. **53**:638, 1974.
2. Bell, J. L., Mason, M. L., Koch, S. L., and Stromberg, W. B.: Injuries of flexor tendons of the hand in children J. Bone Joint Surg. **40A**:1220, 1958.
3. Boyes, J. H.: Flexor tendon grafts in the fingers and thumb: an evaluation of end results, J. Bone Joint Surg. **32A**:489, 1950.
4. Boyes, J. H.: Flexor tendon grafts in the fingers and thumb, J. Bone Joint Surg. **53A**:1332, 1971.

5. Bunnell, S.: Repair of tendons in the fingers and description of two new instruments, Surg. Gynecol. Obst. **26**:103, 1918.
6. Chaplin, D. M.: The vascular anatomy within normal tendons, divided tendons, free tendon grafts, and pedicle tendon grafts in rabbits, Br. J. Bone Joint Surg. **55B**:369, 1973.
7. Entin, M. A.: Flexor tendon repair and grafting in children, Am. J. Surg. **109**:287, 1965.
8. Entin, M. A.: Philosophy of tendon repair, Orthop. Clin. North Am. **4**:859, 1973.
9. Entin, M. A.: Repair of flexor tendons in severely injured hands, Accident Surg. **2**:355, 1964.
10. Hage, J., and Dupuis, C. C.: The intriguing fate of tendon grafts in small children's hands and their results, Br. J. Plast. Surg. **18**:341, 1965.
11. Harrison, S. H.: Delayed primary flexor tendon grafts, Plast. Reconstr. Surg. **43**:366, 1969.
12. Hunter, J. M.: Artificial tendons—early development and application, Am. J. Surg. **109**: 325, 1965.
13. Hunter, J. M., and Salisbury, R. E.: Flexor tendon reconstruction in severely damaged hands, J. Bone Joint Surg. **53A**:829, 1971.
14. Iselin, M.: "Delayed emergency" in fresh wounds of the hand, Proc. R. Soc. Med. **51**: 713, 1958.
15. Kleinert, H. E., Kutz, J. E., Ashbell, S. T., and Martinez, E.: Primary repair of lacerated flexor tendons in no-man's-land, J. Bone Joint Surg. **49A**:577, 1967.
16. Lindsay, W. K., and McDougall, E. P.: Direct digital flexor tendon repair, Plast. Reconstr. Surg. **26**:613, 1960.
17. Littler, J. W.: Free tendon grafts in secondary flexor tendon repair, Am. J. Surg. **74**:315, 1947.
18. Madsen, E.: Delayed primary suture of flexor tendon cut in the digital sheath, J. Bone Joint Surg. **52B**:264, 1970.
19. McCash, C. R.: The immediate repair of flexor tendons, Br. J. Plast. Surg. **14**:53, 1961.
20. McCormack, R. M., Demuth, J. R., and Kindling, P. H.: Flexor tendon grafts in less-than-optimum situation, J. Bone Joint Surg. **44A**:1360, 1962.
21. Peacock, E. E.: Some technical aspects and results of flexor tendon repair, Surgery **58**: 330, 1965.
22. Posch, J. L.: Primary tenorrhaphies and tendon grafting, procedures in hand injuries, Arch. Surg. **73**:609, 1956.
23. Pulvertaft, R. G.: Problems of flexor tendon surgery of the hand, J. Bone Joint Surg. **47A**: 123, 1965.
24. Pulvertaft, R. G.: Reparative surgery of flexor tendon injuries in the hand, J. Bone Joint Surg. **36B**:689, 1954.
25. Pulvertaft, R. G.: Tendon grafts for flexor tendon injuries in the fingers and thumb, a study of technique and results, J. Bone Joint Surg. **38B**:175, 1956.
26. Rank, B. K., and Wakefield, A. R.: Flexor tendon repair in the hand, Aust. NZ J. Surg. **19**:239, 1949-50.
27. Salvi, V.: Delayed primary suture in flexor tendon division, Hand 3:181, 1971.
28. Smith, J.: Blood supply of tendon, Am. J. Surg. **109**:272, 1965.
29. Verdan, C. E.: Half a century of flexor tendon surgery, J. Bone Joint Surg. **54A**:472, 1972.
30. Verdan, C. E.: Primary repair of flexor tendons, J. Bone Joint Surg. **42A**:647, 1960.
31. Verdan, C. E., Crawford, G. P., and Martini-Benkeddache, Y.: The valuable role of tenolysis in the digits. In Cramer, L. M., and Chase, R. A., editors: Symposium on the hand, Vol. 3, St. Louis, 1971, The C. V. Mosby Co.
32. Verdan, C. E., and Michon, J.: Le traitement des plaies des tendons flechisseurs des doigts, Rev. Chir. Orthop. **47**:285, 1961.
33. Wakefield, A. R.: The treatment of tendon injuries in children, Presented at the Annual Meeting of the American Society for Surgery of the Hand, Chicago, January 17, 1964.
34. White, W. L.: Secondary restoration of finger flexion by digital tendon grafts, Am. J. Surg. **91**:662, 1956.

16. Palmar fingertip use of silicone rubber followed by free tendon grafting

modification of the Hunter technique

Spencer A. Rowland, M.D.

The principles and techniques concerning the use of silicone rubber rods followed by free tendon grafting has been well documented by others in the literature.[1, 3-6] Modification of Dr. Hunter's technique is being presented because I believe that the modified technique will give as equally a satisfactory result as his method. It differs principally in the following ways.

The silicone rubber prosthesis extends from the fingertip to the palm rather than extending to the lower part of the forearm as described by Hunter. If there is thick unyielding scar in the palm of the hand, this modified method cannot be used as the scar must be bipassed as in Dr. Hunter's technique. The advantage of the proximal palmar anastomosis is that the more classical tendon graft may be performed using the shorter palmaris longus tendon graft from the forearm rather than going to the leg for the longer toe extensor or the plantaris tendon that adds operative time, wound exposure, scars, and a longer tendon graft.

The silicone rubber prosthesis is sutured at both ends, while Dr. Hunter leaves the tendon free in the forearm. The purpose of suturing both ends of the prosthesis is not to produce active finger flexion, but is twofold. First, the proximal end of the prosthesis is prevented from wandering aimlessly in the palm on passive flexion, which may cause tissue irritation. Second, by splitting the proximal profundus tendon and passing the prosthesis into the tendon, the sheath forms into the tendon itself, which later allows the free tendon graft to be passed from its distal bony insertion into the tendon without leaving the newly-formed tendon sheath.

Technical points concerning the suturing of the ends of the prosthesis include the following. The distal end of the silicone prosthesis is brought over the volar plate and under the stump of the flexor digitorum profundus to bone so that the future gliding tendon sheath will form over the volar surface of the distal finger joint, lessening the chance of adherence of the future tendon graft to the volar plate. The sutures used are heavy 3-0 monofilament nylon reinforced by lighter

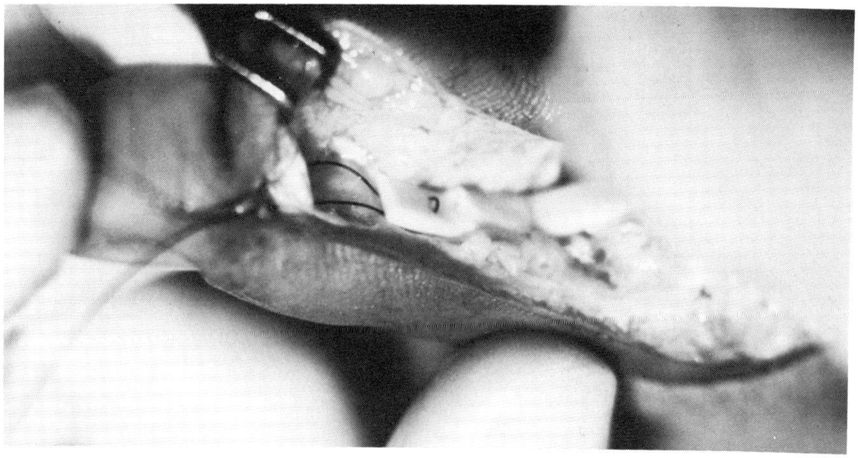

Fig. 16-1. The distal anastomosis is made by bringing the silicone prosthesis under the flexor digitorum profundus to its bony insertion as the secondary tendon graft will be into bone rather than to tendon.

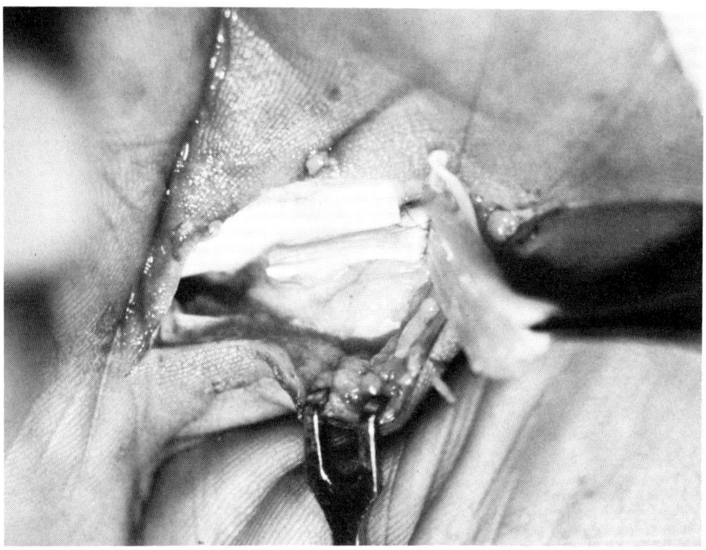

Fig. 16-2. The profundus tendon is split and the prosthetic implant is passed into the tendon.

5-0 monofilament nylon on the sides of the tendon and prosthesis (Fig. 16-1). The proximal anastomosis is performed by first splitting the profundus tendon (Fig. 16-2), and then drawing the tendon into the fish-mouth incision (Fig. 16-3). Suturing is performed with 5-0 monofilament nylon. The purpose of using the weaker suture is that if a suture breaks, it is better that the proximal prosthesis becomes free. The stronger distal anastomosis must not break because it is the continued passive motion of the prosthesis caused by the full passive flexion of the finger that forms the columnar cells within the sheath.[4-6] In my experience,

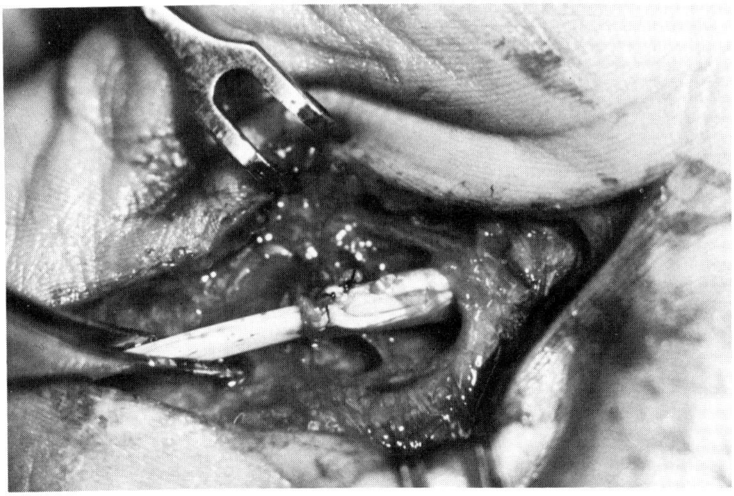

Fig. 16-3. With the split ends of the profundus tendon around the prosthetic implant, the new sheath will form into the tendon.

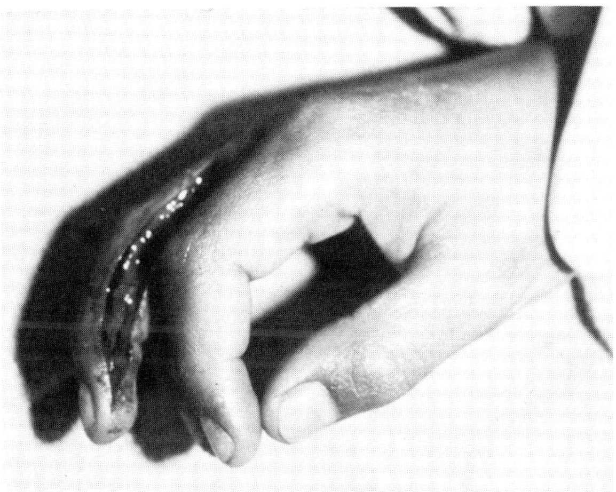

Fig. 16-4. The silicone prosthesis should be sutured under some tension so that the profundus tendon can be pulled forward with passive extension of the finger.

the poorer results have occurred in those patients in whom the distal anastomosis broke, disallowing the continued passive flexion of the prosthesis in the fibrous sheath or in those patients where the prosthesis buckled because the pulleys were too tight (or the prosthesis was too large) preventing the desired passive gliding motion. Another point to be emphasized when suturing both ends of the prosthesis is that it be done with enough tension on the prosthesis to permit some finger stance (Fig. 16-4). This allows the profundus tendon to be pulled forward on passive extension of the finger and when the prosthesis is pushed back with

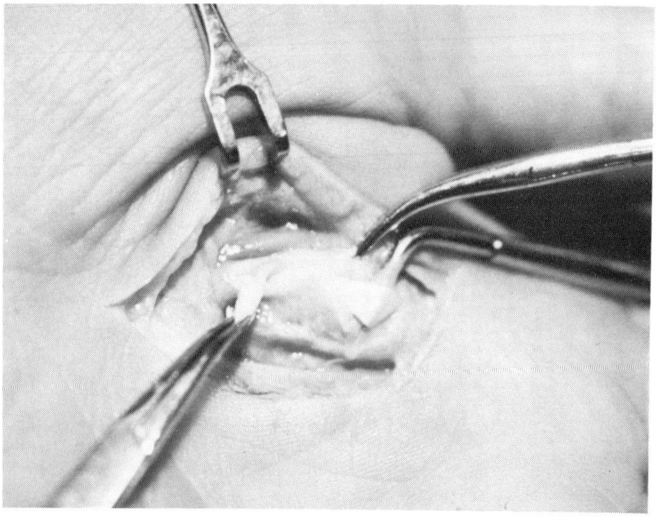

Fig. 16-5. If the sheath is thick and unyielding at the proximal anastomosis, it must be excised to allow for maximum excursion of the flexor digitorum profundus tendon.

Table 3. Results of nineteen consecutive patients using the Hunter tendon prosthesis

						Tip pulp from distal palmar crease	
Case	*Name*	*Age*	*Finger*	*Injury*	*Grade**	*Passive*	*Active*
1	R. S.	20	Index	Saw	5	0	0
2	M. S.	46	Index	Knife	2	0	0.6 cm.
3	B. F.	40	Little	Saw	5	1 cm.	2 cm.
4	C. T.	28	Long	Glass	2	0	0.6 cm.
5	D. S.	12	Long	Glass	4	0	0
6	J. R.	20	Index	Knife	2	0	0.6 cm.
7	G. G.	30	Little	Knife	2	0	0†
8	R. C.	16	Index	Tire rim explosion	5	0	0
9	N. A.	23	Long	Glass	2	0	0
10	C. P.	15	Ring	Saw	5	2.8 cm.	2.8 cm.
			Little	Saw	5	2.8 cm.	3.3 cm.
11	J. L. M.	31	Index	Crushing	5	2.8 cm.	3.0 cm.
12	S. M.	16	Ring	Crushing	4	0	4.5 cm; needed pulley when blocked 1.8 cm.

*Of the seven remaining patients, one patient removed cast and was lost to follow-up; two patients had stage one only and were lost to follow-up; one patient developed infection and subsequently had an amputation; two patients had anastomosis in the forearm because of palmar scarring; and one patient with proximal interphalangeal joint damage had a subsequent arthrodesis.

†Patient had a persistent flexion contracture measuring 55° at the distal joint and 35° at the proximal interphalangeal joint.

passive finger flexion, the tendon retracts. Passive motion is started as soon as the tissues allow it, usually 3 to 5 days postoperatively.

The silicone prosthesis is left in for a shorter period of time than has been suggested by Dr. Hunter. It is my belief that the prosthesis, acting as a foreign body, can cause adverse irritation the longer it is present. Experimental animal studies have shown that the inner lining of columnar cells and the outer layer of the thick fibrous sheath matures in about 6 weeks.[3, 4] Animal experimentation also shows that the longer the prosthesis is present, the thicker the outer fibrous sheath becomes.[3] For that reason, the patient is seen 6 weeks postoperatively. If tissues are soft and supple and there is a maximum range of passive finger motion, the second stage free tendon graft is scheduled.

The final point that differs from Dr. Hunter's technique is the method of the proximal anastomosis of the tendon graft to the flexor digitorum profundus. If the sheath formed about the tendon prosthesis and the proximal profundus tendon is soft and supple and there is good excursion of the profundus tendon, the proximal end of the tendon graft is passed down the sheath into the profundus tendon and then out the side of the tendon, as in Pulvertaft's method, without disturbing the sheath about the tendon (Fig. 16-5). However, if the profundus tendon is tethered with excessive scar around the sheath, the scar must be removed to allow for the maximum excursion of the profundus tendon. If the lumbrical muscle is scarred down, it is excised. If it is healthy in appearance and not tethered with scar, it is left alone. The remainder of the operation differs little from any conventional tendon graft procedure.

RESULTS

The results of nineteen consecutive patients were reported in Philadelphia on March 15, 1974, and Table 3 shows the results. Grading of the injuries was done according to Dr. Hunter's modification of Dr. Boyes' classification.[2, 6]

Grade 1 (good)	Good soft tissues, supple joints, and no significant scarring.
Grade 2 (scar)	Deep cicatrix, resulting from injury or previous surgery, as well as mild soft tissue contractures that, in a few instances, were severe enough to require preliminary plastic procedures.
Grade 3 (joint)	Limitation of passive joint motion, usually in the proximal interphalangeal joint, sufficient to require mobilization by traction and dynamic splinting.
Grade 4 (nerve)	Nerve damage with associated trophic changes in addition to scarring of the tendon bed and joint stiffness.
Grade 5 (multiple)	Soft tissue scarring or joint changes in more than one digit, or a combination of injuries in a single digit of such character that Grades 2, 3, and 4 did not apply.

I believe that if active flexion approached that of passive flexion in the severely injured fingers, then a satisfactory result from the tendon surgery had been obtained.

CONCLUSION

In conclusion, a method has been presented that differs from Dr. Hunter's technique in four basic areas:

1. A silicone rubber prosthesis extends from the fingertip to the palm, rather than extending into the forearm.
2. The silicone prosthesis is sutured at both ends rather than being left free at the proximal end.
3. The silicone prosthesis is left in for a shorter period of time.
4. Proximal anastomosis of the second stage is modified to take full advantage of the sheath if scarring about the proximal end is not excessive.

References

1. Bassett, C. A. L., and Carroll, R. E.: Formation of tendon sheath by silicone rod implants. In Proceedings of the American Society For Surgery of the Hand, J. Bone Joint Surg. **45A**:884-885, June, 1963.
2. Boyes, J. H.: Flexor tendon grafts in the fingers and thumb: an evaluation of end results, J. Bone Joint Surg. **32A**:489, 1950.
3. Farkas, L., McCain, W. G., Sweeney, P., Wilson, W., Hurst, L. W., and Lindsay, W. K.: An experimental study of the changes following silastic rod preparation of a new tendon sheath and subsequent tendon grafting, J. Bone Joint Surg. **55A**:1149-1158, 1973.
4. Hunter, J.: Artificial tendons—early development and application, Am. J. Surg. **109**:325-338, 1965.
5. Hunter, J. M., and Salisbury, R. E.: Flexor tendon reconstruction in severely damaged hands, J. Bone Joint Surg. **53A(5)**:829-858, 1971.
6. Hunter, J. M., and Salisbury, R. E.: Use of gliding artificial implants to produce tendon sheaths, Plast. Reconstr. Surg. **45**:564-572, 1970.
7. Mayer, L.: Reconstruction of the digital tendon sheath, J. Bone Joint Surg. **18**:607-616, 1936.
8. Urbaniak, J. R., Bright, D. S., Gill, L. H., and Goldner, J. L.: Vascularization and gliding mechanism of free flexor tendon grafts inserted by silicone rod method, J. Bone Joint Surg. **56A(3)**:473-481, April 1973.

17. Avulsion of the insertion of the flexor digitorum profundus tendon associated with fracture of the distal phalanx

a brief review

Patrick R. Robins, M.D.
James H. Dobyns, M.D.

Closed fingertip injuries involving avulsion of the insertion of the flexor digitorum profundus (FDP) tendon associated with fracture of the palmar base of the distal phalanx are confusing and may contribute to the delayed diagnosis and unsuccessful treatment of this injury. The mechanism, incidence, and management of avulsion injuries of the FDP tendon have been well documented in recent years.[2, 3, 5-7] The authors of these papers and several textbook authors have noted that bone fragments of varying size can accompany the flexor tendon insertion injuries.

We wish to emphasize some of the puzzling fracture variations of this common tendon injury and to clarify the diagnostic and management pitfalls by discussing four cases that illustrate the range of possibilities.

CORRELATIVE ANATOMY OF FDP INSERTION AND MECHANISM OF INJURY

The FDP tendon is composed of superficial and deep fibers (Fig. 17-1). The superficial fibers, when traced distally from the level of the bifurcation of the corresponding superficialis tendon, gradually diverge from the midline furrow toward the margins of the tendon. Opposite the terminal interphalangeal joint, these superficial fibers diverge more acutely to insert on each side of the ventral lateral surface of the base of the distal phalanx, thus exposing the deeper fibers, which are attached more distally and centrally on the palmar aspect of the shaft of this bone. In the terminal phalanges, the roughening for flexor tendon attachment is limited proximally by a transverse long ridge. The insertion of the flexor tendon fibers is primarily diaphyseal, extending more than half way from the articular margin to the tuft of the distal phalanx. In the adult, as compared with the

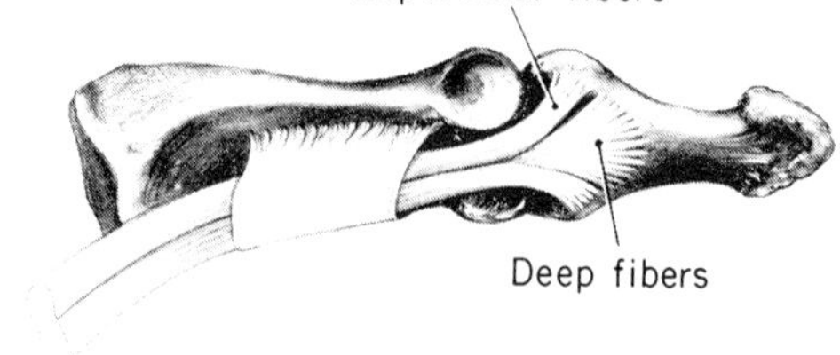

Fig. 17-1. Insertion of flexor digitorum profundus tendon on distal phalanx.

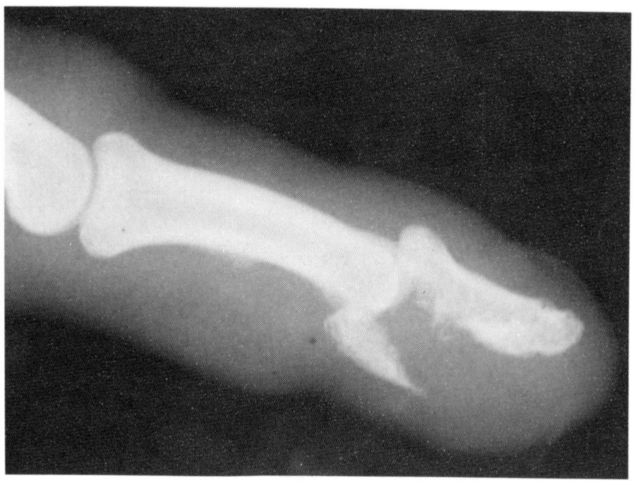

Fig. 17-2. Fracture of distal phalanx with involvement of flexor profundus function (patient 1).

child, the flexor tendon of the terminal phalanx reaches much more distally than does the corresponding extensor tendon.[9]

McMaster[8] has shown that a normal tendon generally ruptures at the musculotendinous junction or at the insertion of the tendon into bone. If neither of these weaker regions gives way, but the force is unrelenting, rupture occurs further distal than the insertion, further proximal than the musculotendinous junction, or through tendon substance. In practice, rupture that occurs further distal than the insertion is more common and accounts for avulsion-fracture injuries.

The course and attachments of the profundus tendon proximal to the distal phalanx have been described and illustrated.[2] Briefly, each profundus tendon possesses a short vinculum near the distal interphalangeal joint and a long vinculum near the proximal interphalangeal joint. Each tendon is contained within the fibrous flexor tunnels of the proximal and middle phalanges. Rupture of the insertion of the tendon may easily strip both vincula and other supportive peritendinous tissues, and the tendon may come to reside in the proximal half of the digit or even in the palm.

The less independent action of extension of the flexed fourth finger has been noted by Gunter[6] and Carroll and Match,[5] and this action may explain the many closed flexor tendon injuries to this finger.

Case material

Patient 1 suffered a fracture of the base of the distal phalanx. The fragment involved the palmar 50% of the base and 50% of the articular surface (Fig. 17-2). In such an injury, the flexor tendon has to be either still attached to the palmar fracture fragment or avulsed from both fragments. Because of the gap between fragments and the proximal displacement of the smaller, palmar fragment, it was believed that the FDP was still attached to this fragment. There was, of course, no active flexion of the distal phalanx, but a painful tugging at the site of the palmar fragment when flexion was attempted further suggested persisting tendon attachment to the avulsed fragment. This case is typical of FDP avulsion including a large bone fragment, with the tendon still attached to the fragment. To establish the degree of tendon injury, as well as to restore normal joint architecture, open exploration and repair were recommended. This patient then returned to his original treating facility, and further results are not known. If, as anticipated, the FDP remained attached, open reduction and fixation of the fracture fragment should restore both bony and tendon continuity with relative simplicity.

Patient 2 was seen in the emergency room after a gasoline engine backfired while he was attempting to start it, the jolt pulling the handle from the fully flexed fingers of his right hand. Physical examination revealed no active flexion of the distal interphalangeal joint of the fourth finger, and the fingertip was fixed in full extension. Roentgenograms revealed a fracture of the palmar aspect of the base of the distal phalanx, involving the joint surface (Fig. 17-3, *A*). After an unsuccessful attempt at closed reduction of the fragment, the patient underwent surgery. Exploration revealed that the fracture fragment constituted about one half of the width of the articular surface and about one half the length of the distal phalanx. The palmar plate was attached to the fragment. Further search revealed that the FDP tendon was totally stripped from the distal phalanx and from the fragment, and was lying just inside the distal pulley. Treatment consisted of retrieving the avulsed tendon, reducing the fracture, maintaining its position with Kirschner wire fixation (Fig. 17-3, *B*), and suturing the tendon end to the adjacent periosteum and fibrous tissue. Two months after the operation, the fracture was healed and the FDP tendon was functioning.

Patient 3 was involved in an automobile accident and sustained multiple injuries. One of the injuries was to the tip of a ring finger (Fig. 17-4). The small chip fracture at the palmar base of the distal phalanx could represent a rather innocuous fracture, but there was the additional clinical finding of loss of flexor profundus action at the distal phalanx. Roentgenographic evidence of a dorsal subluxation of the major fragment also was present, but such subluxation can occur with or without FDP tendon avulsion and indicates only a loss of the volar bony and ligamentous support apparatus of the joint. Exploration revealed that the profundus tendon was attached to the small fragment but was detached from the distal phalanx. The smaller fragment was excised, and the tendon was reattached to the distal phalanx. Follow-up at 18 months revealed return of normal profundus function. In published reports and in the authors' experience, these smaller chips are the more common of the fractures associated with this injury. Furthermore, the level of the chip as noted on the roentgenogram may indicate the position of the avulsed tendon. The site may vary from just off the normal insertion to the distal palm.

Patient 4[4] suffered a fractured and displaced large fragment of bone that represents the palmar base of the distal phalanx. In addition, the flexor profundus tendon was avulsed from this palmar fragment, with still another smaller fragment attached to the tendon. The smaller fragment was visualized near the base of the finger, indicating the position of the avulsed tendon. Apparently, the large palmar fragment was excised at one surgical episode. At a second operation, the FDP tendon was retrieved and reinserted. Three months later, the patient had 35° of voluntary flexion in the distal joint.

A

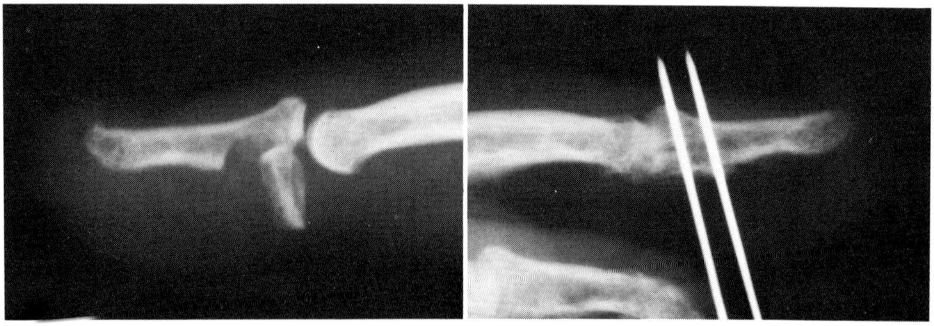

B

Fig. 17-3. **A,** Fracture of palmar base of distal phalanx; flexor profundus tendon stripped from distal phalanx and fragment. **B,** Postoperative open reduction, tendon reattachment (patient 2).

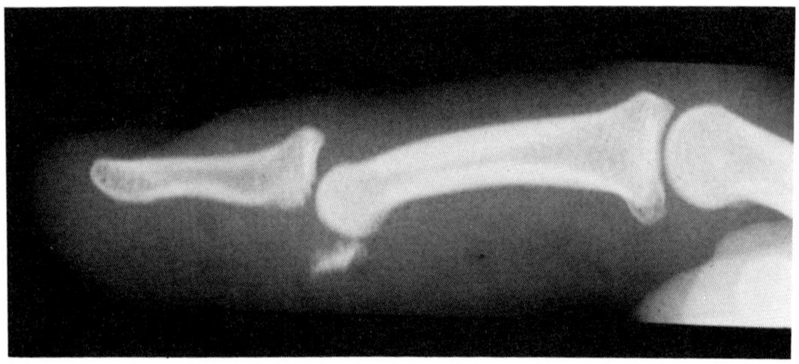

Fig. 17-4. Displaced fracture of base of distal phalanx; flexor profundus tendon attached to fragment (patient 3).

DISCUSSION

The serious problem of an avulsed flexor profundus tendon is intensified when there are associated fractures. There is not only the additional problem of management of the fracture, which may involve a large amount of the articular surface of the distal interphalangeal joint, but also the possibility that the fracture may obscure the avulsed tendon. A clue to the avulsed FDP tendon is the roentgenographic finding of small bone flecks in unusual sites because they have remained attached to the tendon fibers. However, this is not a completely reliable clue because the tendon frequently strips off the fractured fragment without any ossific debris accompanying it. The critical test of any fracture of the palmar surface of a distal phalanx is the demonstration of strong and nearly complete active flexion of the distal phalanx. If this cannot be demonstrated, exploration should be carried out on the presumption that the flexor profundus tendon has been avulsed from the distal phalanx and possibly from the fracture fragment. Böhler[1] has noted that this occurs in 50% of such instances; that is, the avulsed tendon has torn free from the fracture fragment. Our cases do not permit an estimate of percentages, but this possibility seems common and should be anticipated.

The anatomy of the flexor digitorum profundus insertion and the clinical types of cases suggest the following relationships between FDP avulsion and fracture fragments.

1. FDP avulsion with no fracture—both the superficial and the deep fibers strip from the distal phalanx.
2. FDP avulsion with large fracture fragment—the superficial and deep fibers hold long enough for bone to fracture. Either or both fiber groups may remain on the fragment or strip off.
3. FDP avulsion with small fracture fragment—the deep fibers strip but the superficial fibers hold long enough for bone to fracture. The superficial fibers then may remain on or strip from the fragment, but frequently displace the fracture fragment to varying positions in the finger.
4. FDP avulsion with large and small fragment fractures—the large fracture fragment occurs first, followed by stripping of the deep distal fibers, then followed by fracture of the small fragment, probably because the large fragment cannot be displaced proximally without encountering considerable resistance from volar plate, collateral ligaments, and distal pulley. The superficial and proximal fibers may remain with this fragment or may strip free.

SUMMARY

Avulsion of flexor tendons from their insertions without accompanying bone is well known and apparently is the most common type of this injury. The more confusing types in which fracture fragments accompany the tendon are categorized by the authors into large fragment, small fragment, and multiple fragment groups. The fragment size is correlated wilth the mode of insertion of the flexor tendon. Each fragment group can be subdivided on the basis of retention or stripping of the tendon insertion. Treatment depends on the certain determination of which possibilities exist. Appropriate management of both the fracture and the tendon avulsion is then accomplished. Four cases are presented to demonstrate that varieties of this clinical spectrum do exist.

References

1. Böhler, J.: Cited in Carroll, R. E., and Match, R. M.: Avulsion of the flexor profundus tendon insertion, J. Trauma **10**:1109, 1970.
2. Boyes, J. H.: Bunnell's Surgery of the hand, ed. 4, Philadelphia, 1964, J. B. Lippincott Co., p. 470.
3. Boyes, J. H., Wilson, J. N., and Smith, J. W.: Flexor-tendon ruptures in the forearm and hand, J. Bone Joint Surg. **42A**:637, 1960.
4. Bunnell, S.: Surgery of the hand, ed. 2, Philadelphia, 1948, J. B. Lippincott Co., p. 667.
5. Carroll, R. E., and Match, R. M.: Avulsion of the flexor profundus tendon insertion, J. Trauma **10**:1109, 1970.

6. Gunter, G. S.: Traumatic avulsion of the insertion of flexor digitorum profundus, Aust. NZ J. Surg. **30**:1, 1960.
7. Haldeman, K. O., and Soto-Hall, R.: Injuries to muscles and tendons, J.A.M.A. **104**:2319, 1935.
8. McMaster, P. E.: Tendon and muscle ruptures: clinical and experimental studies on the causes and location of subcutaneous ruptures, J. Bone Joint Surg. **15**:705, 1933.
9. Wilkinson, J. L.: The insertions of the flexors pollicis longus and digitorum profundus, J. Anat. **87**:75, 1953.

18. Flexor tenolysis

Lawrence H. Schneider, M.D.
James M. Hunter, M.D.

Successful repair of divided tendons, as measured by return of gliding function, is a great challenge to the surgeon because of the nature of tendon healing. The very process in which an injured tendon heals also causes it to adhere (or heal) to its surrounding bed. These adhesions prevent the smooth gliding of the tendon, which is necessary to produce movement of the fingers. The presence of local tissue injury secondary to the original traumatizing force or that injury added to the wound by the treating surgeon further complicates healing and increases the incidence and density of tendon adhesions. The surgeon's objective, therefore, is to create an environment in which the repaired tendon can heal with a minimal amount of tissue reaction and then, after an initial period of protection, institute physical measures to mobilize the repaired tendon, stretching adhesions created by the natural healing process. The difficulty in achieving this goal is evidenced by the great variability in the end results after tendon repair. While the surgical literature is replete with various authors expressing their preference for their own particular technique of tendon repair, it is apparent that there is no substitute for thorough anatomic knowledge combined with gentle technique so as not to cause further damage to these delicate tissues. This is not a simple proposition. Experimenters have shown that even the passage of a wire suture through an intact tendon will cause significant adhesion formation.[6] Every site where the tissue forceps punctures the tendon surface is a site for potential adhesion formation.[8]

The prevention of the development of limiting adhesions is the ideal and many approaches that seek this goal are being explored.[1, 5, 7] Once significant adhesions have formed, however, and physical therapy measures fail, the surgeon must resort to direct attack, tenolysis, in an effort to mobilize the involved tendon. The magnitude of this procedure must never be minimized and can even be more formidable than the original repair.

Procedures surrounding the actual surgery are at least as important as the lysis itself in achieving success in this frustrating problem. The period after tendon surgery is devoted to the application of physical measures concentrating on the recovery of active motion at the involved joints. Active motion exercises are carefully taught and these procedures are combined with the use of wood blocks and splint devices when indicated.

Because active motion is based on the ability of the repaired tendon to glide smoothly through its bed, the formation of nonpliable adhesions causes a number of patients to be unable to achieve full gliding even with the most conscientious postoperative program. These patients present with a varying degree of deficiency in range of active motion and, having reached a plateau in their progress through exercise, become candidates for tenolysis, assuming that the flexor tendon is intact and the involved joints are not stiff. Other preoperative criteria to be considered are the importance of the shortage in range of motion that is present in relation to the age, occupational needs, and desires of the patient. The sensory status of the involved finger as well as the degree of circulatory sufficiency is of prime importance. An atrophic, cold finger is a poor one even if range of motion is satisfactory. A finger having undergone multiple insults may better be treated, at times, by arthrodesis or amputation. A review of our cases reveals that there can be no absolute indications set forth in regard to the advisability of tenolysis in any one case because of the great variability in patient factors.

As recommended,[2] we wait a minimum of 3 months after repair and about 6 months after tendon grafting before embarking on this surgery. This time period allows for improvement through exercise while wound healing progresses, joints are mobilized, and tendon circulation reestablished. As tenolysis of necessity devascularizes the tendon area treated, rupture through the lysed area can occur in the postoperative period. Delay is felt to reduce the incidence of this disastrous complication.

TECHNIQUE OF THE OPERATION

Active participation of the patient in the surgery, we believe, is the key to improved results in flexor tenolysis. This is achieved through the use of local anesthesia supplemented by an intravenous analgesic-tranquilizer combination drug.[4] The addition of the medication provides sedation for the patient and has increased tourniquet tolerance to over 1 hour. Easily awakened, the patient cooperates dynamically in the surgery. The surgeon can be certain that the tendon has been completely freed and that the motor muscles can actively pull the finger fully into flexion. Most of our patients have been prepared for two-stage flexor tendon reconstruction[3] and, if direct evaluation shows that successful lysis is unfeasible, we proceed immediately with staged flexor reconstruction implanting the silicone rubber artificial tendon as the first stage. This can be combined, when necessary, with pulley reconstruction, nerve repair, and joint release.

The involved flexor system is approached through an ample zigzag incision, long enough, if necessary, to uncover the entire length of the flexor tendon, all limiting adhesions are methodically excised, and care is taken to define the borders of the tendon, a task that is not simple in heavily scarred area. Filmy, nonlimiting adhesions are, if possible, left intact. The retinacular pulley system is preserved with great care. During the surgery, the patient is constantly undergoing active reevaluation while each area of adhesion is attacked. When maximum flexion has been actively recovered, the tourniquet is released and hemostasis achieved. After closure, a dorsal plaster splint is provided and the dressing placed so that immediate flexion can be performed within the bandage to maintain the gliding allowed by the lysis. The patient then enters into the postoperative phase in which active motion exercises play a major role.

It is at this stage that the services of a hand therapist are often vital. Instruction in active exercise, usually begun prior to lysis, is resumed along with the appropriate application of straps, blocks, and spring splints, if needed. The importance of the input in time and effort by the patient in the quest for improved function cannot be overstressed. The patient's responsibilities along these lines are also reinforced during this postoperative period. Because of the danger to the integrity of the lysed tendon, no heavy work is allowed until 8 weeks postoperative.

RESULTS OF FLEXOR TENOLYSIS

A review of our cases of flexor tenolysis was made for the years 1969 to 1973 to coincide with the use and development of our dynamic technique. Sixty-eight operative procedures were performed with 60 patients available for follow-up. These patients presented with a total of 72 flexor systems involved as several patients presented with more than one finger involved. We have adopted a classification similar to the one of Verdan[9]:

5 Excellent	Gained normal range of motion.
4 Good	Gained ability to flex within 1 inch of the distal palmar crease and with flexion deformity less than 30° (total of joints).
3 Fair	Gained 30° of flexion over preoperative state without increase of flexion deformity.
2 Poor	No improvement.
1 Worse	

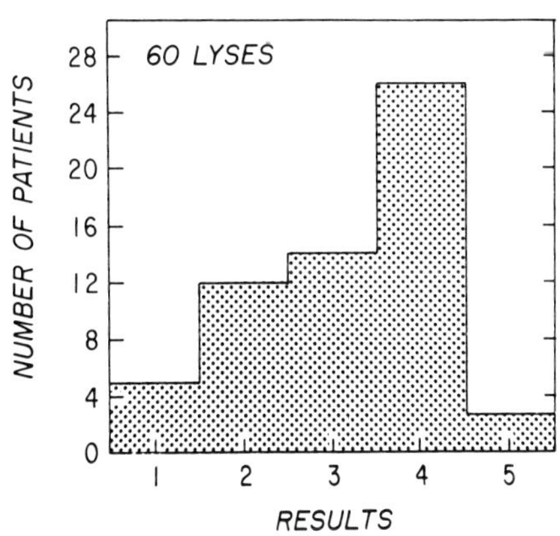

Fig. 18-1. In 60 flexor tenolyses, 29 patients or 48% of the total achieved good or excellent results.

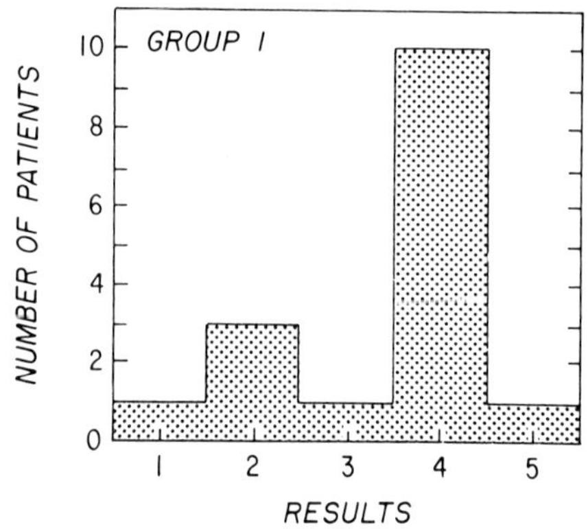

Fig. 18-2. Results of flexor tenolysis in Group I patients, those with failure of direct repair.

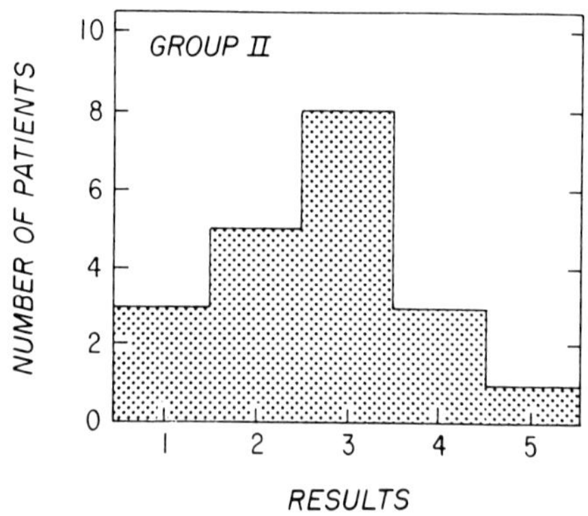

Fig. 18-3. Results of lysis in Group II patients, those who had undergone flexor tendon grafting.

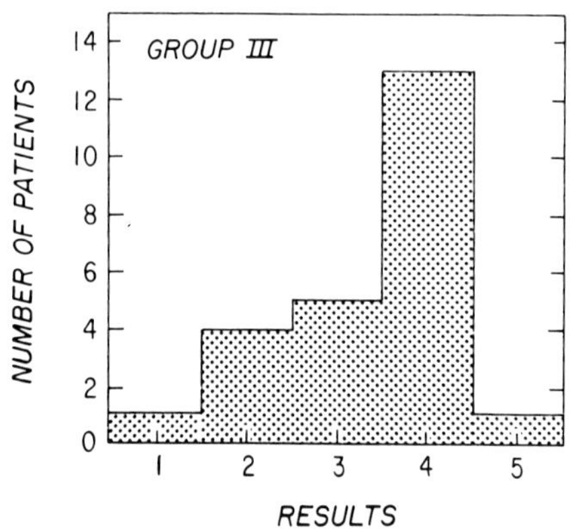

Fig. 18-4. Results of flexor lysis in Group III patients, those who had flexor tendon adhesions of various etiologies.

By these criteria 48% of our patients were in the good and excellent groupings. An additional 24% of patients were graded as having achieved fair improvement so that a total of 72% achieved improvement with tenolysis (see Fig. 18-1).

To better evaluate our results, the patients were grouped according to the etiology of their tendon adhesions:

Group I	Laceration with failed direct tendon repair	16 patients
Group II	Laceration with failed tendon graft	20 patients
Group III	Other causes of tendon adhesions	24 patients
	Infections 3 patients	
	Lacerations 4 patients	
	Crushing injuries 13 patients	
	Gunshot wounds 4 patients	

When charting results by these groups, the following is observed (see Figs. 18-2 to 18-4).

It should be noted that very few patients will gain a completely normal finger after lysis. There were, however, many more good results when lysis followed direct repair than when lysis was used after tendon graft. This would be expected when one considers the nature of direct repair as compared with the more extensive procedure of tendon grafting. Three of our five worst results came in the group that required lysis after tendon graft. Group III patients are not comparable to the other groups because of the nonspecific nature of the injury to the tendon that caused the onset of adhesions. These were all incomplete injuries as far as tendon integrity was concerned and were frequently accompanied by fractures. As a general rule the results in these patients paralleled the extent of damage inflicted on the involved tendon system and the accompanying tissues.

In our experience tenolysis has been found to be a useful tool in the treatment of the adherent flexor tendon and 72% of our patients improved in their range of motion after the procedure. It is a serious undertaking as the five failures in our series will attest. Four of these patients suffered rupture of the profundus tendon in the recovery period; one, a Group I patient, was salvaged by the staged tendon reconstruction method; one in Group II underwent amputation. The remaining two patients with ruptured tendon grafts accepted a rather poor finger. A fifth patient from Group III opted for amputation when lysis failed to improve his finger function.

It should be reiterated that this review consists of a selected group of patients. Not all patients with nongliding flexor tendons will come to lysis. Many patients, with a result that their surgeons regard as a failure, will refuse tenolysis. There is another group denied lysis because, after evaluation, it is felt that arthrodesis of a severely flexed proximal interphalangeal joint or even amputation is a better reconstructive program for their needs. In our series another group was removed to have staged flexor tendon reconstruction when it became apparent to us at attempted lysis, under our dynamic anesthesia technique, that lysis would not offer a feasible solution to the problem.

In summary, flexor tenolysis can be a useful salvage procedure when tendon adhesions prevent gliding of the flexor tendon system and conservative measures, stringently applied, fail to bring improvement in function. The operative procedure is a serious undertaking and may even be of greater magnitude than the tendon repair itself. Ample exposure and patient cooperation during the surgery have been helpful to us. A diligent postoperative program is essential if any degree of success is to be expected.

References

1. Bora, F. W., Jr., Lane, J. M., and Prockop, D. J.: Inhibitors of collagen biosynthesis as a means of controlling scar formation in tendon injury, J. Bone Joint Surg. **54A:**1501-1508, 1972.
2. Fetrow, K. O.: Tenolysis in the hand and wrist, J. Bone Joint Surg. **49A:**667-684, 1967.
3. Hunter, J. M., and Salisbury, R. E.: Flexor tendon reconstruction in severely damaged hands, J. Bone Joint Surg. **53A:**829-858, 1971.
4. Hunter, J. M., Schneider, L. H., Dumont, J., and Erickson, J. C.: A dynamic approach to problems of hand function, Clin. Orthop. **104:**112-115, 1974.
5. Ketchum, L. D.: Effects of triamcinolone on tendon healing and function, Plast. Reconstr. Surg. **47:**471-482, 1971.
6. Lindsay, W. K., and Thomson, H. G.: Digital flexor tendons: An experimental study, Br. J. Plast. Surg. **12:**289-316, 1960.
7. Peacock, E. E., Jr., and Madden, J. W.: Some strides on the effects of B-aminoproprionitrile in patients with injured flexor tendons, Surgery **66:**215-223, 1969.
8. Potenza, A. D.: Critical evaluation of flexor tendon healing and adhesion formation within artificial digital sheaths, J. Bone Joint Surg. **45A:**1217-1233, 1963.
9. Verdan, C. E., Crawford, G. P., and Martini-Benkeddache, Y.: The valuable role of tenolysis in the digits. In Cramer, L. M., and Chase, R. A., editors: Symposium on the hand, Vol. 3, St. Louis, 1971, The C. V. Mosby Co., pp. 192-206.

19. Basic considerations for tendon transfer operations in the upper extremity

Robert W. Beasley, M.D.

INTRODUCTION

Tendon transfer operations are performed to restore power or balance to a partially paralyzed hand. This involves the careful detachment of the tendon of a functioning muscle from its insertion and rerouting the tendon to a new insertion without damaging the muscle.

Tendon transfer operations follow the same guiding principle as all reconstructive procedures. *There is a redistribution of remaining functional parts into the best possible working combination.* Nothing is created, but it is simply a better investment of assets. In all but the most minor losses, this requires a simplification of the design of the hand and thus a lower order of function. An effort to accomplish too much with too little is a common basis for disappointing results. *In general, when any of the three major nerves of the arm (median, ulnar, or radial) is lost, an excellent functional restoration can be achieved; but with loss of any two of the three, a substantial functional impairment is inevitable* (Fig. 19-1).

EVALUATION OF THE PATIENT

Planning tendon transfer operations begins with a very careful assessment of the individual patient. An accurate evaluation of the impairment and functional needs is the first consideration. This entails a detailed history and probing questions, because the losses most apparent to the examiner are often not those that most trouble the patient. Also, it includes a consideration of the patient as a whole: attitudes, adaptive abilities, cooperation, and expectations. Examination begins with the hand, as this is the problem about which the patient has come, but much will be learned about the other factors as the examination proceeds.

Examination of the hand must include the condition of joints, state of sensibility and condition of soft tissues, as well as a tabulation of both functioning and nonfunctioning muscles. Grading and plotting all muscles is helpful in

A

B

C

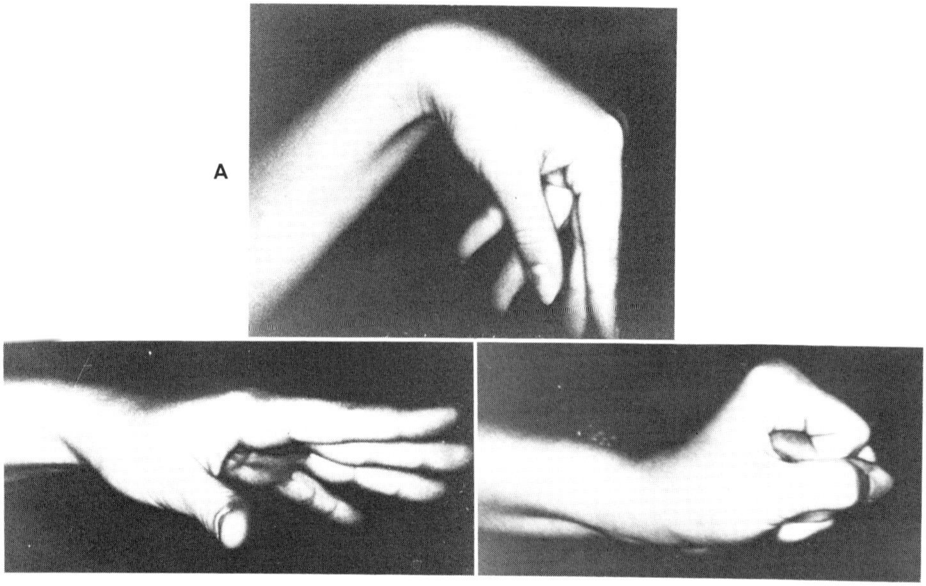

Fig. 19-1. A, Classical radial nerve palsy with loss of wrist and digital extension. **B,** Digital extension restored by transfer of flexor superficialis of ring finger to extensor digitorum communis and flexor superficialis of small finger to extensor pollicis longus. The muscles proper, rather than the tendons, must be carried through the interosseous membrane. (See Fig. 19-4). **C,** Wrist extension restored by transfer of pronator teres to the extensor carpi radialis brevis.

fully appreciating the disorder as well as developing the most realistic plan for reinvesting the functioning unit. In examining muscles, it is important to palpate the muscle for contracture rather than just observing it for its usual actions. Few observed movements result from the action of a single muscle, but result from combinations of stabilizers and antagonists with the prime mover. This accounts for deceptive trick movements and frequent errors of evaluation. Muscle strength is usually graded as zero, trace, fair, good, or normal. Muscles with power less than good are rarely suitable for transfers and spastic muscle can seldom be utilized. Accurate assessment of all these factors is essential to enabling consistently realistic and successful plans.

TIMING THE TRANSFER OPERATION

Having determined that the patient has significant needs and the potential for meeting these needs, the question arises as to when to operate. When there has been irreparable muscle or nerve damage, tendon transfers should be done at the earliest feasible time. They must, however, be preceded by joint mobilization and correction of skeletal derrangement or soft tissue losses, which may include replacement of scar. Of course, as with any elective reconstructive procedure, consideration cannot be given in the presence of any chronic or unhealed wounds.

With a changing condition such as nerve repairs, timing of tendon transfers may be more difficult. In general, one measures the distance from the site of nerve repair to the first muscle innervated by it and looks for evidence of reinnervation at the expected time based on the working rule of an average growth rate of a regenerating nerve of 1 mm. per day. Electromyographic evidence will usually precede clinical evidence of reinnervation by about 6 weeks. Failure to find evidence of reinnervation at the estimated time for appearance leads to consideration of tendon transfers. In general, a muscle that does not have at least useful power 6 months after the first evidence of reinnervation, will never have satisfactory power, and appropriate transfers should be done.

Psychologic factors must be considered. The patient should have a full appreciation of the loss, taking this state as the functional baseline for judging results since total restoration will infrequently be achieved. No patient with a spinal cord injury is a candidate for tendon transfers in the first 6 months after injury. They have overwhelming physiologic and psychologic adjustments that must first be made.

PLANNING THE OPERATION

A precise assessment of the patient's needs and the functioning parts available to meet those needs, is the point of departure for any plan as previously emphasized. The following factors are considered in choosing a muscle for tendon transfer:

1. It must be expendable from its normal function. Obviously we must be certain its intended new use is of more value to the patient than the muscle's normal function (Fig. 19-6, *C*).
2. The muscle must be a functionally independent unit under good volutional control and free of spasticity. One tendon from a muscle having multiple communicating tendons, as the flexor digitorum profundus or extensor digitorum communis, cannot be used for tendon transfers as the remaining tendon slips would checkrein the transferred one.
3. The muscle must have adequate amplitude of excursion for its new function or must cross a controlled joint to enhance its amplitude by tenodesis. For example, no other muscle has the amplitude of the flexor digitorum profundus group, but the effective amplitude of a transfer to it can be increased by wrist flexion with transfers that pass volar to the flexion axis of this joint (Fig. 19-6).
4. The selected muscle must have suitable anatomic location for rerouting its tendon to the new insertion for a straight line of pull between its origin and new attachment. In no case should there be more than one pulley or change of direction in its course.
5. Synergism between the muscle's normal function and intended new one is desirable, facilitating prompt utilization of the transfer, but it is not essential. Any muscle can be reeducated for different function. The diffi-

culty encountered with muscle reeducation in inversely proportional to the benefit derived from the function restored by the transfer (Fig. 19-6).

In planning tendon transfer, it is fundamental that *every joint between the origin of the muscle and its new insertion must be controlled.* This mathematical principle can be stated simply. An uncontrolled multiarticular system submitted to compression (as a finger when the tendons in the sheaths contract) will buckle in a zigzag manner. It follows that when muscles are not available to actively control joints crossed by the transferred tendon, the less important parts must be stabilized in a functional position by arthrodesis. If the system is allowed to buckle, the power of the transferred muscle is dissipated and is ineffective at its new insertion.

Finally, *simplicity of design is the key to success, complexity favoring disappointing results.* An ill-conceived effort to do too much with too little is often the basis for failure in tendon transfer operations.

TECHNICAL CONSIDERATIONS

Planning incisions are necessary for detachment of the tendon, mobilization of the muscle without damage to its neurovascular pedicle, rerouting the tendon, and making its new insertion. With experience, one projects a visual image of the underlying muscles on the skin and draws out appropriate incisions, but one may initially find it advantageous to sketch on the skin the concerned muscles and other structures to ensure optimal planning of incisions to meet all the needs (Fig. 19-2).

IMMOBILIZATION OF THE MUSCLES

Muscles have well-defined neurovascular pedicles that are often not fully appreciated (Fig. 19-3). The muscle must be sufficiently mobilized to permit tendon rerouting in a straight line of pull, but obviously without injury to its neurovascular pedicle (Fig. 19-6, *C*).

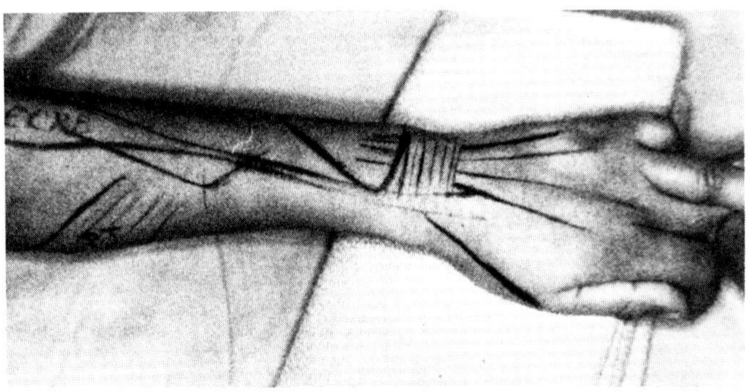

Fig. 19-2. To aid planning of incisions, surface representations of the pertinent structures can be sketched as illustrated here in transfers for a radial nerve palsy.

REROUTING THE TENDON

It is essential for future gliding that tendons be transferred only through mobile tissues such as normal subcutaneous fat. The tendon will initially heal to those tissues in contact with it, but if these tissues are themselves mobile, remodeling of the collagen according to functional demands will follow with tendon mobility. Thus tendon transfers should avoid areas of dense cicatrix, fixed fascia, or bone en route. For example, if the superficial flexor tendons of

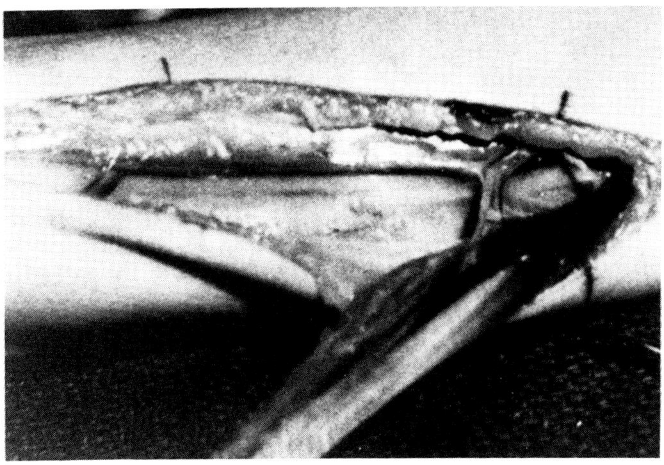

Fig. 19-3. Muscles have well-defined neurovascular pedicles that must be protected by dissection under direct vision. The neurovascular pedicle of the flexor carpi ulnaris is demonstrated.

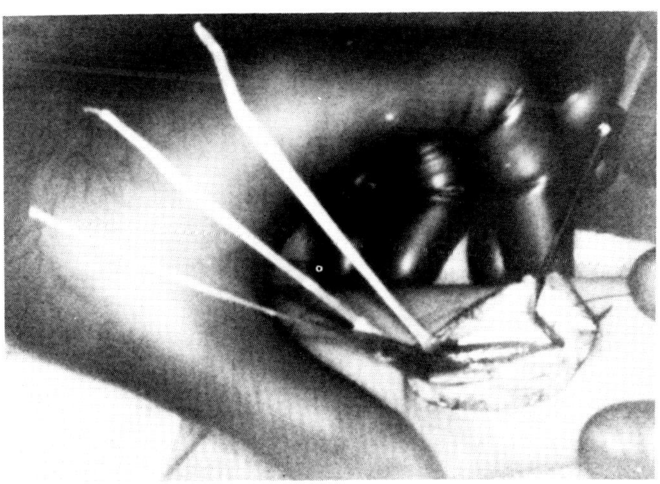

Fig. 19-4. Transferred tendons must not pass in contact with fixed fascia, periosteum, and so forth. In transfers through the interosseous membrane, the muscle proper must pass through the window created in the membrane. Illustrated are the flexor superficialis muscles of the middle, ring, and small fingers passed through the interosseous membrane to the dorsum of the distal forearm.

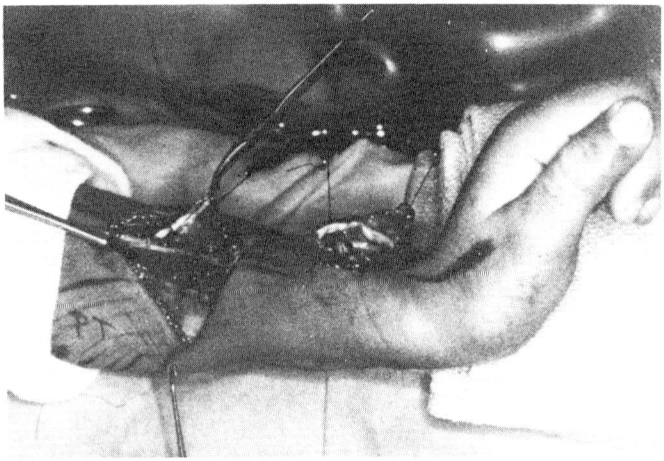

Fig. 19-5. When possible, tendon junctures are placed well under the flap to be in contact with mobile subcutaneous fat rather than incisions to which the tendon will adhere. This is illustrated by transfer of the pronator teres to the extensor carpi radialis brevis in the forearm. Note the extensor carpi radialis is being pulled well anteriorly making the site of suture in a straight line of pull being the pronator teres' origin and insertion of the extensor carpi radialis.

the fingers are to be transferred to the dorsum of the hand via the interosseous membrane, it is essential that the muscles themselves be brought through the narrow, fixed interrosseous space rather than just their tendons (Fig. 19-4). The tendon, in contact with the membrane and periosteum of the ulnar and radius, will almost invariably remain adherent to the fixed structures.

TENDON JUNCTURES

When possible, tendon junctures are done under flaps turned for exposure rather than directly under incisions (Fig. 19-5). This places them in contact with mobile subcutaneous fat to which adherence should be transient. Fixed fascia adjacent to a tendon juncture is excised. Tendons are sutured strongly with nonabsorbable monofilament material. Maximum surface contacts are sought and usually achieved by some form of interweaving technique. Pull-out wire techniques are rarely used today except for insertion of the tendon into bone. The tendons are pulled over to a straight line of pull for the juncture (Fig. 19-5). Any angle will be pulled out with use and result in the transfer's being too slack. When a tendon is being attached to a group such as the four profundi, the transfer is passed through them at the same angle as its rerouting, for a straight line between origin and new insertion (Fig. 19-6, *C* to *E*).

Adjustment of tension in tendon transfers requires much judgment and varies with each situation. Careful observation of the attitude the parts assume in relation to each other and the tenodesis effect on manipulations are the most useful aids. In radial nerve palsy, the digital transfers are done first and transfers to restore wrist extension are done last to allow this observation of the

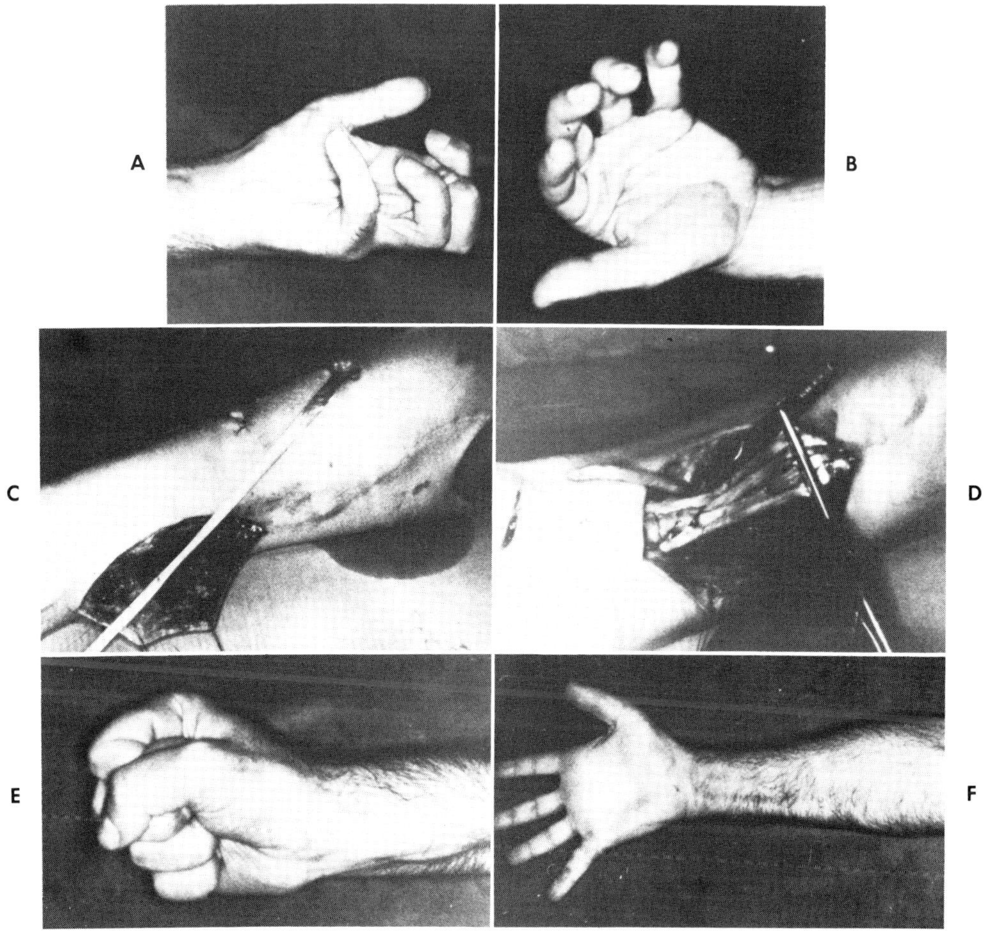

Fig. 19-6. **A,** Maximum finger flexion following infarction of antebrachial musculature with Volksman's ischemic contracture. **B,** Maximum finger extension even with the wrist flexed demonstrates the severe loss of amplitude of the damaged digital flexors. **C,** Extensor carpi radialis longus is detached at its insertion and withdrawn high in the forearm to permit surgical rerouting in a straight line of pull to its new insertion in the profundi. The extensor carpi radialis brevis, the prime wrist extensor, is left undisturbed. **D,** The extensor carpi radialis longus is passed through mobile subcutaneous tissues and woven into the combined flexor digitorum profundi group at the same angle as its rerouting. **E,** Wrist extension enhances, by tenodesis, the amplitude of the transferred extensor carpi radialis longus to give full finger flexion. **F,** With flexion of the wrist just beyond neutral, amplitude of the extensor carpi radialis longus is augmented sufficiently to allow full finger extension.

resulting finger action as the wrist is extended and flexed. Experience shows that transfers to restore wrist extension can seldom be set too tightly. In general, tendon tension of transfers should be a little tight as some rerouting is inevitable and slackens the tension proportionally.

POSTOPERATIVE CARE

Tendon transfers must be protected from disruption until there is sufficient healing to withstand their pull. The period of protective immobilization varies with the stress to which the system will be submitted, but is a minimum of 3 weeks. Tendon transfers to the extensor mechanisms require about 3 additional weeks of some protection as they are opposed by the powerful flexor muscle group. Immobilization, usually by plaster cast or occasionally internal devices, is followed initially by guarded *active* exercises, avoiding passive manipulation.

Children require special consideration with their irresponsibility usually indicating a slightly longer period of immobilization. Children under 4 years of age almost invariably require a long arm cast with the elbow flexed to 90° for protection. Their cleverness at getting out of even these casts is legendary and great care is necessary to maintain protection from their uninhibited use of the part.

Muscle reeducation following tendon transfer is rarely a problem of special effort if the restored function is highly useful. For those of marginal benefit, reeducation may never be fully achieved despite all efforts. Transferred muscles that are synergistic with their new function, such as a wrist extensor for finger flexion, are remarkably adaptable to their new job (Fig. 19-6).

20. Anomalies of muscles and their effect on tendon transfers

Morton Spinner, M.D.

Knowledge of the patterns of variations of musculotendinous units commonly used in tendon transfer procedures can be of immense value to the reconstructive upper limb surgeon. Variations of muscle belly, tendon, or insertion are of common occurrence. Muscles and tendons can be absent, hypoplastic, fused, or reduplicated.

It is my purpose to document the basic patterns of muscle variations that may be uncovered in the operating room. When found, these variations should not deter the treating surgeon. Anomalous muscles and tendons can be utilized for tendon transfers.

VARIATION OF INSERTION

Insertion is the most common of all the different types of musculotendinous anomalies. For example, the versatile extensor carpi radialis longus is an excellent transfer to restore opposition to the thumb[5] (Fig. 20-1) or flexion to the fingers.[7] It is a strong muscle with a long tendon (Fig. 20-2). However, there are considerable variations of the insertion of the extensor carpi radialis longus. Classically, this muscle has a single tendon of insertion that attaches to the base of the second metacarpal on its dorsal surface. It can have two tendons one attaching to the second metacarpal and the other to the third metacarpal base. Similarly, the extensor carpi radialis brevis usually inserts by a single tendon to the third metacarpal but may have two tendons, one inserting at its usual site and an accessory attachment by a separate tendon to the second metacarpal (Fig. 20-3, *A* and *B*).

On rare occasions the extensor carpi radialis longus may have three tendons of insertion and no extensor carpi radialis brevis.[6] Because the extensor carpi radialis brevis is the key wrist neutral dorsiflexor, it is important to preserve its function. If it is absent, then one should not remove the extensor carpi radialis longus from the dorsum of the wrist. If there is any question about these two extensors, they can be identified in the midforearm and at their insertion. A

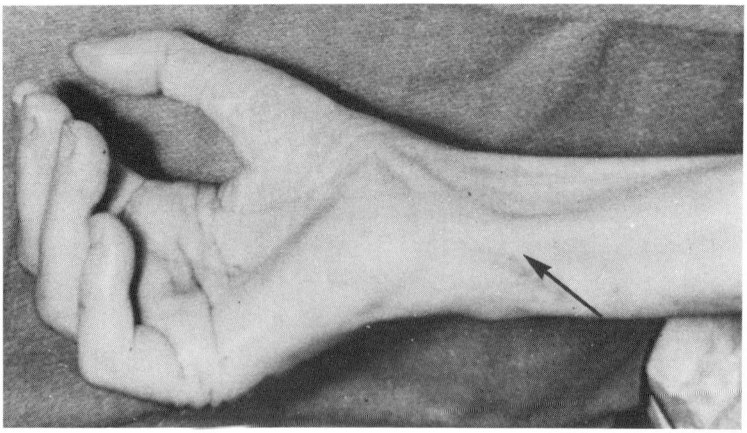

Fig. 20-1. Note the course of the extensor carpi radialis longus lengthened with a tendon graft to the thumb. It is routed subcutaneous over the distal ulnar border of the forearm (arrow).

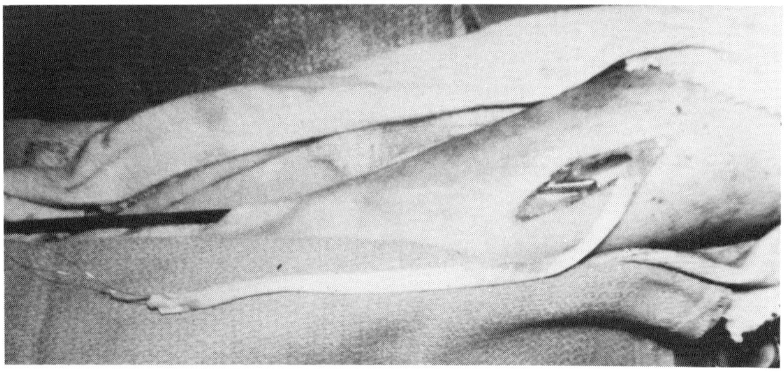

Fig. 20-2. The extensor carpi radialis longus has a long tendon. It is seen prior to its subcutaneous rerouting. It can be transferred as necessary around the radial or ulnar border of the forearm.

A

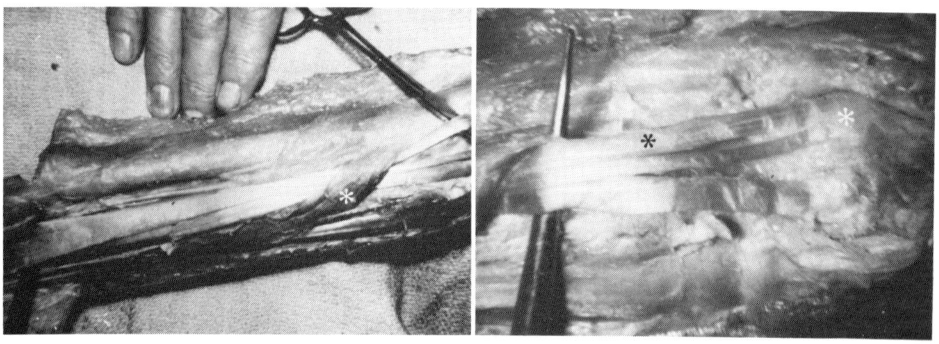

B

Fig. 20-3. A, Right forearm anatomical specimen. The hemostat is under the tendon of the extensor carpi radialis longus. Two tendons of the extensor carpi radialis brevis pass deep to the outcropping muscles of the thumb (asterisk). **B,** Close-up of the dorsoradial aspect of the hand. Two tendons are inserting into the base of the second metacarpal (white asterisk). The more radial tendon (black asterisk) is the tendon of the extensor carpi radialis longus. Of the two tendons of the extensor carpi radialis brevis, one inserts into the second metacarpal while the other attaches to the third.

radioulnar imbalance in dorsiflexion of the wrist postoperatively can thus be avoided. It should be noted that the extensor carpi radialis longus is the more radial of the two and it has the longer tendon. The musculotendinous junction of extensor carpi radialis brevis is much more distal than that of the longus. It is frequently found at the level in the distal third of the forearm where the superficial radial nerve passes from volar to the dorsoradial aspect of the forearm from deep to the brachioradialis tendon.

Other variations of the extensor carpi radialis longus have been reported—reduplication,[8] an extensor carpi radialis intermedius, and an extensor carpi radialis accessorius.[6] The latter muscle arises from the lateral epicondyle of the elbow and attaches to the first metacarpal, proximal phalanx, or adjacent thumb soft tissues (abductor pollicis brevis, flexor pollicis brevis, or first dorsal interosseus). Partial or complete fusion of the brachioradialis and the extensor carpi radialis longus also has been described.

Awareness of these variations is important in facilitating a tendon transfer procedure utilizing the extensor carpi radialis longus. Delivering this tendon from under the outcropping muscles in the distal forearm is made easier by identifying the extensor carpi radialis longus and brevis proximally and distally. The tendon can be delivered into the proximal wound by detaching the single or double insertion (Fig. 20-3, *A*).

At times even without these anomalies being present there exists either a firm synovial attachment or tendinous connections between the two radial wrist extensors within the second extensor compartment and under the outcropping muscles. To deliver the tendon of the extensor carpi radialis longus proximally it is then necessary to separate the tendon of the longus from the brevis in its distal 4 cm. to 5 cm. It then can be rerouted radially to attach it to the flexors anteriorly, or it can be lengthened with a graft and passed ulnarly to the thumb

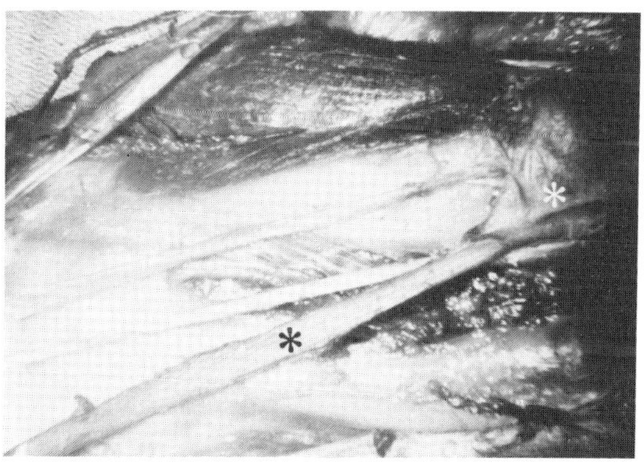

Fig. 20-4. Close-up of the dorsoradial aspect of the hand of another anatomical specimen. The extensor digitorum communis tendon to the index finger (black asterisk) is retracted. Bifid extensor indicis proprius tendons are demonstrated, attaching to both the radial and ulnar aspects of the extensor hood mechanism (white asterisk) of the index finger.

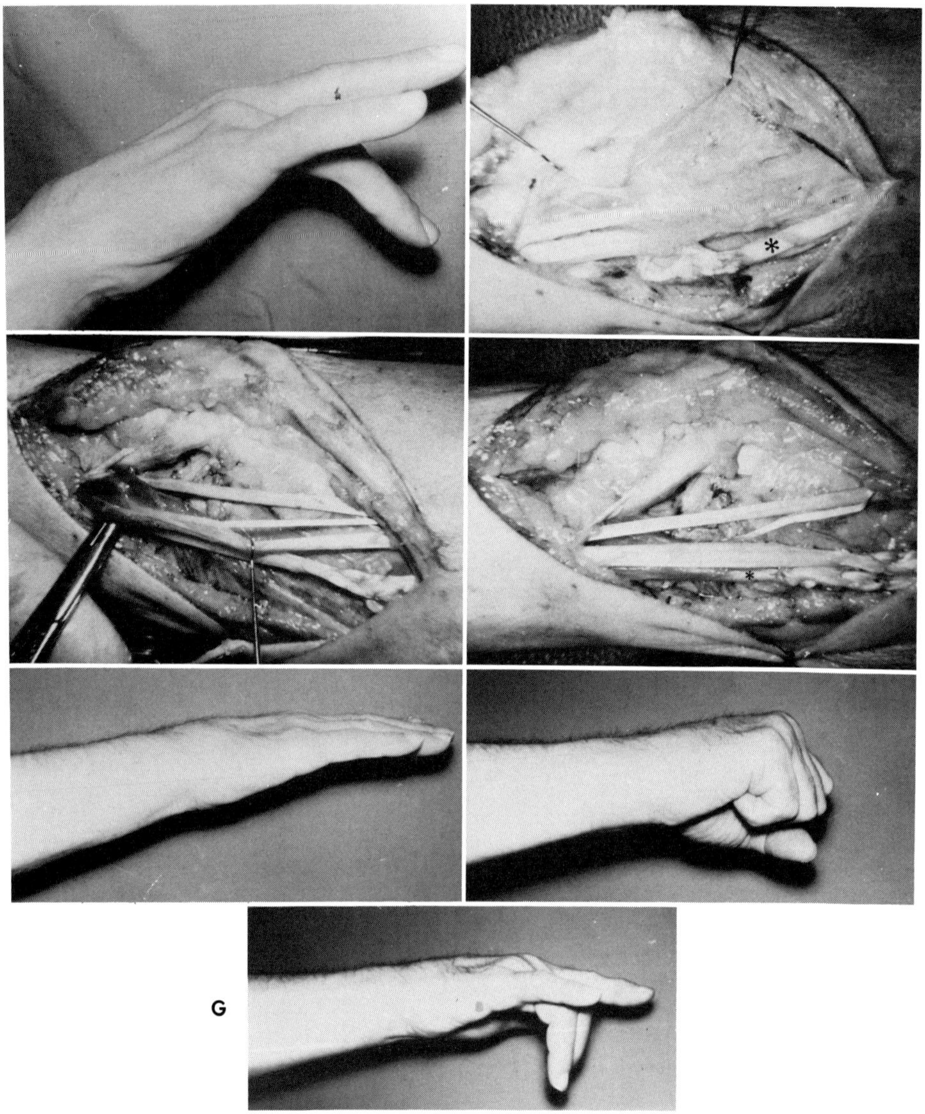

Fig. 20-5. A, A 46-year-old butcher sustained a spontaneous rupture of the common extensor tendon to the right ring finger over a bony prominence that was secondary to an old fracture-subluxation of the wrist. **B,** The ruptured extensor tendon of the ring finger (asterisk) is visualized. **C,** The hemostat is under the extensor indicis proprius. The hook demonstrates the bifid tendon of this muscle. The distal ring finger ruptured tendon stump has been woven into the intact common extensor tendon of the long finger. **D,** The tendon transfer is completed. One tendon of the bifid extensor indicis proprius has been sutured to the ruptured extensor communis tendon of the ring finger. **E,** Full extension of the fingers and **F,** full flexion was obtained postoperative. **G,** The patient could still utilize the remaining extensor indicis proprius tendon slip to extend the index finger and the extensor digiti quinti to extend the little finger.

for opposition. Similarly lengthened with multistrand grafts, it can be passed distally through the intermetacarpal spaces, then anterior to the intermetacarpal ligaments to be attached to the proximal phalanx or extensor hood mechanism for intrinsic muscle replacement.

VARIATIONS OF TENDON

The extensor indicis proprius usually attaches by a single tendon to the extensor hood mechanism on the ulnar side of the common extensor tendon. On occasion this tendon may be bifid attaching to the extensor mechanism at the metacarpophalangeal level of the index finger both radial and ulnar to the common extensor tendon (Fig. 20-4). When this is found one of the bifid tendons can be used for tendon transfer (Fig. 20-5).

Variations in tendons occur on the ulnar side of the dorsum of the hand as well. These become important when transferring the extensor digiti quinti. It has a double tendon in 84% of limbs. It can even have a triple tendon (Fig. 20-6). This latter variation has been reported in 7% of hands.[9] The presence of these variations is important when reestablishing the balance in the digitis, as in an ulnar clawhand as recommended by Fowler (Fig. 20-7).[4]

VARIATIONS OF MUSCLE BELLY

The extensor indicis proprius most recently has been recommended by Burkhalter for opponensplasty.[2] There are numerous variations of the extensor indicis

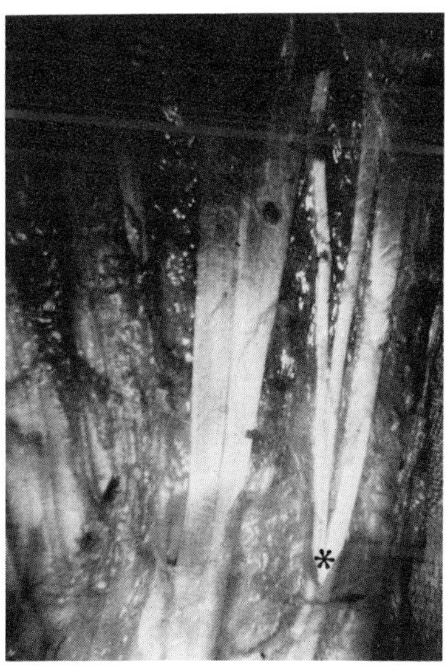

Fig. 20-6. The dorsoulnar aspect of an anatomical specimen of a right hand. The extensor digiti quinti (asterisk) has three tendons that pass through the fifth extensor compartment of the wrist. The radial slip attached to the ring finger while the two ulnar tendons passed to the little finger.

A B C D E F

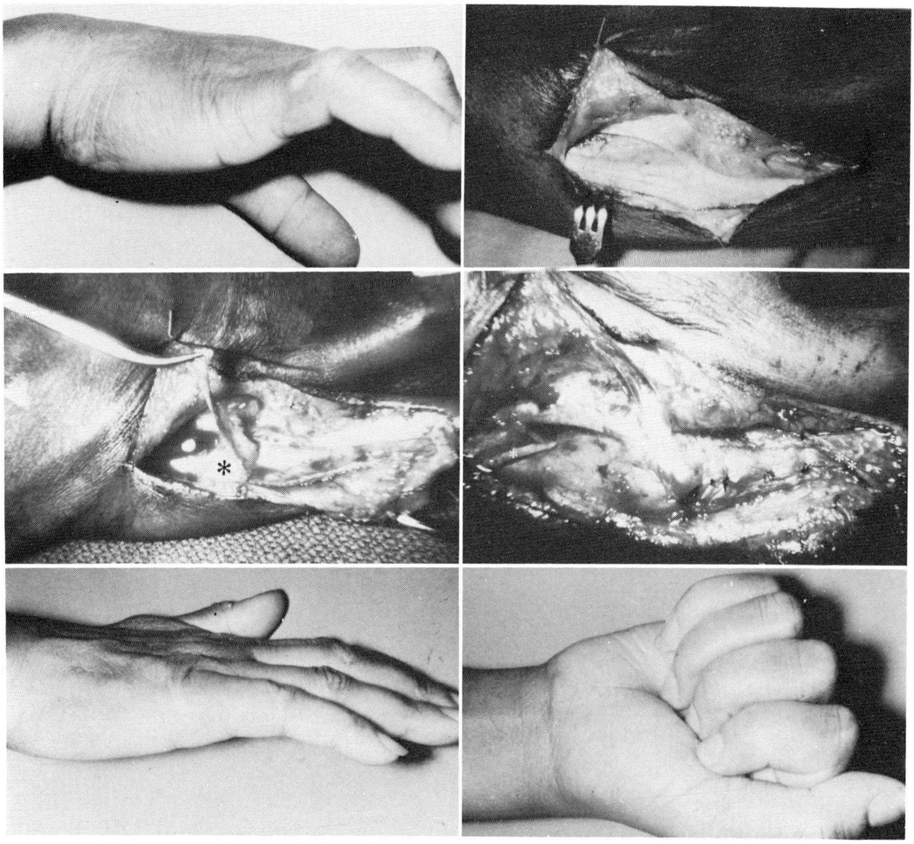

Fig. 20-7. A, A 50-year-old woman with an ulnar claw of the right hand. **B,** Note the numerous tendons attaching to the extensor hood mechanism of the little finger. **C,** Extra length of the extensor digiti quinti (asterisk) for Fowler transfer has been obtained by mobilizing a portion of extensor hood mechanism (in the hemostat). **D,** The extensor hood mechanism has been repaired over the proximal phalanx. One slip of the digiti quinti to the little finger (single white asterisk) has been passed through the intermetacarpal space and anterior to the intermetacarpal ligament to be sutured to the extensor hood mechanism distally (two white asterisks) at the proper tension. **E,** Postoperative extension attitude of the hand reveals the clawing to have been corrected. **F,** Full flexion of the digits has been maintained.

proprius. One that I recently encountered was an extensor indicis proprius with an extensor medius proprius. Both were utilized for the tendon transfer to obtain opposition (Fig. 20-8).

Musculotendinous units may be absent completely. On occasion just the muscle or its tendon may be absent.

A musculotendinous unit may be *hypoplastic.* A hypoplastic flexor digitorum superficialis of the little finger is present in 5% of hands. Laceration of just the flexor digitorum profundus of the little finger may be observed with inability to flex not only the distal interphalangeal joint but the proximal interphalangeal joint as well.[3] This is probably due to an underdeveloped flexor digitorum

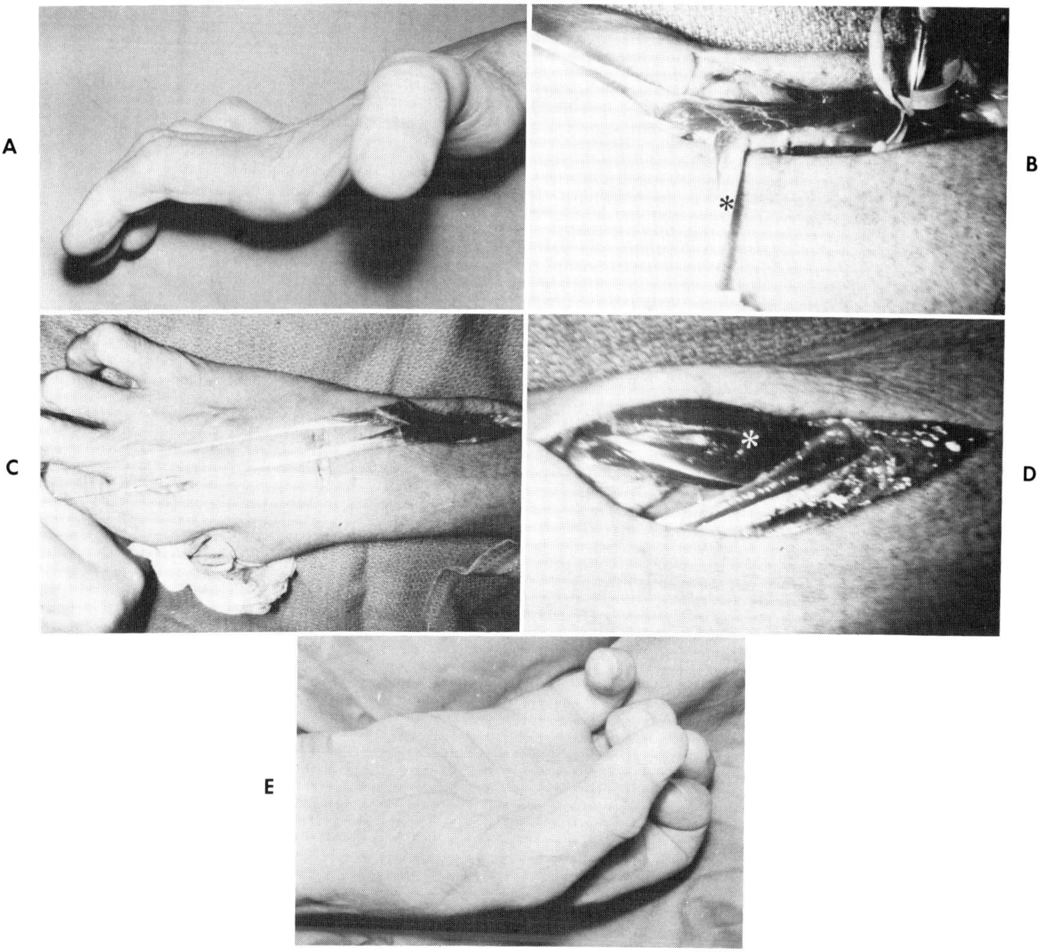

Fig. 20-8. A, A 56-year-old man with a combined median and ulnar nerve paralysis of his right hand. **B,** For the opponensplasty procedure the anomalous musculature is observed on the dorsoulnar aspect of the distal forearm. The extensor indicis proprius tendon (asterisk) has been brought out of the forearm incision. Another muscle, the extensor medius proprius, (in the distal rubber band) is seen passing into the dorsum of the hand. **C,** A distinct view of the anomalous muscle, the extensor medius proprius is seen with the extensor indicis proprius. **D,** Both muscles (asterisk) have been transferred around the ulnar border of the distal forearm. **E,** Postoperative opposition of the thumb is strong. In addition to the transfer the metacarpophalangeal joint of the thumb was arthrodesed.

superficialis. This can be tested by keeping the index, long, and ring fingers in full extension and asking the patient to flex the little finger. A hypoplastic flexor digitorum superficialis is demonstrated if the patient can flex the proximal interphalangeal joint of the little finger. The mechanism for this response is probably on the basis of checkreining the lacerated flexor profundus. Its lumbrical is also weakened. The extensor force of the cut flexor digitorum profundus

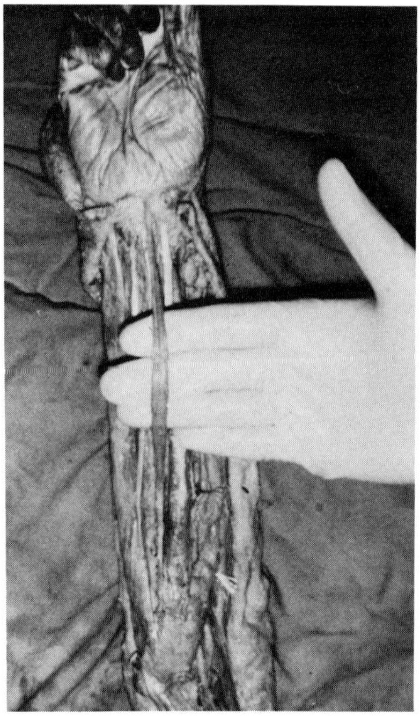

Fig. 20-9. Right forearm anatomical specimen. The muscle of this palmaris longus is seen in the midforearm. It arises by a short tendon from the medial epicondyle and distally has a short tendon of insertion.

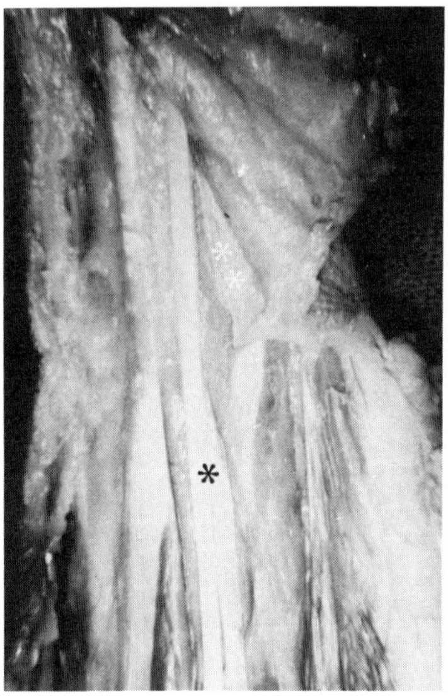

Fig. 20-10. Left forearm anatomical specimen. The palmaris longus is bifid (black asterisk). The ulnar tendon of the bifid palmaris longus attaches distally to the forearm antebrachial fascia (two white asterisks) while the radial one passes to the palmar aponeurosis.

through the lumbrical to the extensor mechanism is thus blocked. The hypoplastic flexor digitorum superficialis can then flex the proximal interphalangeal joint of the little finger when the adjacent fingers are held in extension.

TENDON GRAFT DONOR VARIATIONS

Variations of the palmaris longus occurs in 12% of upper limbs. Its total absence is most frequent. The palmaris longus muscle usually arises proximally from the medial epicondyle. On occasion it may arise and insert by a tendon with its muscle in the midforearm (Fig. 20-9). Awareness of a variation of this type is important for the palmaris longus tendon is often a source of a tendon graft. Knowledge of the occurrence of this anomaly can avoid the frustration of obtaining a short unusable tendon graft when the belly of the palmaris is observed extending into the distal third of the forearm. The extreme of this variation occurs when the entire palmaris attaches as a muscle to the flexor retinaculum and arises as a tendon from the medial epicondyle.

Another variant is a bifid palmaris longus, which occurs in 3% of limbs. One tendon frequently attaches to the palmar aponeurosis and the other one attaches to the antebrachial fascia in the distal forearm (Fig. 20-10). This clinically is of importance when one is obtaining a palmaris longus tendon graft. Knowledge of the accessory antebrachial attachment and the bifid tendon allows accurate retrieval of the palmaris longus tendon with its bifid without damaging the tendon graft.

In conclusion, the existence of a particular anomaly cannot in most instances be determined before surgery. Therefore, in planning for a specific operative procedure one should include a review of the possible variations that may be encountered. Reference books, specifically dealing with this subject, like Le Double,[6] Testut,[11] Macalister,[8] Shäfer et al.,[10] and Anson[1] are highly recommended. Analysis of this type will enable the surgeon to recognize and manage the unexpected. This additional preoperative preparation can only yield the best possible end-result for the patient and satisfaction for the treating surgeon.

References

1. Anson, B.: An atlas of human anatomy, Philadelphia, 1963, W. B. Saunders Co.
2. Burkhalter, W., Christensen, R. C., and Brown, P.: Extensor indicis proprius opponensplasty, J. Bone Joint Surg. **55A**:725, 1973.
3. Dolich, B. H., Schultz, R. J., and Kaplan, E. B.: The posttraumatic "lumbrical plus" finger: etiology and treatment, Bull. Hosp. Joint Dis. **34**:107, 1973.
4. Enna, C. D., and Riordan, D. C.: The Fowler procedure for correction of the paralytic claw hand, Plast. Reconstr. Surg. **52**:352, 1973.
5. Henderson, E. D.: Transfer of wrist extensors and brachioradialis to restore opposition of the thumb, J. Bone Joint Surg. **44A**:513, 1962.
6. Le Double, A. F.: Traité des variations du système musculaire de l'homme, Paris, 1897, Schleicher.
7. Littler, J. W.: Principles of reconstructive plastic surgery, In Converse, J. M., editor: Reconstructive plastic surgery, Philadelphia, 1964, W. B. Saunders Co., p. 1635.

8. Macalister, A.: Additional observations on muscular anomalies in human anatomy (third series), Tr. Royal Irish Academy **25:**1, 1875.
9. Schenck, R. R.: Variations of the extensor tendons of the fingers. Surgical significance, J. Bone Joint Surg. **46A:**103, 1964.
10. Shäfer, E. A., Symington, J., and Bryce, T. H., editors: Quain's Elements of anatomy, ed. 2, Vol. 4, Part 2, New York, 1923, Longman, Inc.
11. Testut, L.: Les anomalies musculaires chez l'homme, Paris, 1884, Masson & Cie Editeurs.

21. Surgical treatment of the clawhand

Richard J. Smith, M.D.

Paralysis of the intrinsic muscles of the fingers will cause deformity, weakness, and asynchronous metacarpophalangeal and interphalangeal joint motion. Active control of lateral deviation of the fingers is also affected. In planning treatment for the hand with intrinsic muscle paralysis, each of these factors must be evaluated; each may demand correction.

Deformity. In the normal hand, the tendons of the interosseus and of the lumbrical muscles (plus the abductor digiti quinti and flexor digiti quinti brevis) form the *lateral bands* at either side of the metacarpophalangeal joint. *Transverse fibers* from the lateral band arch over the dorsum of the proximal phalanx at its middle third and serve as the principal and primary flexors of the metacarpophalangeal joint.

Extension of the metacarpophalangeal joint is achieved entirely by the long extensors: the extensor digitorum communis, the extensor indicis proprius, and the extensor digiti quinti proprius. Each of these tendons is surrounded by a sling of sagittal fibers that passes between the metacarpophalangeal joint capsule and the lateral band to insert at the lateral edge of the volar plate and onto the periosteum at the base of the proximal phalanx. The *sagittal bands* lift the proximal phalanx into extension.[23] If intrinsic muscle function is eliminated because of paralysis, the extensor tendons lift the proximal phalanx unrestricted and unbalanced by opposing flexors. The volar plate is stretched, the metacarpophalangeal joint hyperextends, and the sagittal bands tether the extensor tendons to the metacarpophalangeal joint.[20] Both the excursion and the force of the extensor tendon distal to the metacarpophalangeal joint are thus limited.

The *oblique fibers* of the lateral bands that spiral over the distal third of the proximal phalanx and the *central slip* of the extensor tendon insert at the base of the middle phalanx and contribute to proximal interphalangeal joint extension. The *terminal tendon* is formed at the distal third of the middle phalanx and is the ultimate confluence of the intrinsic muscles and extensor tendons. It extends the distal interphalangeal joint. Therefore, if the intrinsic muscles are paralyzed, and if the distal excursion and force of the long extensors is diminished because of metacarpophalangeal joint hyperextension, interphalangeal joint extension is

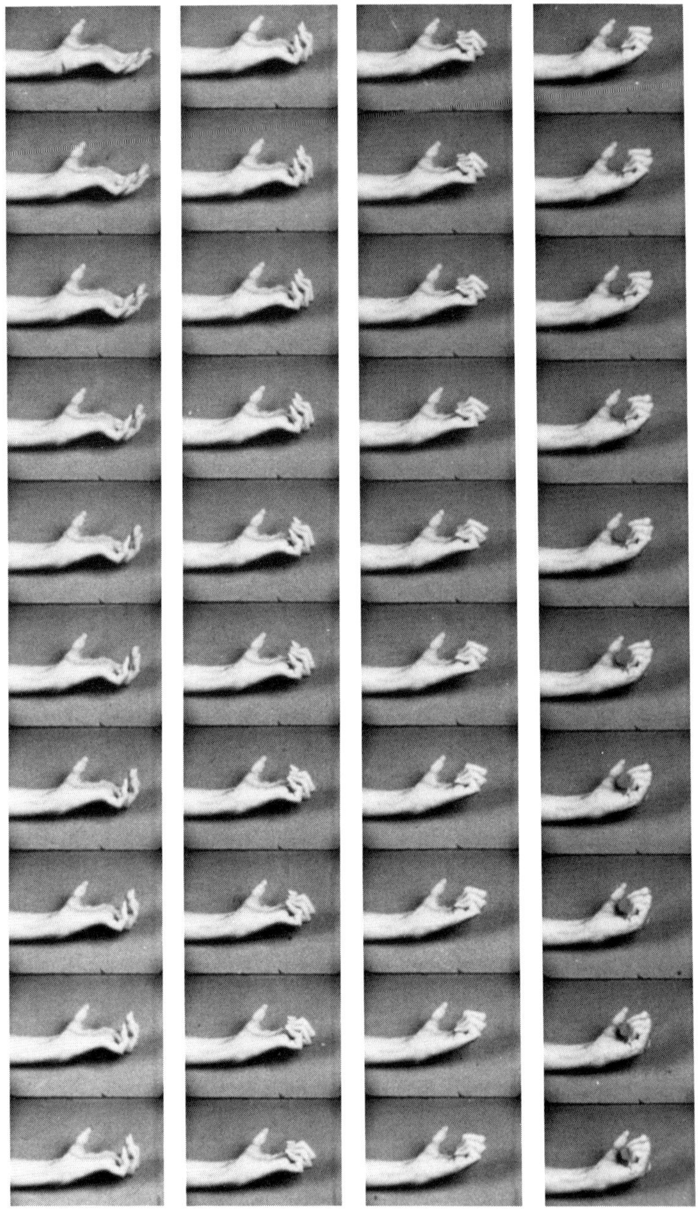

Fig. 21-1. Copy of a 16 mm motion picture strip of a patient with intrinsic palsy flexing her fingers. Notice how the fingers flex from the clawed position. Proximal and distal interphalangeal joints flex first. Only after full interphalangeal joint flexion has been achieved does flexion occur at the metacarpophalangeal joints.

A B C D

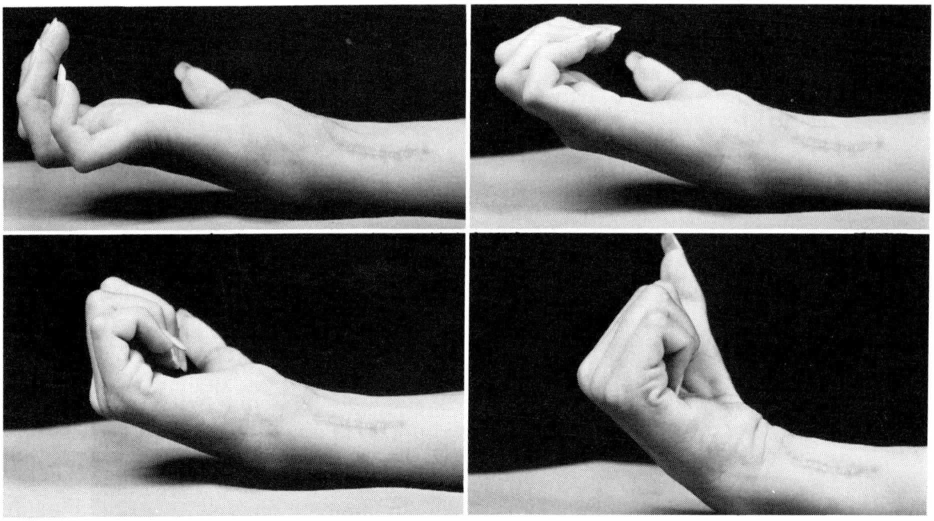

Fig. 21-2. Still photographs taken in rapid succession of a patient with complete intrinsic palsy flexing her fingers. An opposition tendon transfer had previously been performed. **A,** With attempts at full extension all fingers are clawed and the wrist is mildly palmar flexed. **B,** Flexion is initiated at the proximal and distal interphalangeal joints. The metacarpophalangeal joints remain extended. **C,** After the interphalangeal joints are fully flexed, the metacarpophalangeal joints are flexed by the flexor digitorum profundus and superficialis. **D,** The fingers now tightly clench within the palm through the action of the flexor digitorum profundus and superficialis. Note that with strong flexion, the flexor superficialis of the ring finger that had been transferred to the thumb for opposition becomes active.

weakened. The flexor digitorum superficialis and flexor digitorum profundus will curl these joints into moderate flexion.[24] The finger will claw (Figs. 21-1 and 21-2). In a subconscious attempt to gain greater power and excursion of the long extensors of the interphalangeal joints, the patient will palmar flex the wrist (Thomas' sign),[18] which merely exaggerates the metacarpophalangeal joint hyperextension deformity.

If the flexor digitorum superficialis (FDS) and flexor digitorum profundus (FDP) are paralyzed in addition to the intrinsics, as with high ulnar and median nerve palsy, the long extensors have no effective interphalangeal joint antagonist and can then fully extend all the joints of the fingers. In these patients there is no deformity (Fig. 21-3, *A*). In contrast, if the FDS and FDP are tight, as in Volkmann's ischemic contracture, the claw deformity will be most severe since the wrist and interphalangeal joints will be drawn into extreme palmar flexion (Fig. 21-3, *B*).

In patients with normal median nerve function but with paralysis of the ulnar innervated muscles, there will be clawing of only the ring and little fingers. The radial two lumbricals are innervated by the median nerve and can prevent deformity of the index and middle fingers.

Weakness. Considering their small size, the intrinsic muscles of the fingers

A 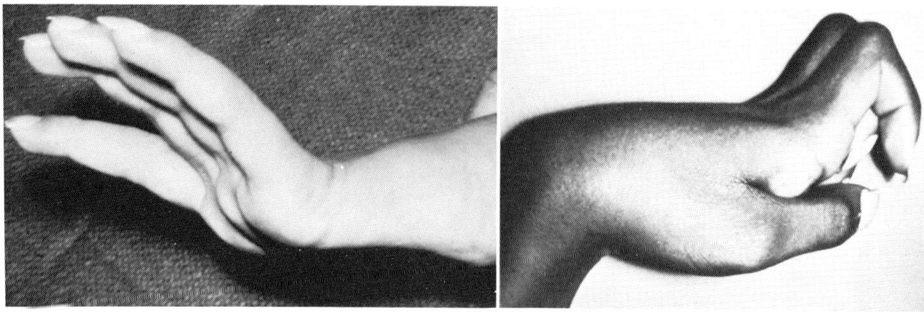 B

Fig. 21-3. The degree of clawing that occurs with intrinsic palsy is dependent upon the integrity and tone of the flexor digitorum profundus and superficialis. **A,** This patient has total absence of the intrinsic muscles of the hand and of the flexor digitorum profundus and superficialis. The fingers do not claw despite metacarpophalangeal hyperextension. Full extension of the interphalangeal joints can be achieved through the common extensor tendons. **B,** With Volkmann's ischemic contracture of the finger and wrist flexors, associated with intrinsic paralysis, the claw deformity is most severe. The common extensor tendons are unable to overcome the force of the tightened flexors at the interphalangeal joints.

might be thought to contribute little to the power of grip. Surprisingly, the grip strength of the hand with total intrinsic muscle palsy is often decreased by as much as 60% to 80% when compared with the normal side.[7, 18] Whereas the excursion of a muscle is proportionate to the length of its fibers, its strength is related to the effective cross sectional area of its fibers. A workman with intrinsic palsy may thus be seriously handicapped by the weakness following loss of intrinsic muscle power.

Asynchronous motion. Although a supple metacarpophalangeal joint can be flexed fully in the absence of active intrinsic muscles, this flexion occurs only after the interphalangeal joints are fully flexed. The fingers curl into the hand (Figs. 21-1 and 21-2). Grasping a large object is difficult as the arc described by the flexing fingertips remains small. Simultaneous flexion of the metacarpophalangeal joint with the interphalangeal joints is necessary for normal prehension of a large sphere. Similarly, many types of fine pulp-to-pulp or pulp-to-side pinch require extension of the interphalangeal joints while the metacarpophalangeal joints are flexed.[14] Without intrinsic muscle function this control is lost, and a small coin must be retrieved from a flat surface by awkward tip-to-tip pinch that often proves frustrating or ineffective. When the ability to perform simultaneous MP flexion–IP flexion or MP flexion–IP extension is lost with intrinsic palsy, prehension is seriously compromised for both small and large objects (Fig. 21-4).

Loss of abduction-adduction control. The shape of the metacarpophalangeal joints causes the fingers to automatically diverge with extension and converge with flexion. The collateral ligaments tighten when the fingers are flexed and prevent both active and passive lateral deviation in this position. In extension, however, these ligaments are slack. The interossei, the abductor digiti quinti,

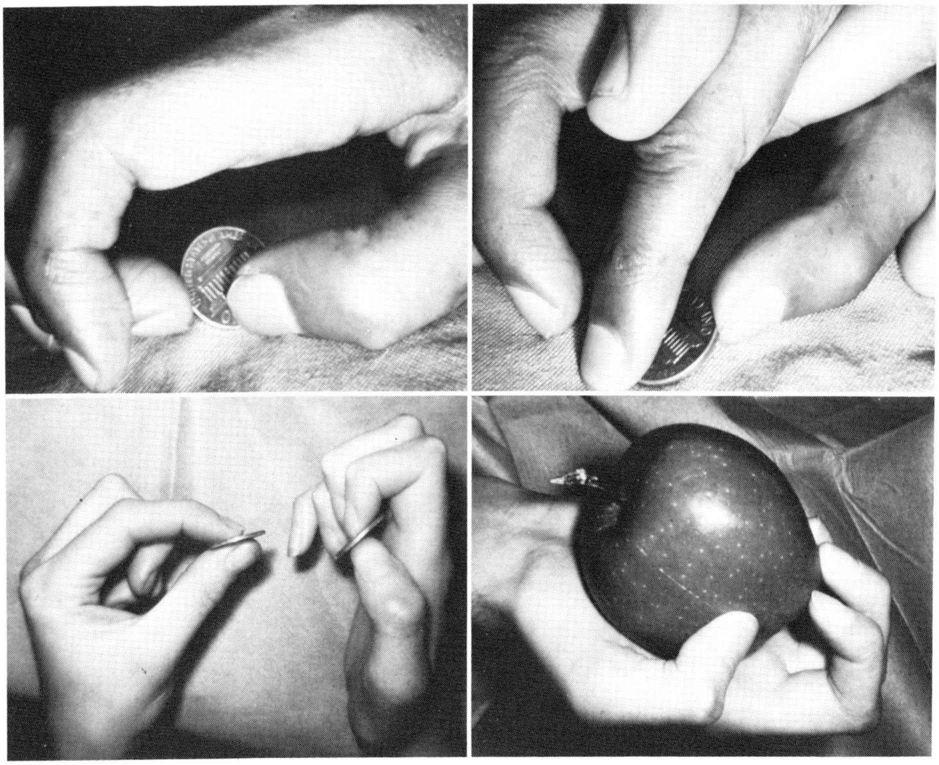

A B C D

Fig. 21-4. In the hand with intrinsic paralysis, prehension is awkward. **A,** Retrieval of small objects from a table top is difficult if the ability to simultaneously flex the metacarpophalangeal joint and extend the interphalangeal joints is lost. **B,** If the metacarpophalangeal joint is held passively flexed, the interphalangeal joints can extend and the small coin can readily be retrieved. **C,** Without simultaneous metacarpophalangeal flexion and interphalangeal extension, pulp-to-pulp pinch (as seen in the left hand) is difficult. Small objects are held with tip-to-tip pinch (as seen on the right) and are less secure. **D,** With intrinsic muscle paralysis the fingers push a large object from the hand before it can be surrounded and grasped.

and the flexor digiti quinti brevis are the only muscles that can actively control lateral deviation. With intrinsic muscle paralysis, this control is lost. Consequently, there is weakness of pinch and of three-point chuck grip. Absence of lateral motion in the ulnar two fingers is less disabling and is manifest mainly by abduction of the little finger in extension (Wartenberg's sign)[18] caused by the unopposed ulnar and dorsal traction of the extensor digiti quinti proprius upon the fifth metacarpophalangeal joint.

TREATMENT OF THE HAND WITH INTRINSIC MUSCLE PARALYSIS

There are many methods by which the hand with intrinsic palsy may be treated. Each method has as its goal correcting the disability that results from one or more of the abnormalities already noted:

1. Claw deformity
2. Loss of grip strength
3. Asynchronous motion
   a. Loss of simultaneous MP flexion–IP flexion
   b. Loss of simultaneous MP flexion–IP extension
4. Loss of abduction-adduction control

Ideally, we would like to correct all these abnormalities. Practically, however, we must determine which features are most disabling in the patient we are to treat. We must then choose the procedure that is most applicable considering the disability and the cause of the intrinsic paralysis.

The procedures that have been recommended in the treatment of fingers with intrinsic muscle palsy may be classified into three groups: (1) procedures to prevent or correct metacarpophalangeal joint hyperextension; (2) procedures to provide active flexion of the metacarpophalangeal joints, or simultaneous flexion of the metacarpophalangeal and extension of the interphalangeal joints; and (3) procedures to restore abduction of the index finger. Rarely should a surgical procedure be performed unless all joints are supple. Splints, serial casts, physical therapy, or capsulectomy may be employed to loosen tight ligaments. Tendon transfers may be performed only when the passive joint motion achieved would be considered satisfactory for good function if it could be performed actively.

Procedures to prevent or correct metacarpophalangeal joint hyperextension

With intrinsic muscle paralysis, full proximal interphalangeal joint extension can usually be achieved if metacarpophalangeal joint hyperextension is prevented. With longstanding posterior interphalangeal flexion deformity, however, the central slip of the common extensor tendon may become so attenuated and lengthened over the dorsum of the proximal interphalangeal joint that the common extensor tendon can no longer extend the middle phalanx even if MP hyperextension is prevented. The competence of the central slip can be tested by passively holding the metacarpophalangeal joint in flexion and requesting the patient to actively extend the proximal interphalangeal joint. If full extension is possible, one may expect that preventing MP hyperextension will correct the claw deformity. Under such circumstances, one of the following methods of treatment may be employed to correct the deformity.

Splints. The *dorsal knuckle bender* is an "active" splint constructed with padded bars over the dorsum of the metacarpal shafts and proximal phalanges and counterpressure in the palm of the hand just proximal to the metacarpophalangeal joints. Rubber bands are applied to provide gentle pressure over the proximal phalangeal bar. With appropriate tension on the rubber bands, full metacarpophalangeal joint extension can be achieved.[9] The splint suffers from being somewhat bulky, cumbersome, and conspicuous. It can correct the claw deformity, may mildly increase the strength of grip (proportionate to the tension on the rubber bands), and provides independent MP flexion regardless of IP position. It does not affect the abduction or adduction of the fingers.

A

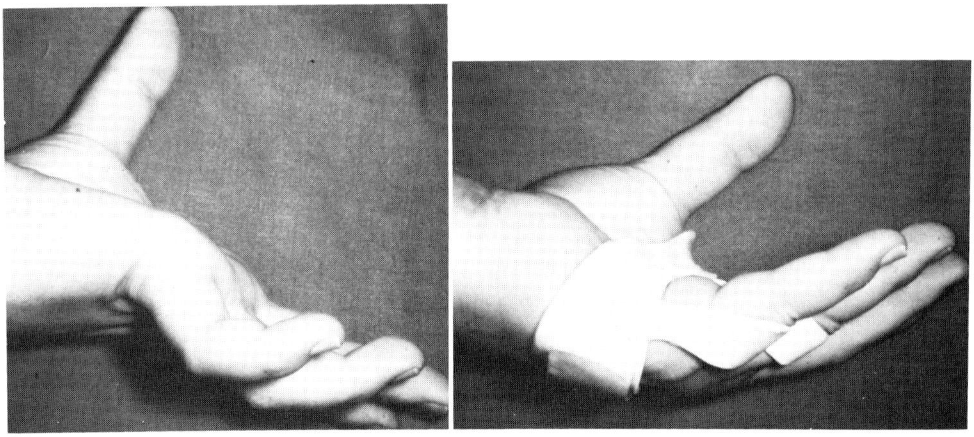

B

Fig. 21-5. A, This patient has a claw deformity of the ring and little fingers due to a low ulnar nerve palsy. **B,** A dorsal static splint prevents metacarpophalangeal joint hyperextension and corrects the deformity. This achieves the same effect as a volar capsulorrhaphy.

The *lumbrical bar* is a small static dorsal splint that prevents hyperextension of the metacarpophalangeal joints. It may be placed to hold these joints in about 25° of flexion. (The term "lumbrical bar" is somewhat of a misnomer as MP flexion is not primarily produced by the lumbricals.[17]) The splint is light, less awkward, and less conspicuous than the knuckle bender. Although it corrects the claw deformity, it does not increase grip strength or aid in MP joint flexion (Fig. 21-5).

Surgical procedures to prevent MP joint hyperextension. Many surgical procedures have been recommended to prevent hyperextension of the proximal phalanx. These include the insertion of a dorsal bone block, tightening of the volar plate, and the construction of a volar check ligament.

The dorsal bone block procedure[19] has fallen into disfavor. Failure following resorption of the bone block and joint complications resulting from osteotomy of the articular cartilage of the metacarpal head are such that the procedure is rarely used today.

Volar capsulorrhaphy[26] was recommended by Zancolli (Fig. 21-6, *A*). Through a volar incision, the proximal pully is opened and the flexor tendons are retracted. A transverse incision is made in the volar plate under the metacarpal head, and two longitudinal incisions are made distally from the margins of the transverse incision. The volar plate is then advanced proximally and is resutured into its new position to produce a mild flexion contracture of the metacarpophalangeal joint. With MP hyperextension prevented, interphalangeal joint extension can be achieved through the central slip. The claw deformity is corrected.

Several modifications of Zancolli's technique have been suggested to prevent gradual stretching of the resutured capsule and recurrence of the deformity.[7, 9, 15] Excision of an ellipse of skin and subcutaneous tissue 1.5 cm. wide from the midpalm may prevent stretching of the resutured capsule postoperatively. Some

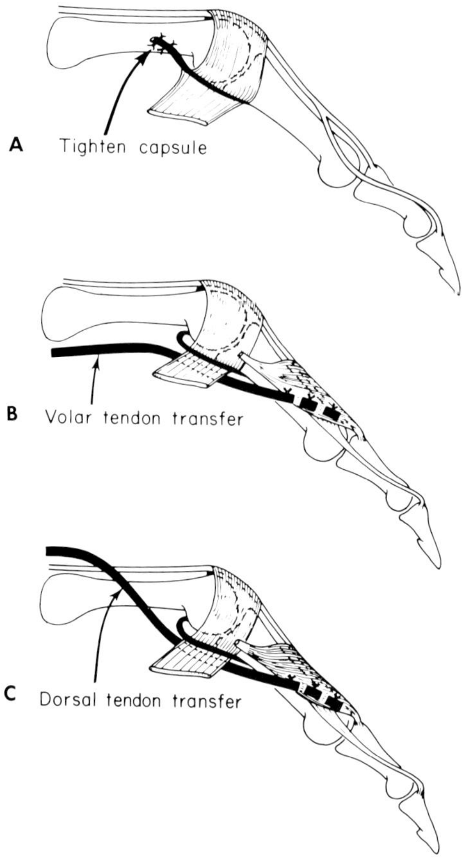

Fig. 21-6. Diagrams of three means by which clawed fingers may be surgically treated. **A,** The volar capsule may be tightened to correct metacarpophalangeal joint hyperextension. **B,** A tendon transfer may be passed through the carpal canal, volar to the deep transverse metacarpal ligament and sutured to the lateral band. **C,** A tendon transfer may be passed from the dorsum of the hand, through the intermetacarpal spaces, then volar to the deep transverse metacarpal ligament and finally to the lateral side of the finger and the lateral band.

have advised inserting the advanced volar plate into the metacarpal neck by use of a pull-out wire. The flexed proximal phalanx is held in place with a dorsal splint for a minimum of 6 weeks, during which time the interphalangeal joints are actively exercised. This volar plate advancement also may be combined with a pully advancement (described below).

The metacarpophalangeal joint may be held in flexion by means of a tenodesis. Parkes[21] attaches a tendon graft proximally to the transverse volar ligament and distally attaches it to the lateral band of each finger. Riordan[22] divides the extensor carpi radialis longus and the extensor carpi ulnaris longitudinally from their insertion to the juncture of the middle and distal thirds of the forearm. One half of each of the divided tendons is further split longitudinally. Each of the four tendon strands to be transferred is still attached at its metacarpal insertion. The free ends are then passed between the metacarpals, volar to the deep transverse metacarpal ligament, and sutured to the radial lateral bands of the clawed fingers.

These procedures all correct the claw deformity. They restore full interphalangeal joint extension through the extensor digitorum communis if its central slip is not stretched and if the proximal interphalangeal joint remains mobile. These procedures do not increase the power of grip. They do not provide simultaneous MP flexion-IP flexion or MP flexion-IP extension. None provides active lateral deviation of the fingers. In addition, the volar capsulorrhaphy or checkrein reconstruction often produces a mild to moderate flexion contracture of the metacarpophalangeal joint. This is not usually disabling. Many patients, however, find the contracture disconcerting and assume the distressing habit of attempting to gradually stretch the reconstructed volar plate or check ligament by passive extension exercises.

To their advantage, these operations do not require the transfer of a muscle-tendon unit. They are therefore of great advantage in patients with diffuse paralysis of the upper limb with claw deformity and with few motors available for transfer. In the case of severely clawed ring and little fingers with low ulnar nerve palsy, a volar capsulorrhaphy may be indicated at the time of nerve repair. The deformity is corrected, and interphalangeal joint contracture with resulting attenuation of the central slip is prevented while the patient awaits reinnervation of the intrinsic muscles to these digits.

The middle-aged working man with an ulnar (and median) nerve injury may not develop severe clawing because of the thickness and strength of his volar plates. His chief complaint is likely to be weakness of grip and pinch. Capsulorrhaphy or construction of volar check ligaments would appear to offer little help. Any patient whose complaints of awkwardness of pinch or grasp are caused by lack of independent MP joint flexion may find the results of these surgical procedures somewhat disappointing. Lastly, those patients in whom IP joint extension cannot be achieved even when the MP joints are flexed, may be somewhat disappointed by the results of capsulorrhaphy. Such patients have had weakening of the extensors of the proximal interphalangeal joints that demands correction by active transfers.

Surgical procedures to provide active flexion of the metacarpophalangeal joints (and extension of the interphalangeal joints)

Many procedures have been described to enable the patient with intrinsic palsy to actively flex the metacarpophalangeal joints. Most of these procedures also restore active interphalangeal joint extension. Active control of the metacarpophalangeal (and interphalangeal) joints may be achieved through tendon transfers or through an active tenodesis (a tenodesis that is under the active control of a more proximal joint). In all these procedures, the tendon passes volar to the deep transverse metacarpal ligament. With few exceptions the tendon is attached distally to the lateral bands.

The Bunnell pully advancement.[9] The Bunnell pully advancement is the only one of this group of surgical operations that is neither tendon transfer nor tenodesis. The principle of the procedure is to alter the mechanics of flexion of the FDP and FDS in such a way that they become active flexors of the metacarpophalangeal joint. Each side of the proximal pully is split 1.5 cm. to 2.5 cm., up to the middle of the proximal phalanx "until the pull of the flexor tendon flexes the metacarpophalangeal joint 'well.'"[9] The split flap of proximal pully is not excised but is allowed to remain in place so that the flexor tendons do not become scarred or adherent to the overlying skin. The flexor profundus and superficialis will bowstring. These bowstringing tendons will flex the proximal phalanx by the force they exert at the pulley underlying the neck of the proximal phalanx. Thus, the moment arm at the proximal phalanx will be increased. The pully advancement procedure will not be effective when the MP joint is hyperextended, because the tendons must bowstring across a partially flexed MP joint before they can function.[4] Thus the procedure does not initiate MP joint flexion with a claw deformity. For this reason, some authors[15] use the pully advancement procedure only in conjunction with volar capsulorraphy (Zancolli's procedure).

The pully advancement procedure may increase the power of MP joint flexion, but only with an accompanying decrease of power of IP flexion. Certainly the strength of the long flexors is not increased by pully advancement; their power is merely distributed to all three joints of the finger. The procedure does not restore independent MP flexion-IP flexion. It does not control active lateral deviation of the fingers.

The pully advancement procedure appears most valuable in conjunction with volar capsulorrhaphy. As capsulorrhaphy requires division of the proximal pully, the Bunnell pully advancement adds very little in operating time and has the advantage of restoring synchronous MP flexion–IP flexion to improve prehension. Pully advancement should not be performed without capsulodesis since it is ineffective with MP hyperextension and there is a risk of ulnar deviation of the fingers if the bowstringing flexor tendons subluxate ulnarly and the volar plate is not firmly fixed.

The Stiles tendon transfer.[25] This procedure is mainly of historical interest. Stiles reported two cases in which the flexor superficialis was split and passed dorsally. One half of each portion of the split superficialis was sutured to the extensor digitorum communis. In neither case was a follow-up reported. Bunnell performed the procedure with unsuccessful results and then modified it.

The Stiles-Bunnell tendon transfer.[9] With Bunnell's modification of Stiles' procedure, the split flexor superficialis is passed to the dorsal surface of the transverse fibers of the intrinsic apparatus of each finger. Split superficialis of index was transferred to the radial sides of the index and the middle fingers; split superficialis of the middle finger was transferred to the ulnar sides of the index, middle, and ring fingers; split superficialis of the ring finger was transferred to the radial sides of the ring and little fingers; the entire superficialis of the little finger (it is the smallest) was transferred to the ulnar side of the little finger. Bunnell had hoped to provide both ulnar and radial deviation to each of the fingers by this transfer in addition to correcting the clawing. The operation requires the use of all four superficialis tendons. Multiple split tendons

A

B

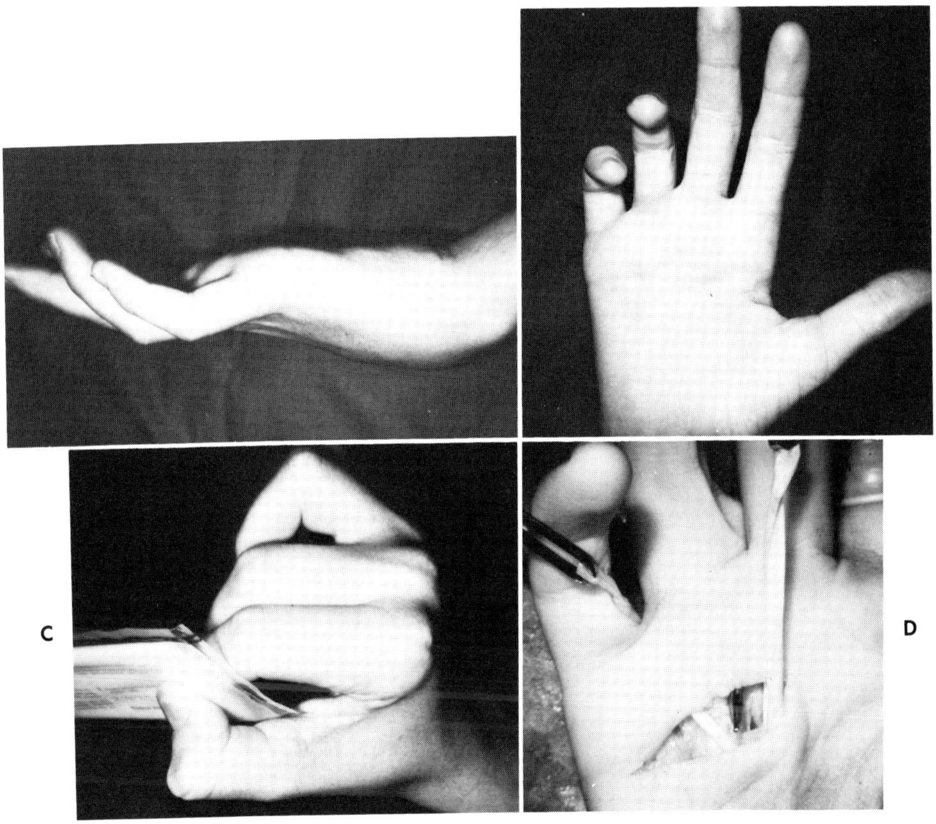

C

D

Continued.

Fig. 21-7. This patient with a low irreparable ulnar nerve palsy, causing claw deformity of the ring and little fingers and an awkward grip was treated by a modified Stiles-Bunnell procedure. **A,** With attempts at complete extension of the fingers, the ring and little fingers claw and the wrist palmar flexes. **B,** Atrophy of the hypothenar muscles is seen. There is no deformity of the index and middle fingers because of intact median nerve innervated lumbricals. **C,** With atrophy of the first dorsal interosseus muscle, pinch is weak and the middle finger and ring finger must support the index finger to prevent it from deviating ulnarly. The patient also demonstrates a strongly positive Froment's sign of the thumb indicating weakness of the adductor pollicis. **D,** Flexor superficialis has been divided opposite the neck of the proximal phalanx of the middle finger. The tendon is split longitudinally. Half has been passed along the lumbrical canal of the little finger. A curved hemostat has been bluntly tunnelled volar to the deep transverse metacarpal ligament and will guide the other strand of the superficialis along the lumbrical canal.

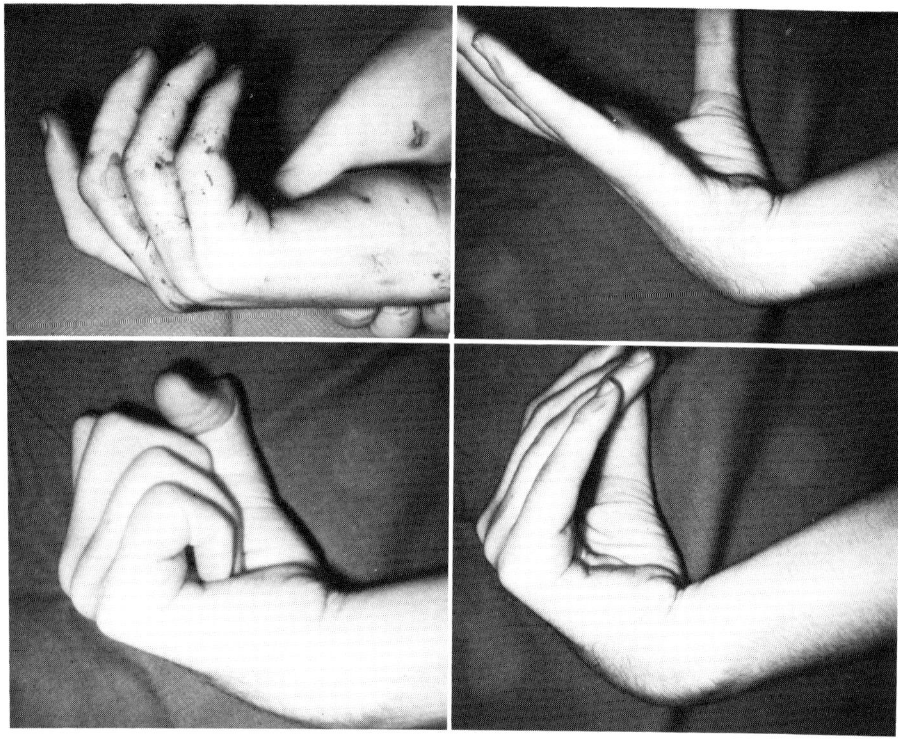

Fig. 21-7, cont'd. E, The two strands of the flexor digitorum superficialis are sutured to the radial lateral band of the ring and little fingers. At the completion of the surgery, the metacarpophalangeal joint of the little finger is in 80° of flexion, that of the ring finger in slightly less flexion when the wrist is held in a neutral position. The fingers are splinted in this position for 4 weeks. **F,** Several months later there is full extension of the fingers even with the wrist palmar flexed. **G,** The patient is now able to assume the intrinsic-plus position. The transferred tendons are working actively as is demonstrated by function of the transfer even with the wrist palmar flexed. **H,** There is full flexion of all fingers. Although the power of grip is not changed, the deformity and mechanics of finger motion have been corrected and hand function is improved.

crisscross throughout the palm. Each finger is left without a superficialis and each has transfers to both lateral bands. There is great risk of adhesions within the palm and of overcorrection of the deformity in each of the operated fingers.[1] Too many tasks appeared assigned to each of the transferred superficialis tendons. The original Stiles-Bunnell procedure was modified not only by Bunnell but by others.

Modified Stiles-Bunnell tendon transfer.[22] One or two superficialis tendons are removed (usually from the middle and ring fingers), split, and rerouted along the lumbrical canal to the transverse fibers of the radial lateral band (Fig. 21-7). Some authors recommend that the transfer to the index finger be passed to its ulnar side rather than to its radial side. Thus, the index and middle fingers will be apposed for better three point chuck grip. The modified Stiles-Bunnell procedure does not increase the strength of grip of the hand. Although flexion power of the metacarpophalangeal joints is increased, it is at the expense of loss of flexion power of the proximal interphalangeal joints of the donor fingers. However, when successful, the modified Stiles-Bunnell procedure corrects the deformity, restores synchronous MP flexion–IP flexion and MP flexion–IP extension, and also controls lateral deviation of the fingers.

Occasionally, particularly with hands that are hypermobile and with leprosy patients, a secondary swan-neck deformity of overcorrection may develop several years after surgery. This deformity is the result of simultaneously decreasing the power of PIP joint flexion and increasing PIP joint extension. In addition, the modified Stiles-Bunnell procedure is out of phase relative to IP joint motion. A muscle that previously flexed the interphalangeal joint must now extend it. There is also the risk that the transferred motor may not be able to adapt to its new function. The Stiles-Bunnell procedure should not be used in cases of high ulnar nerve palsy, because the superficialis muscle is essential for flexion of the ulnar digits. The procedure cannot be used in cases of high ulnar and median nerve palsy, because the superficialis muscle is paralyzed in these cases.

To its credit, the procedure is a direct one, relatively simply done, with few visible scars and with little chance of adhesions. When successful, it can improve all facets of the disability of intrinsic paralysis except for the loss of grip strength. The swan-neck deformity occasionally seen may be avoided by dividing the donor superficialis tendon opposite to the neck of the proximal phalanx. Most often, the superficialis stump will then adhere to adjacent tissues, preventing posterior interphalangeal hyperextension in the donor finger. Splitting one donor superficialis into four segments, rather than utilizing two donor tendons, may also avoid overcorrection by diminishing the power of the transferred tendons. In cases of isolated low ulnar nerve palsy, superficialis of the middle finger may be used as the donor to the ring and little fingers.

Considering its advantages and shortcomings, the modified Stiles-Bunnell procedure would appear *not* to be indicated in the hands of patients with wrist flexion contracture, leprosy, fingers that are hypermobile, intrinsic palsy as a result of high ulnar or ulnar and median nerve palsy, intrinsic palsy due to laceration of the ulnar and median nerves along with the flexor tendons at the wrist, or in those patients whose chief complaint is loss of power of grip. It appears well suited to the treatment of intrinsic palsy in which the chief complaint is deformity, and awkwardness of prehension and grip due to lack of synchronous MP flexion–IP flexion and MP flexion–IP extension.

Riordan tendon transfer.[22] Riordan has recommended transferring the flexor carpi radialis (FCR), elongated with a brachioradialis tendon graft, through the intermetacarpal spaces and lumbrical canals to the lateral bands of the palsied fingers (Fig. 21-6, *C*). This transfer has the potential advantage of being in phase with interphalangeal joint extension. As noted earlier, patients with intrinsic palsy often develop wrist palmar flexion deformity. Transfer of FCR decreases this tendency.

Potential disadvantages of this procedure include the prolonged route of the transfer-graft through the intermetacarpal spaces, risking adhesions. In cases of high median and ulnar nerve palsy, the flexor radialis may not be functioning. Multiple forearm scars might be objectionable in some younger patients.

The Riordan transfer is most valuable in the treatment of intrinsic palsy accompanied by a palmar flexed wrist, injury to the flexor tendons, and in those patients in whom increased strength of grasp is a primary requirement along with correction of deformity and prehension. The use of a powerful wrist

A

B

C

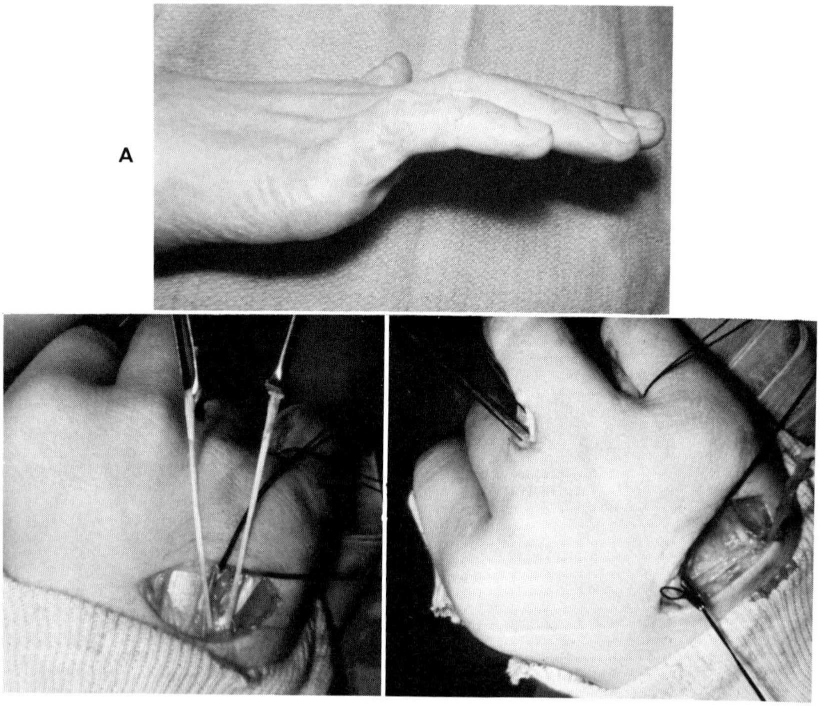

Fig. 21-8. This man with a low ulnar nerve palsy has clawing of the ring and little fingers and weakness of abduction of the index finger. He was treated with a transfer of extensor digiti quinti proprius (Fowler transfer) to correct the clawing of the ring and little fingers, and transfer of extensor indicis proprius to improve index abduction. **A**, Clawing of the ring and little fingers is seen. **B**, Extensor digiti quinti proprius is freed from the metacarpophalangeal joint and split longitudinally into two parts. Before removing the extensor digiti quinti, one must be certain that the extensor digitorum communis to the little finger is functional. **C**, A curved hemostat is tunnelled from the radial lateral band of the recipient fingers, volar to deep transverse metacarpal ligament, and through the intermetacarpal spaces. The tunnel is made quite wide in the intermetacarpal area. Guide sutures direct the split extensor digiti quinti through the new route.

flexor as a motor may significantly increase the power of grip in the operated hand.

The Fowler tenodesis.[22] For the treatment of intrinsic paralysis, Fowler has recommended suturing two tendon grafts through a hole in the dorsal carpal ligament and then tunneling the four tendon ends through the intermetacarpal spaces and the lumbrical canals to the lateral bands. When the wrist flexes, the tendon grafts are tightened and active MP flexion–IP extension is achieved. This is an *active* tenodesis operation.

No active motor is transferred in the Fowler tenodesis, making it valuable in the hand with multiple muscle weakness. As the procedure requires active wrist flexion to be effective, it would have little value in the presence of poor

D E

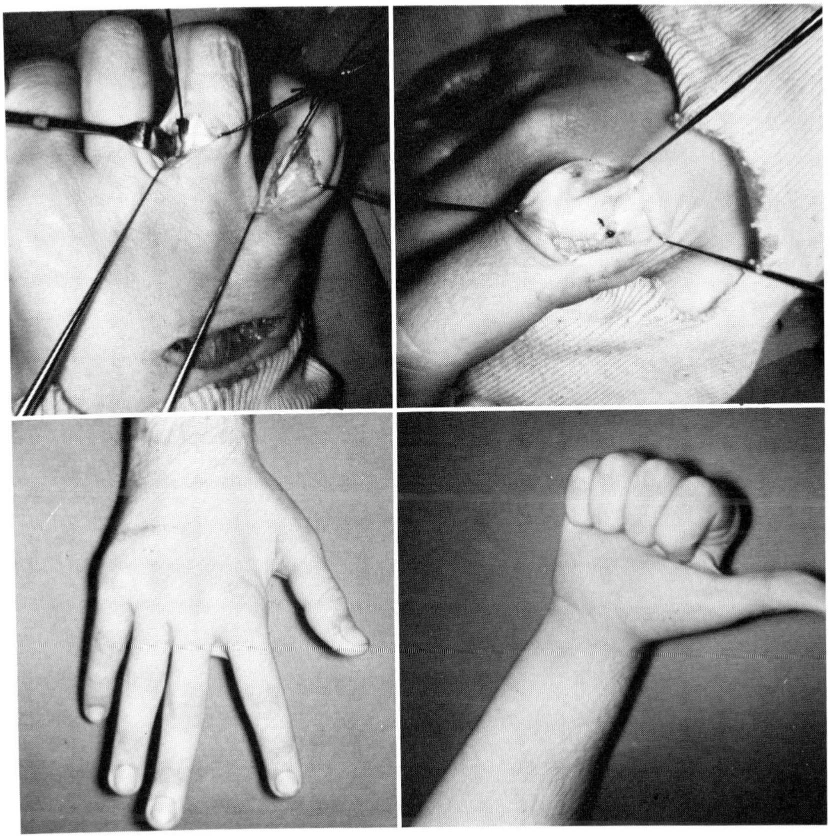

F G

Fig. 21-8, cont'd. D, The split flexor superficialis is sutured to the radial lateral bands while holding the wrist in mild dorsiflexion and the metacarpophalangeal joints in acute flexion. **E,** The extensor indicis proprius has been detached from its insertion, rerouted, and sutured to the tendon of the first dorsal interosseus muscle. **F,** Postoperatively, clawing has been corrected in the ring and little fingers and independent metacarpophalangeal joint flexion can be achieved. Active abduction of the index finger is restored. **G,** Full flexion of the fingers is preserved.

wrist motor control or with a patient with a hyperflexed wrist. Theoretically, strength of grasp may be improved since the power of the wrist flexors is indirectly transmitted to the metacarpophalangeal joints. Thus, ideally, the Fowler tenodesis can improve strength, decrease deformity, and restore more normal MP-IP joint kinetics in the palsied hand without detaching an active motor. In fact, however, the proximity of the sutured grafts to the axis of motion of the wrist joint have led many to believe that the grafts usually work as checkreins to prevent MP hyperextension and are under little active control.

Extensor proprius tendon transfer (Bunnell proprius transfer,[9] Fowler tendon transfer[22]). In this procedure the extensor digiti quinti (EDQ) and extensor indicis proprius (EIP) tendons are split longitudinally and pass through the intermetacarpal spaces and along the lumbrical canal to the lateral bands. EIP is transferred to the index and middle fingers and EDQ to the ring and little fingers (Fig. 21-8).

This is an active transfer that can correct the claw deformity not only by flexing the MP joints and extending the IP joints, but also by removing an MP extensor from the index and little fingers—the donor fingers. There is so little power to these two transferred muscles that grip strength is rarely significantly altered. The transfer is *out of phase* at the MP joint and runs the risk of not adapting to its new position. Utilizing the split EIP to correct the clawing of the index and middle fingers precludes its transfer to provide good abduction to the index finger. Also, EDQ is frequently the only effective extensor of the little finger as the extensor digitorum communis (EDC) is often vestigial in this area.

For these reasons, the extensor proprius tendon transfer is perhaps best used in isolated ulnar nerve palsy in which clawing of the ring and little fingers is severe, in which there is extensive scarring at the volar aspect of the wrist and/or hand, and in which clinical examination reveals a good EDC to the little finger. In these cases a dorsal transfer for adduction of the thumb, transfer of EIP to the radial side of the index finger, and transfer of the extensor digiti quinti proprius (EDQP) for clawing of the ring and little fingers may all be performed at the same time with good functional results.

Brand intrinsic transfers.[2, 4] Brand, working mainly with lepers, has used the extensor carpi radialis brevis (ECRB) or extensor carpi radialis longus (ECRL), elongated with a "four tailed" plantaris graft dorsally, through the intermetacarpal spaces and through the lumbrical canals of the middle, ring, and little fingers and ulnar side of the index finger to the lateral bands (Fig. 21-9). This transfer lessens the chance of swan neck overcorrection often found in the Bunnell transfer. It also increases the strength of grip by transferring a strong wrist motor for MP joint flexion. Brand has specifically recommended attaching the transfer to the ulnar side of the index finger so patients may more readily use the apposed index and middle fingers in eating rice. As with all dorsal-to-volar tendon transfers and tenodeses, when the tendon is transferred to the ulnar side of the index finger the deep transverse metacarpal ligament serves as an excellent pully to keep the transfer volar to the axis of MP joint motion (Fig. 21-6, *C*). There is no deep transverse metacarpal ligament to the radial side of the index finger to serve as a pulley.

Potential disadvantages of the Brand procedure include the risk that removing a strong wrist dorsiflexor may increase the propensity of the patient to palmar flex the wrist. In addition, as with all dorsal to volar transfers, they are most effective with wrist palmar flexion. This increases the chances of further wrist deformity. For this reason Brand has modified his procedure and suggested a

A

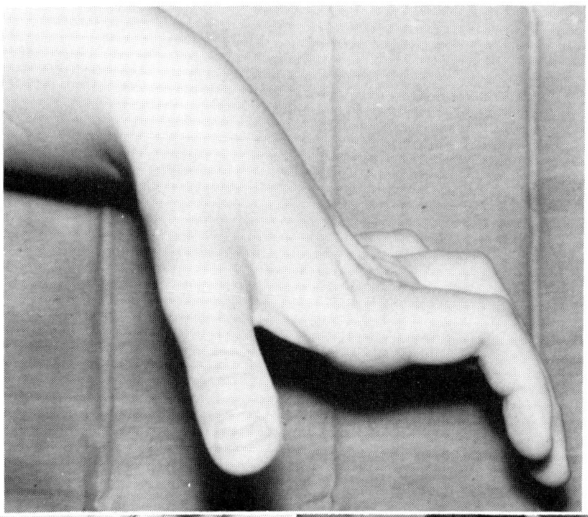

B

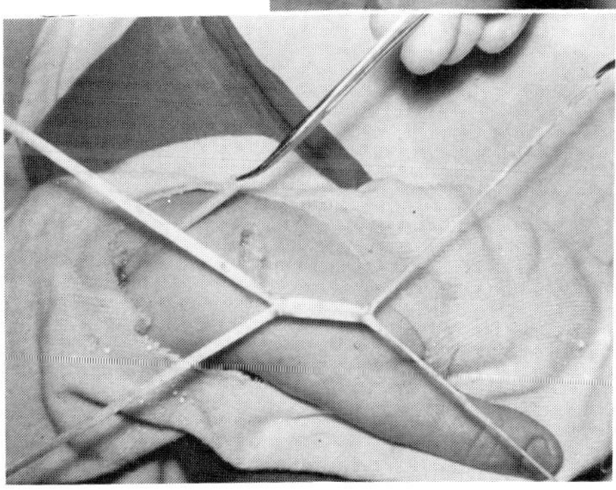

C

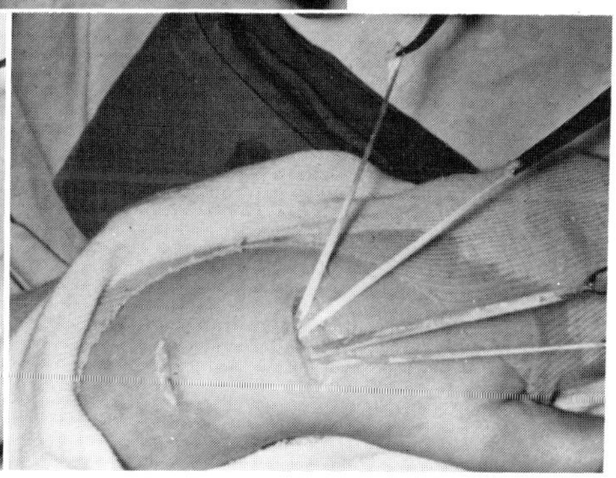

Continued.

Fig. 21-9. This patient with intrinsic muscle palsy is treated with a Brand dorsal intrinsic transfer. **A,** There is clawing of all four fingers with palmar flexion of the wrist when she attempts to extend the interphalangeal joints. **B,** Extensor carpi radialis brevis is detached from its origin. A plantaris tendon graft is removed from the leg and split into four parts, two proximally and two distally. **C,** The central segment of the plantaris graft is sutured to the extensor carpi radialis brevis and the four "tails" are seen at the level of the bases of the metacarpals. From here, they are tunnelled between the metacarpals, volar to the deep transverse metacarpal ligament, and then sutured to the radial lateral bands of the middle, ring, and little fingers and to the ulnar lateral band of the index finger.

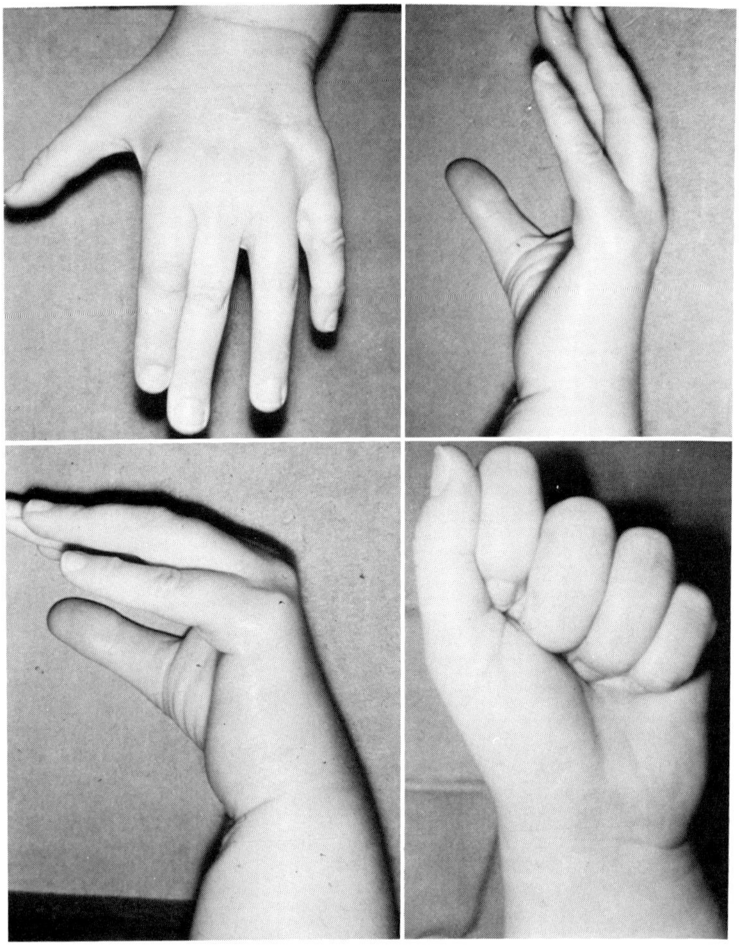

D E F G

Fig. 21-9, cont'd. D, The index and middle fingers are closely apposed because the tendons were transferred to the adjacent sides of these two digits. **E,** Clawing has been corrected. **F,** The transfer works actively. Even with the wrist in neutral position the patient is able to assume the intrinsic-plus position. **G,** Full flexion is preserved.

volar route transfer. Either ECRL or brachioradialis is used as a motor and again elongated with a "four tailed" plantaris graft. It is passed volarly through the carpal canal and attached to the lateral bands of the respective fingers (Fig. 21-6, *B*). Again, mechanics and strength of grasp is improved and deformity is corrected. The transfer, however, increases the mass of tissue in the carpal canal and risks possible carpal tunnel syndrome. In cases of low median nerve palsy in patients with leprosy this risk is of little significance.

The Brand transfers (as the Riordan transfer) appear ideal for patients who require increased power of flexion as well as correction of their deformity and synchronous joint motion. In a patient with leprosy or diffuse muscle weakness caused by other neurologic diseases the added risk of adhesions of the multiple tendon grafts through the intermetacarpal spaces or carpal canal is probably justified to increase grip strength. For the patient with peripheral ulnar nerve injury, however, whose complaints are usually lack of independent MP flexion and the claw deformity, the more direct modified Bunnell procedure would appear to be preferable.

Burkhalter transfer.[10, 11] Burkhalter has recommended that tendon transfers to the fingers be inserted not onto the radial lateral band or dorsal transverse fibers but rather directly into the proximal phalanx. Specifically, he has described using ECRL or brachioradialis prolonged with a free graft of palmaris longus or plantaris through the intermetacarpal spaces and lumbrical canals into the proximal phalanges. Essentially, this is similar to the Brand transfers except for the site of insertion.

A bony attachment of a tendon transfer minimizes the danger of swan-neck deformity. IP extension could be achieved through the common extensor tendon. Transfer to the proximal phalanx would be inadvisable if the dorsal expansion were attenuated at the PIP joint preventing full PIP extension when the MP joint is held flexed. This attachment would appear ideal for those cases with hypermobile proximal interphalangeal joints.

Brooks-Jones transfer.[5] Brooks and Jones have described using the flexor carpi radialis (FCR) elongated with toe extensor tendon grafts through the carpal canal and attached to the proximal pullies. Such an attachment is similar to the Burkhalter bone attachment. It is probably easier to perform than a bony attachment, but risks loosening of the pully.

Zancolli "lasso" operation.[27] In order to achieve flexion of the proximal phalanx in the clawhand, Zancolli has described passing the flexor superficialis of each finger through its pully, 1.5 cm. distal to the proximal pully edge. The cut tendon end is then looped superficial to the pully and sutured to itself in the distal palm. A lasso ("lazo") of superficialis flexes the proximal phalanx through its pully. The operation is similar to the Stiles-Bunnell procedure with attachment of the transfer to the pully rather than to a lateral band.

Lennox transfer. Fritschi[12] has noted that Lennox uses the palmaris longus as a motor elongated with a plantaris "four tailed" graft through the carpal tunnel to the lateral bands as an effective means of correcting the claw deformity in highly mobile leper hands. Fritschi also notes that in lepers the fascia lata serves as an excellent tendon graft. It is doubtful that the palmaris longus would provide sufficient power or excursion to rival the more standard transfers and tenodeses with traumatic ulnar and median nerve injuries. In addition, palmaris longus tendon usually is affected by distal ulnar and median nerve injuries.

Transfers for abduction of the index finger

As noted above, most tendon transfers and tenodeses that restore metacarpophalangeal joint flexion are sutured to the radial sides of the middle, ring, and little fingers and to the ulnar side of the index finger. Thus, the fingers are drawn together after these operations. For strong pinch, however, radial deviation of the index finger must be restored. (Thumb adduction is also of prime importance but will not be covered in this chapter.)

Of the many tendon transfers recommended, all suture the transferred tendon either to the lateral band at the proximal third of the proximal phalanx or into the lateral side of the proximal phalanx itself. The muscles recommended to replace the paralyzed first dorsal interosseus have included extensor indicis proprius,[6] extensor carpi radialis longus (with a tendon graft),[17] extensor pollicis brevis,[16] extensor digiti quinti proprius,[28] and flexor digitorum superficialis.[8, 13, 16] In performing this transfer, one must avoid providing too much power of radial deviation, as ulnar deviation through the multiple slip intrinsic transfers may be insufficient to restore the index to its neutral position. The most popular of the transfers is probably the extensor indicis proprius. The tendon must be freed proximally and redirected from the wrist, taking a straight course to its site of insertion. Although some have feared that detaching extensor indicis proprius may rob the index finger of its independent extension, this is rarely the case. The index finger extends independently of the adjacent fingers principally because its tendons are not bound to those of its neighbors with juncturae teninae.

DISCUSSION AND CONCLUSIONS

We often hear that if many procedures are described for correction of a pathologic condition, none is effective. Such is not the case with the treatment of the intrinsic palsied hand. The intrinsic muscles of the hand are essential for the normal balance, kinetics, power, and position of the fingers.[23] There are many causes of intrinsic palsy. The disability resulting from each may be quite different. Thus the treatment also varies.

Several considerations influence our choice in selecting a proper plan of treatment for the hand with intrinsic palsy.

1. With a distal irreparable ulnar nerve lesion the modified Stiles-Bunnell procedure may be preferable if power loss to an assistive hand is not a major complaint and if clawing and asynchronous MP-IP motion prove bothersome. If clawing is not severe, transfers to the radial side of the hand for abduction of the index finger and adduction of the thumb may suffice.
2. With low irreparable median and ulnar nerve palsy resulting from trauma that has divided the superficialis tendons, a dorsal route Brand or Riordan transfer appear preferable for clawing. EIP is transferred to the first dorsal interosseous for index finger abduction.
3. For irreparable high ulnar and median nerve palsies, a volar route Brand transfer appears preferable. This should be performed after appropriate transfers for flexion of the fingers and thumb.

4. With distal ulnar palsy and moderate scarring at the volar side of the wrist and hand, the EDQ proprius transfer (Fowler or Bunnell) plus EIP transfer to first dorsal interosseus appears advantageous.
5. Volar capsulorrhaphy with Bunnell pully advancement appears advisable to correct clawing and to improve MP-IP integrated joint flexion in the presence of diffuse muscle palsy with few motors available. Fowler's tenodesis operation may also be performed here.
6. The Riordan tendon transfer appears advisable in the presence of wrist flexion deformity.
7. The Brand dorsal route transfer appears preferable after severe Volkmann's ischemic contracture with extensive scarring of the volar aspect of the forearm.

Regarding the techniques of tendon transfers and the selection of the procedure to use, several points deserve emphasis.

1. The volar route transfers require immobilization of the wrist in palmer flexion for several weeks postoperatively. These transfers can therefore be performed simultaneously with median and ulnar nerve repair, with opponensplasty, and with repair of flexor tendons. The transfer is more direct than a dorsal route transfer and does not risk adhesions in the intermetacarpal spaces.
2. With dorsal route transfers, wrist palmar flexion potentiates interphalangeal joint extension. These functions are usually synergistic and easily learned. Dorsal route transfers avoid the risk of causing carpal tunnel syndrome. The potential risk of adhesions between the metacarpals must be considered.
3. Power of grip may be improved by transferring a wrist flexor or extensor, or brachioradialis to flex the MP joint. FDS and extensor proprius tendons will not increase the power of grip.
4. If the interphalangeal joints cannot be extended when the MP joint is stabilized in flexion, tendon transfers should be attached to the dorsal apex of the proximal interphalangeal joint or the conjoined lateral band. In these patients, transfers to the proximal phalanx are insufficient to achieve IP extension.
5. In cases of progressive disease such as leprosy, intrinsic transfers should be performed on all four fingers, including those that may not (as yet) be paralyzed. If not, the unoperated digits may feel weak and may later develop paralysis and deformity.[12]

As with all other reconstructive procedures of the hand, there is no one *best operation*. Selection must be based upon the disability, the disease, and an analysis of the anatomic abnormalities of the entire limb. A successful intrinsic tendon transfer will work actively to restore agility, versatility, and often strength to the clawhand.

References

1. Brand, P. W.: Capsulodeses and pully advancement for correction of claw finger deformity (Discussion), J. Bone Joint Surg. **54A**:1470-1471, 1972.
2. Brand, P. W.: Deformity in leprosy. In Cochrane, R. G., and Devey, T. F., editors: Leprosy in theory and practice, ed. 2, Bristol, Eng., 1964, Wright & Sons, Ltd., pp. 447-492.
3. Brand, P. W.: Paralytic claw hand with special reference to paralysis in leprosy and treatment by the sublimis transfer of Stiles and Bunnell, J. Bone Joint Surgery **40B**: 618-632, 1958.
4. Brand, P. W.: Tendon grafting illustrated by a new operation for intrinsic paralysis of the fingers, J. Bone Joint Surg. **43B**:444-453, 1961.
5. Brooks, A. G. and Jones, D. S.: A new tendon transfer for the paralytic hand, Abstract submitted to ASSH, personal communication, 1974.
6. Brown, P. W.: Reconstruction for pinch in ulnar intrinsic palsy, Orthop. Clin. North Am. **5**:233-342, 1974.
7. Brown, P. W.: Zancolli capsulorrhaphy for ulnar claw hand, J. Bone Joint Surg. **52A**: 868-877, 1970.
8. Bruner, J. M.: Tendon transfer to restore abduction of the index finger using the extensor pollicis brevis, Plast. Reconstr. Surg. **3**:197-201, 1948.
9. Bunnell, S.: Surgery of the intrinsic muscles of the hand other than those producing opposition of the thumb, J. Bone Joint Surg. **24**:1-31, 1942.
10. Burkhalter, W. E.: Restoration of power grip in ulnar nerve paralysis, Orthop. Clin. North Am. **5**:289-303, 1974.
11. Burkhalter, W. E., and Strait, J. L.: Metacarpophalangeal flexor replacement for intrinsic paralysis, J. Bone Joint Surg. **55A**:1667-1676, 1973.
12. Fritschi, E. P.: Reconstructive surgery in leprosy, Baltimore, 1971, Williams & Wilkins, Co., pp. 42-82.
13. Goldner, J. L.: Deformities of the hand incidental to pathological changes of the extensor and intrinsic muscle mechanisms, J. Bone Joint Surg. **35A**:115-131, 1953.
14. Landsmeer, J. M. F.: Power grip and precision handling, Ann. Rheum. Dis. **21**:164-170, 1962.
15. Leddy, J. P., Stark, H. H., Ashworth, C. R., and Boyes, J. H.: Capsulodesis and pully advancement for the correction of claw finger deformity, J. Bone Joint Surg. **54A**: 1465-1471, 1972.
16. Littler, J. W.: Tendon transfers and arthrodeses in combined median and ulnar nerve paralyses, J. Bone Joint Surg. **31A**:225-234, 1949.
17. Long, C., and Brown, M. E.: Electromyographic kinesiology of the hand: muscles, moving the long finger, J. Bone Joint Surg. **46A**:1683-1706, 1964.
18. Mannerfelt, L.: Studies on the hand in ulnar nerve paralysis, Acta Orthop. Scand. Supp. 87, 1966.
19. Mikhail, I. K.: Bone black operation for claw hand, Surg. Gynecol. Obstet. **118**:1077-1079, 1964.
20. Mulder, J. D., and Landsmeer, J. M. F.: The mechanism of claw finger, J. Bone Joint Surg., **50B**:664-668, 1968.
21. Parkes, A. R.: Paralytic claw fingers—a graft tenodesis operation, The Hand **5**:192-194, 1973.
22. Riordan, D. C.: Surgery of the paralytic hand. In A.A.O.S. Instructional Course Lectures, vol. 16, St. Louis, 1959, The C. V. Mosby Co., pp. 79-90.
23. Smith, R. J.: Balance and kinetics of the fingers under normal and pathological conditions, Clin. Orthop. **104**:92-111, 1974.
24. Smith, R. J.: Intrinsic muscles of the fingers: function, dysfunction, and surgical reconstruction. In A.A.O.S. Instructional Course Lectures, vol. 24, St. Louis, 1975, The C. V. Mosby Co.
25. Stiles, H. J., and Forrester-Brown, M. F.: Treatment of injuries of the peripheral spinal nerves, London, 1922, H. Frowde, p. 166.

26. Zancolli, E. A.: Claw-hand caused by paralysis of the intrinsic muscles, J. Bone Joint Surg. **39A**:1076-1090, 1957.
27. Zancolli, E.: Correccion de la "garra" digital por paralisis intrinseca; la operacion del "lazo," Acta Ortop. Latinoamericana **1**:65-72, 1974.
28. Zweig, J., Rosenthal, S., and Burns, H.: Transfer of the extensor digiti quinti to restore pinch in ulnar palsy of the hand, J. Bone Joint Surg. **54A**:51-59, 1972.

22. Restoration of partial or complete loss of elbow flexion by muscle and tendon transfers

J. Leonard Goldner, M.D.

Absence or weakness of elbow flexion results in serious loss of hand and forearm function. The muscles that control flexion of the forearm are the biceps humerus, the brachialis muscle, the brachioradialis, and the radial and ulnar forearm flexors because of their two joint span. If the biceps and brachialis are paralyzed, and if the shoulder girdle muscles and the brachioradialis are normal, elbow flexion is possible if the forearm is in pronation. Resistance against gravity is minimal, however, and reinforcement, if possible, is desirable.[1]

ETIOLOGY OF ELBOW FLEXION WEAKNESS OR LOSS

Anterior horn cell paralysis caused by poliomyelitis was the most common cause of denervation of the elbow flexor muscles.[11] The incidence of this disease is low in the United States, but in certain parts of the world may still account for absence of elbow flexion. Trauma to nerve roots or to the brachioplexus, or direct injury to the musculocutaneous nerve may result in partial or complete loss of function of the elbow flexor muscles.[3] In situations such as these, accurate manual muscle testing is necessary and electromyography is used to determine presence or absence of denervation potentials. Not only must a decision be made to do the transfer, but timing must also be considered.

Birth defects may result in partial or complete absence of elbow flexion because of cervical root damage that may affect the shoulder girdle as well as the arm and forearm muscles.

Inflammatory conditions such as brachial plexusitis (Spillane or Parsonage-Turner syndrome) may cause a muscle deficiency requiring reinforcement of muscles that flex the elbow.

Direct muscle damage or loss of muscle mass caused by open trauma requires consideration of muscle replacement or tendon transfer.

FUNCTIONAL ANATOMY

Flexion of the elbow joint is essential for maximum hand function. The biceps muscle has a unique double origin with the long head stabilizing the humerus in the glenoid, and the short head contributing to stabilization of the scapula. The direction and mechanics of insertion of the biceps tendon into the tubercle of the radius provides supination, stabilization of the radius and ulna with the humerus, and flexion of the forearm.[1] The coracobrachialis muscle adds strength to elbow flexion and reinforces the biceps during heavy lifting. The brachioradialis muscle because of its attachment to the outer lower humerus pronates and supinates the forearm as well as functioning as a flexor. This muscle does not provide full strength in elbow flexion, but does supplement the action of both the brachialis and the biceps.

Flexion of the elbow is augmented by action of the forearm flexor muscles that originate from the medial condyle of the humerus, and the forearm extensor muscles that originate from the lateral humeral condyle. Strong elbow flexion is accomplished with the forearm in supination, the fingers and wrist relaxed, and the arm stabilized against the trunk. If additional elbow strength is required, it is added by wrist flexion that activates the flexor carpi ulnaris, flexor carpi radialis, and palmaris longus as all of these muscles cross the elbow joint. Additional elbow flexion strength is obtained by flexion of the fingers. The added burst of energy obtained by forcibly flexing the fingers into the palm results in stabilization of both the forearm flexors and extensors, and in turn, provides more force to the already flexed forearm.

The concept of using forearm muscles to improve elbow flexion depends on this double action of the forearm muscles. As the muscle origins are advanced proximally, the substitution pattern adds strength to elbow flexion.[17] The patient must realize that maximum flexion is obtained by utilizing the wrist and finger flexors as well as stabilizing the wrist and finger extensors.

METHODS OF RESTORATION OF ELBOW FLEXION

Steindler described elbow flexorplasty, a procedure based upon the use of two-joint forearm muscles such as the flexor carpi ulnaris, the flexor carpi radialis, and the palmaris longus. Also, a single-joint muscle such as the pronator radii teres augments flexion of the forearm if the muscle origin is advanced proximally. Steindler advanced the forearm muscles and the medial epicondyle to the medial aspect of the humerus to provide elbow flexion.[17] This alteration utilizes the concept of Blix's curve, which relates muscle length and strength so that forearm muscles will function as flexors of the elbow in addition to providing flexion of the wrist joint. Increased muscle tension and shortening, provided that the tension is not excessive, will increase muscle strength.

Also, elbow flexion in an extremity without nerve or muscle damage can be strengthened by voluntary flexion of the fingers and by stabilization of the wrist joint in acute flexion or extension. Augmentation of elbow flexion in these instances depends on the attachments of the extensors or flexors of the fingers to the medial and lateral condyles of the humerus.

The procedure as described by Steindler resulted in advancement of the flexor mass to the medial side of the humerus. Pronation of the forearm occurred because of tension on the pronator radii teres. Improvement of elbow flexion was possible but the pronation deformity was somewhat disabling.[17]

Bunnell modified the Steindler flexorplasty by elongating the forearm muscle origins with fascia and by attaching the muscle origins and the fascia to the lateral aspect of the humerus just proximal to the elbow joint. This modification provided elbow flexion and supination rather than excessive pronation.[3] The transferred muscles are placed under sufficient tension to cause a flexion contracture of the elbow of 20° to 30°. This contracture is desirable in initiating flexion. The patients included in the Duke series have all been managed by this modification.

Clark described a transfer of the muscle belly of the pectoralis major anterior to the humerus and attached the elongated muscle belly to the radial tubercle. This transfer provides strength and bulk with a cosmetic improvement as well.[7]

A modification of the Clark procedure utilized the pectoralis major or minor muscle elongated with fascia lata that was attached to the radial tubercle. This provided pectoralis major or minor strength and muscle mass without mobilization of the muscle origin and the risk of damage to the motor innervation. From a biomechanical standpoint, elongation of the origin into the radial tubercle is as effective as is the transplantation of the entire muscle belly.[16]

Zancolli has described modifications of the muscle transfers described by Bost-Schottstadt by isolating the entire latissimus dorsi muscle, mobilizing it on a neurovascular pedicle, and transferring the muscle belly anterior to the humerus.[18] Strength resulting from that isolated transfer is not as great as the combination of forearm muscle flexorplasty and pectoralis major transfer.

Eyler modified the Steindler flexorplasty by using the origins of the flexor carpi radialis, the pronator radii teres, and one half of the flexor carpi ulnaris rather than the entire muscle mass of the latter.[10] This is a less complicated modification, but in my experience does not provide maximum strength. If the forearm flexor muscles are to provide maximum flexion in place of the paralyzed biceps and brachialis muscles and in the absence of a brachioradialis muscle, then the entire flexor carpi ulnaris muscle should be used in conjunction with the other forearm flexors.

Brooks and Seddon modified the pectoralis major transfer by elongating the insertion of the pectoralis major with the paralyzed biceps muscle and tendon as a free graft from the insertion of the pectoral muscle through the attachment of the biceps tendon into the radial tubercle.[2] My limited experience with this procedure has been unsatisfactory because the paralyzed muscle and tendon and its surrounding fascia stretched and elongated several months after the original procedure had been done even though the "graft" had been placed under maximum tension. In my opinion, a large strip of fascia lata should be rolled and one end braided into the pectoralis major insertion and the other end sutured into the tubercle of the radius with a pull-out suture or into the insertion of the biceps tendon into bone.

Carroll presented his experience using the triceps tendon for restoration of elbow flexion.[4] The triceps muscle will provide strong elbow flexion, but certain disadvantages do exist after the extensor power of the triceps is eliminated. The stabilizing effect of the triceps as an extensor, the use of the forearm in extension when gravity is eliminated, and the desirability of triceps function for trunk shifting all suggest that other motors should be selected if they are available.

Bunnell and Carroll have used the sternocleidomastoid elongated by fascia lata for restoration of elbow.[3, 5, 6] When no other muscle motor is available, this substitution pattern should be considered.

The degree of flexion contracture that results after flexorplasty depends on the procedure selected. The original Steindler flexorplasty, if successful, always resulted in a flexion contracture of the elbow joint. I believe that stronger flexion is maintained and frequent elbow flexion is done with greater ease if a contracture of 20° or 30° is permanent.

PRELIMINARY ASSESSMENT AND ORDER OF RECONSTRUCTION OF ELBOW FLEXION

Detailed manual muscle testing and an analysis of individual neuromuscular components must be performed prior to making a final decision concerning flexorplasty. If the forearm muscles rate less than 70% of normal strength, they will not provide a range of elbow flexion in which the forearm can be moved through a complete range of motion against gravity and without resistance. The relatively weak forearm flexors must be supplemented by the pectoralis major muscle. This is essential and successful and should be done without hesitation. The procedures can be carried out at the same operation. However, if the forearm muscles are normal, and if the shoulder is stable, the standard flexorplasty using the forearm muscles only is usually sufficient. If the patient's needs are for maximum strength, then double augmentation using forearm flexors and pectoralis major should be considered.

The extent of muscle weakness, sensory alterations of the extremity, the presence or absence of pain, and upper limb dystrophy all affect the timing of the elbow flexorplasty. Furthermore, the strength of the shoulder girdle muscles as well as those of the hand require preliminary planning about the order of reconstruction. In general, the forearm muscles are advanced for completion of the modified flexorplasty as the primary procedure. If hand function is weak and if, for example, wrist flexors are to be transferred to wrist and digit extensors, then the hand reconstruction should be done as the second stage. Once the forearm flexors are advanced proximally and the elbow contracture occurs, then the tension of the transferred muscle tendon units to the hand can be judged accurately.

If the shoulder girdle is weak and arthrodesis or tendon transfers are required for stabilization, these procedures should be done last. Fusion of the glenohumeral joint as the first procedure will make positioning of the patient on the table for elbow flexorplasty difficult. If the pectoralis muscle is to be used for augmentation, maximum adduction cannot be obtained if arthrodesis of the shoulder has been done.

The details of the operative procedure will be given under the section on patient problems. The procedure used in managing the individual patient will be more meaningful if described in conjunction with individual patient management rather than making generalities that may or may not be applicable in individual situations.

Furthermore, since the complications related to the operative procedures are dependent on preliminary assessment, positioning of the patient, technique of the operation, and postoperative care, these are discussed now as complications that affect the success of the procedures.

COMPLICATIONS TO BE AVOIDED IN OBTAINING RESTORATION OF ELBOW FLEXION

Inadequate tension of the transferred muscle. Ideal tension must be obtained if maximum elbow flexion is to result. Inadequate tension may be due to: (1) insufficient proximal advancement of the forearm muscles attached to the medial epicondyle; (2) insecure attachment of the medial epicondyle and its muscles to the lateral humerus, which can be avoided by taking a relatively large piece of medial condyle, drilling a large hole through the lateral cortex of the humerus, and elongating the muscles with fascia or tendon graft; (3) inadequate advancement of the medial condyle and its attached muscles either medially or laterally, which results in insufficient tension of the forearm muscles and no resulting flexion contracture; and (4) closure of the elbow wound after the tendon transfer has been completed resulting in insufficient tension on the transferred muscle mass because wound closure requires extension of the forearm to at least 90°. If the tendon transfer is sufficiently loose to allow the elbow to be extended easily to 90°, the ultimate strength-tension curve will be insufficient to provide maximum range of flexion and to cause a flexion contracture. The tendon to be transferred should be prepared for insertion into the lateral shaft of the humerus but not actually fixed there until the elbow incision is completely closed except for the lateral superior portion.

Difficult exposure of the medial aspect of the elbow and awkwardness in manipulating and placing the humerus during transfer of the forearm muscles or pectoralis major muscles. If arthrodesis of the shoulder is done as the first procedure, the subsequent operative procedures about the elbow and the hand are difficult to perform and placement of the humerus in a position of flexion and adduction after flexorplasty is difficult. Arthrodesis of the shoulder or tendon transfers should be delayed until elbow flexorplasty has been completed.

Temporary or permanent weakness of the forearm muscle mass or the pectoralis major or latissimus dorsi may occur because of over-zealous mobilization of the muscles to be advanced or transferred. Weakness of the transferred muscles may be temporary or, in certain instances, permanent. Accordingly, a nerve stimulator should be present and should be used frequently throughout the operation to identify major motor branches from the nerves that innervate the muscles or from adjacent nerves. The major nerves involved, such as the median or the nerve to the pectoralis major or latissimus dorsi, should be identified before mobilization of the muscle has been initiated.

Stretch or elongation of the muscle or tendon transfer may occur if the forearm is not protected for an adequate period of time after the transfers have been completed. The minimum time for absolute immobilization of a flexorplasty regardless of which procedure is selected is 4 weeks. However, if latissimus dorsi muscle is used or the pectoralis major muscle belly is reversed and inserted into the arm, active motion can be started at 3 weeks. Tendon transfers and elongation of muscle bellies with fascia lata necessitate protection at night and part-time protection during each day for at least 2 weeks after the initial 4 weeks. Collagen must mature, and the forces of the lever system on the tendon transfers will result in significant stretch of the transferred muscle-tendon unit unless 3 to 6 months of connective tissue maturity is allowed.

Use of muscles of insufficient strength for flexorplasty. Forearm muscles less than 80% of normal should not be used for the primary support in a flexorplasty. A fair muscle may be used if augmentation is to occur from pectoralis major, latissimus dorsi, or brachioradialis that may be functioning already. Use of less than an 80% muscle will be insufficient to provide voluntary flexion of the forearm against gravity through a full range of motion.

The pectoralis major or latissimus dorsi can be done as a second stage operation. If possible, however, the entire operative procedure should be done in one stage. Once the relatively weak forearm muscles are to be augmented by the pectoralis major or latissimus dorsi, then the timing must be established. The accessory transfer will augment weakened forearm flexors and prevent a 60% forearm flexor mass from regressing to 30%, which will occur if reinforcement is delayed for several months or a year.

Absence of a permanent flexion contracture of the elbow may result in less than optimum flexion range and maximum flexion strength. Strong tension on the transferred muscles and an adequate period of immobilization will assure a flexion contracture. Zancolli states that when the entire muscle belly of the latissimus dorsi is transferred as an elbow flexor, the contracture is not a requirement for satisfactory elbow flexion.[18] I have seen this in his motion pictures, but I have not observed it clinically.

Weakening of the forearm flexors may occur if these muscles are used to correct deficiencies from an irreparable radial nerve injury. Transfer of these muscle tendon units to the extensor surface may increase their tension and limit the extent of advancement that can be done when the forearm flexors are moved at a second stage to the lateral border of the humerus. Or, if the forearm flexors are transferred to the extensors, that is, flexor carpi radialis to extensor carpi radialis brevis, pronator radii teres to extensor carpi radialis brevis, and flexor digitorum sublimes to thumb and finger extensors, advancement of the flexor carpi radialis and ulnaris to the humerus may result in increased elevation of the fingers and hand and result in limited finger and wrist flexion. The elbow flexorplasty should be done initially. It is followed several months later by transfer of wrist or finger flexors to wrist or digit extensors in a more consistent and predictable way.

Obstruction of the brachial artery and compression of the median and ulnar nerves will result from the flexorplasty procedure if the muscle mass is not directed under the median nerve and brachial artery when the muscle mass is transferred from the medial condyle to the lateral aspect of the humerus. If the ulnar nerve is not transferred forward, traction or compression of the nerve may occur after the medial muscles are transferred laterally.

Direct damage to ulnar nerve is avoided by meticulous dissection of this nerve as it is being transferred forward and while the medial muscle mass is being mobilized. The motor branches to the flexor carpi ulnaris and flexor digitorum profundi are isolated with a nerve stimulator. The radial nerve is dissected upward and away from the lateral humerus as the medial muscle mass is inserted into the lateral humeral shaft. Damage to the ulnar or median nerves on the inner side of the arm is avoided by making a separate incision when the pull-out suture is passed from lateral to medial through the humerus and out the medial side of the arm. The incision should be sufficiently large to allow the surgeon to see the course of the needles as they pass through the bone and out the skin. In this way the ulnar and median nerves and the brachial artery will not be punctured.

Insufficient muscle mass will not provide adequate elbow flexion. If one half of the flexor carpi ulnaris is left behind, if the forearm flexor muscles are less than 80% strength, or if a supplementary muscle transfer is not added to the less than normal elbow flexors, insufficient elbow flexion strength will result.

Flexion deformities of the fingers may result if the flexores digitorum sublimes and the flexores digitorum profundi are transferred proximally as a part of a forearm muscle mass. These muscle bellies should not be mobilized when the flexorplasty is done.

Insufficient advancement of the flexor muscle mass may be the result of moderate fibrosis preventing easy mobilization, or of reluctance to use the fascia lata graft, which will provide strong anchorage to bone and obviate the risk of advanced muscle mass with a piece of the medial epicondyle slipping distally during the period of immobilization.

PATIENT PROBLEMS—CLINICAL MATERIAL INCLUDING OPERATIVE TECHNIQUES FOR DIFFERENT PROCEDURES

Patient 1

This patient had a brachial plexus injury, with severe involvement of peripheral muscles (Fig. 22-1, *A-C*). The trapezius muscle rated good (80%) as did the serratus muscle. The deltoid, triceps, supraspinatus, and infraspinatus muscles were paralyzed. The pectoralis

A B C

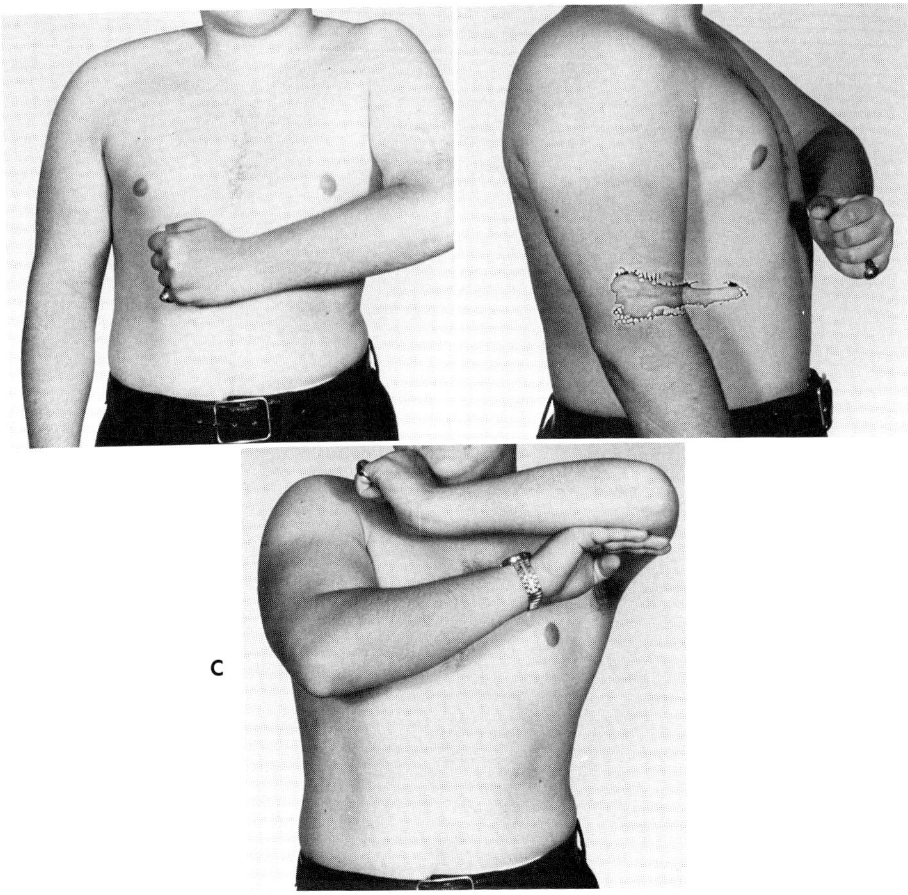

Fig. 22-1. **A**, Flexorplasty has reestablished strong flexion against gravity and fair resistance in a 22-year-old man who had lost all voluntary elbow flexion as a result of a stretch of the left brachial plexus. Note how the patient elevates the wrist and flexes the fingers to increase tension on all muscles that cross the elbow joint. He is able to supinate the forearm. The arm rests across the chest because of weakness of the shoulder girdle muscles and his inability to externally rotate. **B**, The patient is demonstrating active range of flexion against gravity. He is not able to get the hand to the mouth, because of weakness of shoulder abduction and flexion. **C**, When abduction is possible by using the opposite normal extremity, he is able to flex the hand to his mouth and bend the forearm with even greater strength.

muscle was good (80%). Treatment of the hand included arthrodesis of the distal joint of the thumb to eliminate flexion contracture secondary to weakness of the extensor pollicis longus. A forearm muscle flexorplasty was completed using the flexor carpi ulnaris, flexor carpi radialis, and pronator radii teres. These muscles were isolated, mobilized, and elongated with a fascia lata graft. Insertion was from the lateral to medial humerus. Good forearm flexion resulted, but adduction of the humerus against the chest wall was necessary to stabilize the arm and obtain maximum benefit from the transferred forearm muscles. To move the hand to the mouth, the patient used his opposite strong extremity to complete the last part of flexion (Fig. 22-1, *C*). In this position, gravity was at least partially eliminated and the range of flexion was greater than when he moved against gravity; also, the strength improved. Because of shoulder girdle weakness, he could not flex the humerus adequately to elevate the forearm and hand above the waistline.

Patient 2 (Fig. 22-2, *A-C*)

An eighteen-year-old female was affected by anterior poliomyelitis with resulting severe residual paralysis of both upper extremities. The shoulder girdle muscles were weak, the deltoid was 0, the pectoralis major was P+, the external rotators were 0, the trapezius was trace, and the serratus muscles were P.

Elbow function was absent because of complete paralysis of the biceps humerus, the brachialis, and the brachioradialis. Hand function was adequate, as she had good flexores digitorium profundi, and fair flexores digitorium sublimes. The intrinsic muscles were fair.

Plan of treatment. Treatment included flexorplasty of the elbow using either forearm muscles or latissimus dorsi. Because of the extreme weakness about the shoulder, use of latissimus dorsi was not advisable, as the patient would need that muscle for upper extremity stability at a later time. After maximum elbow flexion had been obtained, stabilization of the shoulder joint by arthrodesis would be performed.

The initial operation included isolation of the pronator radii teres, the flexor carpi radialis, and the entire origin of the flexor carpi ulnaris, which were moved from the anteromedial to the lateral humerus. The ulnar nerve was isolated; the origins of the forearm flexor muscles, excluding the flexor digitorum sublimes and the flexores profundi, were mobilized after the motor branches to the flexor carpi ulnaris had been identified and confirmed with a nerve stimulator. Motor branches were dissected into the muscle, and the flexor carpi ulnaris was moved away from its origin with minimal damage to its nerve supply. A fragment of medial epicondyle about 1 cm. × 1 cm. was elevated with the forearm muscle origins.

The soft tissue anterior to the elbow joint was incised and the median nerve and brachial

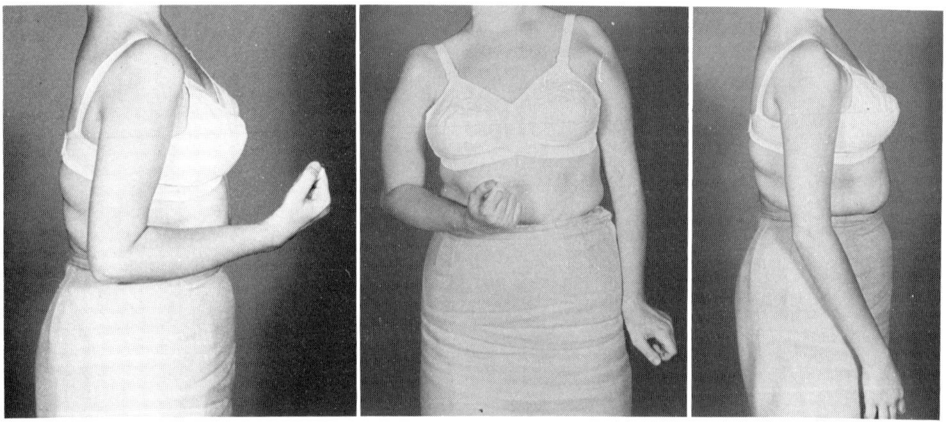

A B C

Fig. 22-2. This patient had paralysis of several muscles about the elbow and the shoulder because of poliomyelitis. She was unable to flex the elbow preoperatively. This range of elbow flexion and supination resulted after flexorplasty has been completed. **A,** After flexorplasty, in spite of the instability of the shoulder because of loss of stabilizers, she was able to flex the elbow through 100°. Reinforcement occurred by flexion of the fingers and the wrist, and by maximum adduction of the humerus against the chest wall. Note the tendency of the humerus to extend posteriorly. **B,** The internal rotation position occurs because of severe weakness of the shoulder girdle muscles. Again, note that the patient flexes the wrist and fingers, and stabilizes the humerus against the chest wall in order to provide maximum elbow flexion. **C,** This extension occurs several months after flexorplasty has been done. The contracture of the elbow of about 30° is usually necessary and desirable to initiate flexion quickly and strongly. This patient's actual range of active motion was about 65°.

artery were elevated and retracted. A short, wide strip of fascia lata was removed from the thigh, the fascia rolled as a tube, and strips were braided into the origin of the forearm flexors. The fascia and the muscle origins were then passed under the median nerve and the brachialis and were pulled to the outer side of the humerus. The radial nerve and the extensor muscle mass were retracted laterally and a large drill hole was made in the shaft of the humerus from lateral to medial. The hole was enlarged in order to accept the fascial graft and the bone fragment. (The necessary length of fascia can be determined after mobilization of the muscles has been completed, and after the forearm muscle mass is moved to the lateral side of the arm.) With the elbow flexed, the length of fascia lata was determined. A second incision was made on the medial side of the arm, so that the ulnar nerve was retracted, the bone exposed, and the No. 0 polypropylene suture, which had been braided through the forearm muscles and the fascia lata, was identified on the long needles passed from lateral to medial.

At this time, bleeding points were coagulated, and the medial and anterior incisions were closed in layers. Deep and subcutaneous sutures of nonabsorbable material were used, and a No. 2-0 polypropylene pull-out suture was placed subcuticular. This skin closure, before placement of the tendon transfer, was essential in order to maintain maximum tension on the forearm muscles. Once the incision was closed, the fascia lata and the muscle mass attached to it were anchored to the humerus with the pull-out suture, and several additional fixation sutures were taken to the muscle mass on the lateral side of the humerus, which anchored this to the periosteum. The bone fragment was inserted into the humerus so that at least one edge was in contact with the shaft.

Postoperative immobilization was obtained by maintaining the elbow at 100° of flexion, the forearm in midposition, and the digits exposed for observation. The humerus was adducted and flexed, and the arm was placed across the chest. This position was essential to prevent the arm dressing from causing traction on the forearm during the early healing period. Immobilization lasted 4 weeks. At the end of that time, a new posterior splint was constructed with the forearm at a right angle. The splint was removed 6 times a day, and the patient was given elbow flexion exercises by doing simultaneous wrist flexion with both hands. During the next 2 weeks, additional elbow extension was allowed, but gravity pull was avoided. No undue stretch was allowed on the forearm muscles or the fascia lata for 8 weeks. Gradual extension was then permitted, and during the next 2 months the forearm reached a point of maximum extension, which was at 30° (Fig. 22-2, *C*). A flexion contracture was desired to provide a mechanical advantage for the action of the transferred forearm flexors and the extensors of the forearm as well, as the latter do participate in elbow flexion once the contracture has occurred.

The patient's ability to flex the elbow voluntarily was evident after the initial immobilization was removed. The range of flexion and the strength against resistance improved rapidly during the subsequent 6 weeks. Her ability to flex the elbow improved after the humerus was stabilized against her chest by someone else, as she did not have sufficient strength to do this herself. A stable shoulder joint was essential for maximum strength of elbow flexion after flexorplasty.

After maximum elbow flexion had occurred and hand strength had been regained, arthrodesis of the glenohumeral joint was done in 15° abduction, 10° flexion, and 10° internal rotation. This provided the patient with even greater ability to flex the elbow because the humerus was stable, the forces applied to the ulna were not dissipated by posterior displacement of the humerus, and efforts at maintaining the humerus against the chest were lessened.

Final treatment was directed toward improved thumb function with an opponensplasty. After the forearm musculature had been relocated and the shoulder fused, treatment of the hand did not directly affect the proximal joints of the extremity.

Several years have passed since this was done, and her extremity function persists (Fig. 22-2, *A-C*).

An alternate flexorplasty is an external device or an external motor. This requires cables, harness, and power pack. The gadget tolerance of most individuals is limited if they are walking. They prefer reasonable assurance that operative tendon transfer and/or joint stabilization will provide them with improved strength and improved activity, and they will usually forgo efforts at utilizing external devices.

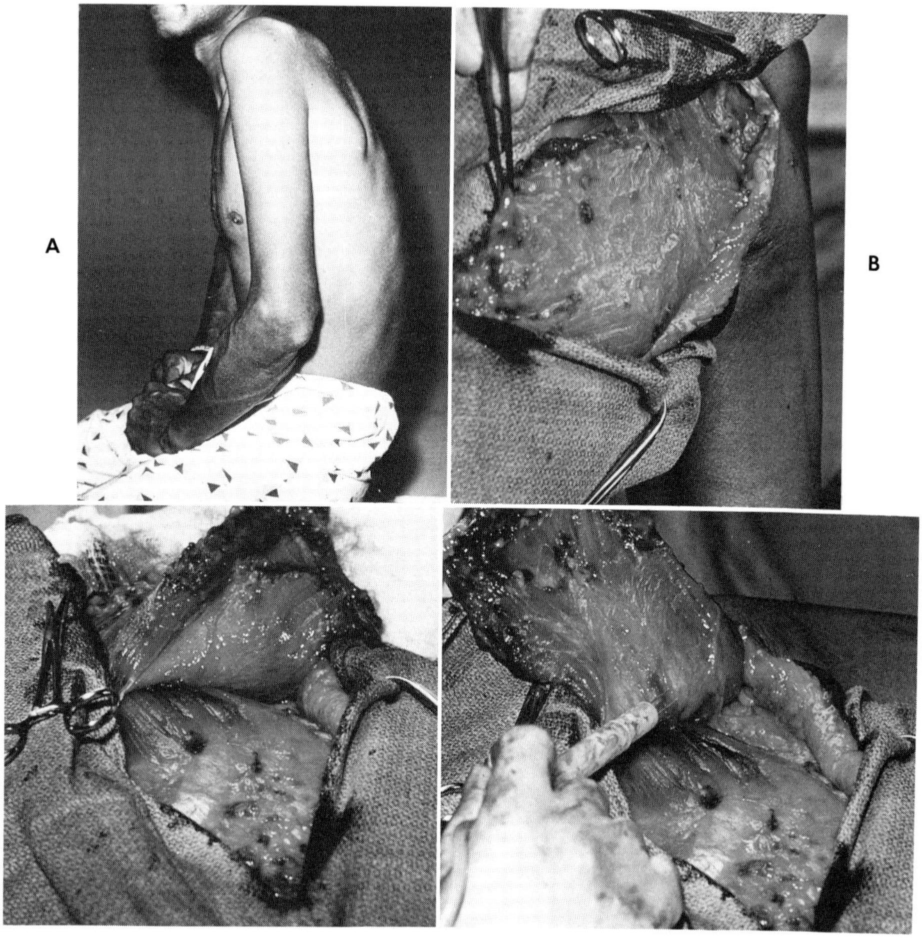

A B C D

Fig. 22-3. A, This patient had a cervical root injury from direct laceration. Elbow flexion was not possible because of paralysis of the biceps, brachialis, and brachioradialis. Restoration of elbow flexion was done by flexorplasty to the outer aspect of the humerus and later was augmented by transfer of the pectoralis major origin. The additional use of the pectoral muscle provided increased strength of elbow flexion and an improved range of motion. The shoulder girdle also required tendon transfers for maximum stability. **B,** The pectoralis major muscle has been exposed and the origin is elevated from the chest wall. The strip of external oblique fascia is left attached to the pectoral muscle to bridge the gap after the muscle is relocated over the biceps muscle in the arm. **C,** The muscle origin of the pectoralis major being elevated from the chest wall, just prior to identification of the nerve to the pectoralis. This particular procedure (Clark) does provide a large mass of muscle to replace forearm flexors. However, elongation of the insertion of the pectoralis major does accomplish approximately the same benefit, with less extensive dissection. **D,** The pectoralis muscle has been dissected from the anterior chest wall and the upper abdominal area. The electrical stimulator is used to identify the nerve to the pectoralis major so that contusion and stretch of this nerve can be avoided. Damage to the nerve results in partial or complete failure of the transfer.

Patient 3

This man had a cervical root injury resulting from a blow from a machete. Elbow flexion was weakened (Fig. 22-3, *A*). At that time (1960) we were utilizing the muscle belly of the pectoralis major. Fig. 22-3, *B-C* show the degree of mobilization of the muscle belly, and also the elongation of the origin by using a strip of the external oblique muscle. The pectoralis major nerve supply was located and preserved. The muscle mass was turned on itself and inserted into the arm, and fascia from the pectoralis major was attached to the radial tubercle by pull-out suture. Immobilization lasted 4 weeks and gradual mobilization was performed during the next 12 weeks. Good elbow function resulted.

Patient 4

This patient had an extensive brachial plexus injury and severe damage to tissues about the hand and forearm. The median nerve injury was treated by neurolysis and repair to decrease pain and improve sensation. The next step was use of the pectoralis major and a graft to bridge the gap from the insertion of the pectoralis to the radial tubercle. The recommendation of Seddon and Brooks was to use the paralyzed biceps muscle-tendon unit as a bridging graft (Fig. 22-4). In this instance, the interposed tissue stretched and strength of flexion was diminished. A graft of fascia lata or a strong intact tendon is recommended rather than the material from the biceps. Use of the muscle belly of the latissimus dorsi, augmented by a new graft from the pectoral to the radial tubercle, did provide adequate elbow flexion.

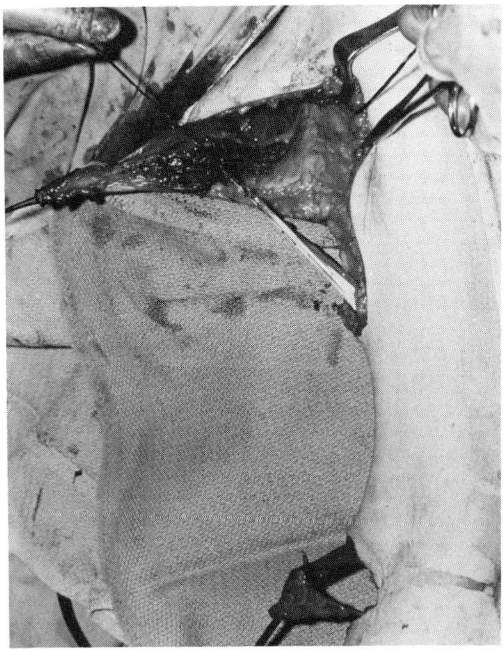

Fig. 22-4. The pectoralis major has been mobilized proximally. The attachment to the humerus has been elevated and rotated toward the midline. The biceps tendon has been isolated at the point of its attachment to the humerus and the muscle belly, distally with its fascial covering, has been isolated. Proximally the long and short heads of the biceps attached to the coracoid have been released, sutured together, and directed toward the pectoralis major. This tissue does serve as a bridge between the pectoralis major and the radial tubercle, but because it is paralyzed and because the tendon and fascia make up less than half of the total material, the likelihood of early loss of tension and stretch is far greater than when fascia lata is used to bridge the gap between the pectoral and radial attachment.

Patient 5

This patient had a traumatic incident that resulted in loss of function of the muscles supplied by the musculocutaneous and radial nerves. The biceps humerus and brachialis were completely paralyzed. The brachialis muscle usually receives a motor branch from the radial nerve and, even though the musculocutaneous nerve is completely out, a trace of elbow flexion persists. In this instance, there was complete absence of brachialis function (Fig. 22-5, *A-E*).

A

B

C

D

E

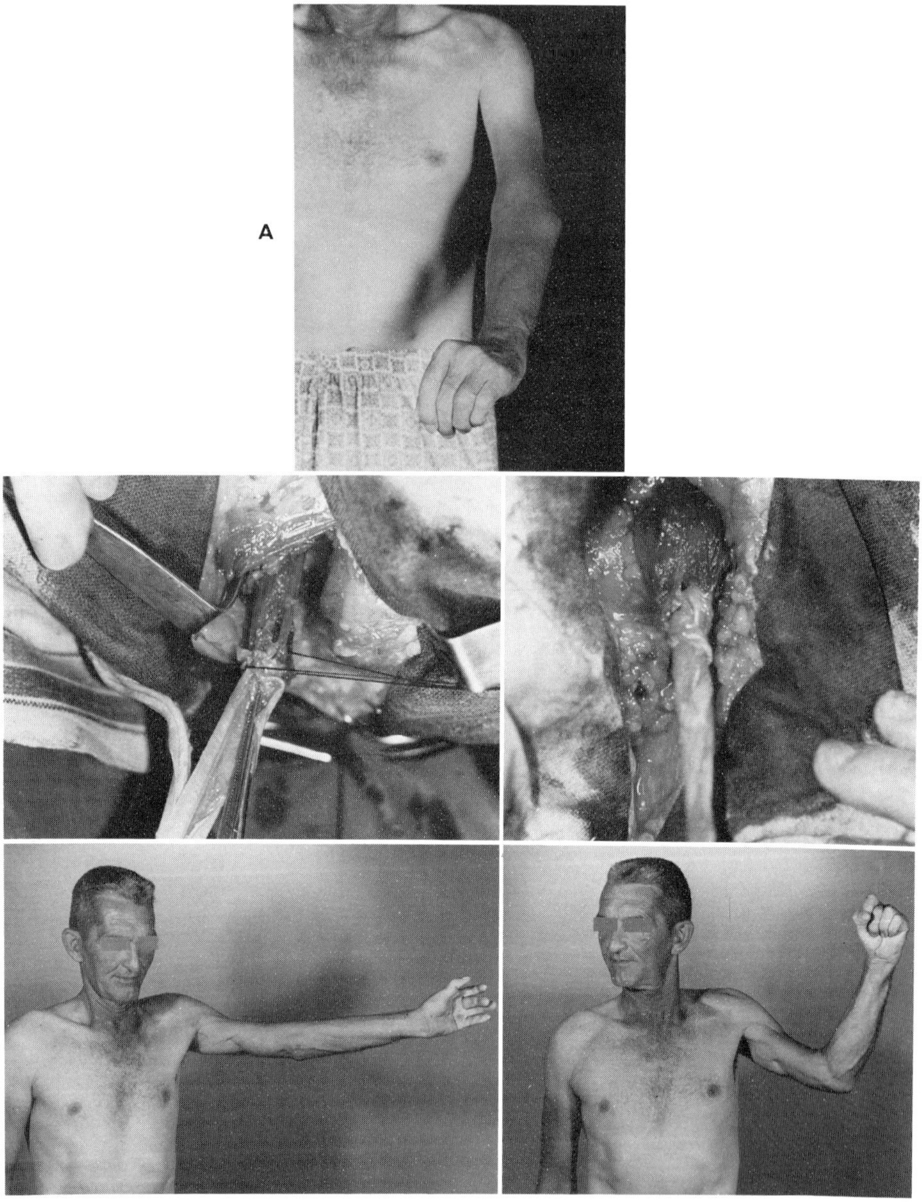

Fig. 22-5. For legend see opposite page.

The patient's original injury and initial reconstructive phase had been managed by a surgeon who was pessimistic about restoration of elbow flexion. Accordingly, the treatment was directed toward restoring hand elevation by doing tendon transfers to restore strength to the muscles supplied by the radial nerve. This included transfer of the pronator radii teres to the extensor carpi radialis longus and brevis, and transfer of flexor carpi ulnaris to the extensor digitorum communis. The patient had regained reasonable extension of the hand and fingers, but only fair extension of the thumb.

The patient had been offered an elbow arthrodesis or an external device. He refused both. The muscle groups available for restoration of elbow flexion were:

1. Forearm flexors, two of which had been transferred to the extensor muscles; The origins could be used proximally but tension of these origins was critical
2. Pectoralis major with free graft elongation to the radial tubercle
3. Latissimus dorsi, muscle belly (Zancolli), or use of latissimus dorsi by elongation of the distal end

---

Fig. 22-5. A, This patient had trauma to the upper humerus, on both the medial and lateral aspects of the arm. His treatment "elsewhere" had included tendon transfers to the hand and thumb as the first stage of reconstruction initially, and a suggestion for arthrodesis of the elbow as a second stage. The patient is attempting to flex the forearm by closing the fingers, elevating the hand, and pronation as well as contraction of the anterior deltoid and pectoralis major. The elbow flexors are not functional. When the patient attempts flexion, the biceps muscle, which was affected directly by fibrosis secondary to the prior trauma, has minimal elasticity remaining. **B,** The pectoralis major insertion has been released from the humerus through an incision that allows mobilization of the distal end of the muscle belly and isolation of the insertion into the humerus through the anterior axillary fold. Incision is curved sufficiently to avoid scar contracture. The nerve supply is identified under the pectoralis major with a nerve stimulator, and the superior fibers are released so that free excursion is possible. A fascia lata graft was removed through a long lateral thigh incision. The thick distal portion as well as the thinner proximal segment were removed. The fascia lata was split into three tails. These were woven into the pectoralis major insertion and sutured individually with nonabsorbable double 0 suture. The graft was then rolled into a tube with the deep surface being superficial and the underlying slick surface of the fascia lata exposed. The fascia is stabilized by a few sutures at the upper and middle thirds, as well as distally. **C,** The pectoralis major muscle proximally with its insertion directed toward the elbow and elongated with the large piece of fascia lata that has been braided into its insertion and rolled on itself. The muscle belly of the pectoral is stretched by the fascia and the fascial graft is placed in a large wide subcutaneous tunnel that extends from the axilla to the elbow. This tunnel is made by a heavy curved forceps that is spread about 4 cm. so that the fascial graft has adequate room for passage and will not impinge on skin ligaments. The elbow incision is made on the anterior medial surface, the radial tubercle is exposed, and a hole drilled into the tubercle. Part of the fascial attachment is pulled through the radius and held distally by a pull-out suture, and the remainder is sutured to the most distal segment of the biceps tendon under maximum tension. The tension can be adjusted by adducting and flexing the humerus. Part of the elbow incision is closed before final fixation of the fascial graft is made into the radius. **D,** The action of the pectoralis major, that caused tenting of the skin over the muscle has been detached from its insertion, elongated with fascia lata, and is now functioning as an adjunct to the flexors of the forearm, is evident. Note the extended position of the wrist, limited extension of the fingers, and the pronated position of the forearm. A fixed flexion contracture of the elbow was mild. **E,** The patient demonstrates isolated flexion of the elbow joint. He closes the fingers and dorsiflexes the wrist, and also contracts the pectoral to obtain maximum range of elbow flexion with maximum strength, which is about 85°. He is able to do this against gravity and strong resistance. The resistance was about 80% of normal when compared with his opposite side. Total range of elbow motion was about 75° actively.

The problem related to flexorplasty was that proximal advancement of the flexor carpi ulnaris and the pronator radii teres would place additional tension on this muscle mass and possibly result in increased contracture of the extensor tendons, thereby limiting flexion of the fingers and the wrist. The flexor capi radialis could be transferred without difficulty, as it had not been moved for restoration of the weakened radial nerve muscles.

Operative procedure. The forearm muscles were mobilized, the ulnar nerve isolated and transferred forward, and, with a segment of the epicondyle and elongation by fascia lata, the origins of the pronator radii teres, flexor carpi ulnaris, and flexor carpi radialis were transferred to the lateral aspect of the humerus and inserted into bone. The tension was not as great as is usually used, because of the prior transfers. Several months after operation, the patient was able to flex against gravity and rated about fair plus. This improvement was of sufficient benefit to the patient to encourage us to proceed with tendon transfer of the pectoralis major elongated with fascia lata to the radial tubercle.

Operative procedure. This operative procedure was done by exposing the humeral insertion of the pectoralis major, isolating the muscle belly proximally for about 4 cm., and not mobilizing it as is done for transfer of the entire muscle belly. A long strip of fascia lata is obtained through multiple incisions, which is split into three segments proximally, and braided into the insertion of the pectoralis major. The tubed fascia lata is then passed subcutaneously through a large wide tunnel to a second incision on the anterior medial surface of the elbow. This tunnel, which extends from the axilla to the elbow, is made by heavy curved forceps that is spread about four centimeters so that the fascial graft has adequate room for passage and will not impinge on skin ligaments. The biceps tendon is isolated and it is followed to the radial tubercle after the median nerve and brachial artery and vein had been isolated and retracted. Nonabsorbable sutures were used proximally and a strong union was secured. A ¼ inch hole was drilled into the tubercle of the radius and No. 0 polypropylene pull-out suture was passed through the hole with long needles. The needles were guided next to the ulna, and thereby avoided the extensor muscle mass, otherwise compression of the motor branch of the radial nerve might have occurred.

Before the pull-out suture is tied in place, the anterior elbow skin incision is closed, so that the elbow can be maintained in the position of about 120° of flexion, against the chest, and internally rotated thereby allowing maximum tension on the pectoralis transfer.

Immobilization lasts 4 weeks in plaster and the patient is then provided with a posterior splint to protect against forcible stretching, and is gradually allowed to extend the elbow during the following 6 weeks. Elbow flexion is practiced each hour during the day by simultaneous contraction of both the right and left pectoralis major, and by closing the fingers and elevating the wrist. The effect of the flexorplasty on this man's tendon transfers to the extensor surface of the hand was minimal because the flexorplasty was not done under maximum tension. If this had been done, wrist and finger flexion would have been limited.

The strength of elbow flexion improved noticeably over a six-month period, and at the end of a year he was flexing against gravity, past right angles, and was able to lift objects weighing more than 10 pounds. This range of motion allowed him to retrain as an electrical appliance repairman and store operator, and to be independent. Elbow arthrodesis would have limited his ability to carry out certain activities that he now does readily each day.

Substitution and augmentation patterns are important to observe. One appreciates the functional alterations that occur when the pectoralis major activates forearm flexion, and, simultaneously, wrist flexors act as wrist extensors. The degree of training necessary to accomplish this is not great. The patients adapt over a period of 2 or 3 months.

Patient 6

This patient received multiple injuries to the left upper extremity. Elbow flexion was weak and a nonunion of the humerus existed. His primary concern related to the weak elbow flexion—part of which was related to the nonunion of the humerus. Restoration of elbow flexion was accomplished by using the pectoralis major muscle belly (Fig. 22-6, *A-C*).[7]

Some patients with brachial plexus injury and residual musculocutaneous nerve deficit need strengthening of elbow flexion. Certain of these patients have

A

B

C

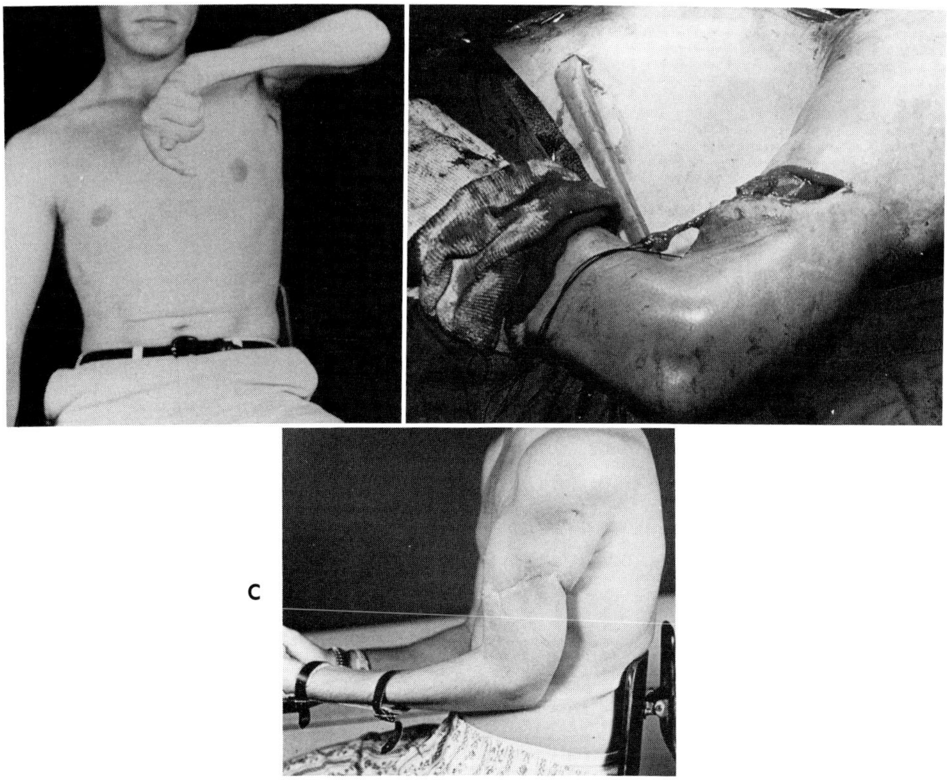

Fig. 22-6. A, This patient had multiple injuries to the left upper extremity. A nonunion of the humerus was present and elbow flexion was weak. He also had partial loss of finger extension and flexion of the index finger. He is shown here flexing the elbow when gravity is eliminated, by holding the forearm parallel with the floor. This action is possible when there is no resistance but not against gravity or resistance. **B,** The absence of muscle in the arm area was a contributing factor to nonunion of the humerus. The pectoralis major was elevated from the abdominal wall and the muscle belly, and its origin transferred to the anterior aspect of the forearm. The old oblique incision, which resulted from the original injury, was used to deliver the pectoral muscle distally. Extreme atrophy of the arm, including the distal portion of the triceps and all of the arm flexors, influenced the decision to move the muscle origin. Note the rubber drain in place on the chest wall and the extension of the pectoralis major by a strip of external oblique fascia of sufficient length to provide insertion of the pectoralis major into the tubercle of the radius. **C,** Postoperative elbow flexion strength against gravity and resistance. The nonunion of the humerus weakened the flexion, because stability was not normal. The patient could lift a 20 lb. weight without difficulty. As this photograph was taken, he was applying downward resistance to the arm in which the pectoral transfer was done by the opposite extremity. The resistance was equivalent to over 40 lbs. The nonunion of the humerus and additional reconstruction of the hand were done at a later time. In this instance, the presence of weak elbow flexion prior to the transfer and the weakness of the forearm flexors made use of the pectoralis major essential. In similar instances, the latissimus dorsi muscle belly could be transferred but the mass of muscle is not as great.

the ability to flex the elbow against gravity but can maintain no resistance and are not able to hold objects weighing more than a few ounces. An example would be a patient with a good plus pectoralis major but weak forearm flexors. The pectoralis major can be used to restore elbow flexion with noticeable strength and the technique would depend on the goal and the requirement for strength. In most instances, the insertion can be elongated with fascia lata and the strength provided by the pectoral muscle is approximately the same as that obtained when the whole muscle belly is dissected and transposed to the upper arm. The muscle origin is detached and maintained in an elongated position by using fascia from the external oblique. The nerve supply of the pectoralis major is identified with a nerve stimulator and the dissection is carried up to that point but not beyond. If the nerve is stretched, function will be lost. The advantage of the procedure is the replacement of the paralyzed muscle mass.

The procedure is done by utilizing a long incision on the anterior chest wall, bypassing the nipple, and locating the incision far enough laterally to provide a cosmetic scar. The dissection is performed down to the external oblique muscles, and a large, wide piece of fascia is dissected up to the pectoralis major muscle mass. The muscle belly is isolated and elevated by blunt dissection, the nerve to the pectoral is identified with the nerve stimulator, and the overlying fascia around the musculotendinous junction is incised and spread so there will be no constriction. The whole pectoral muscle is then mobilized. A recipient bed is prepared in the arm by extensive subcutaneous dissection superiorly and inferiorly. The humerus is maintained at the side and inflexion to decrease stretch on the nerve to the pectoral. At this point, if the shoulder has been arthrodesed initially, the humerus is not easily manipulated and placement of the pectoralis major anterior to the humerus is more difficult than if the joint were flexible.

The external oblique muscle-tendon is delivered at the elbow incision and a hole is drilled into the radial tubercle. Fixation is then the same as that used for anchoring the fascia lata when the insertion of the pectoralis major is utilized. The elbow incision is closed before the insertion is completed and the proximal area on the abdominal wall is closed and drained.

An alternate to the pectoral-flexor mass is use of the triceps, half or full, for elbow flexion and reinforcement by using the insertion of the teres major and latissimus dorsi by elongation and suture into the pectoralis major or into the triceps, whichever is being used.

In other cases, the triceps is used as an elbow flexor by detaching it distally, mobilizing it proximally, elongating it if necessary, and attaching it directly to the radial tubercle after passing it forward on the lateral side.

Another choice is the sternocleidomastoid. This must be elongated and fixed to the ulna or the radial tubercle. Any of these transfers is more desirable than an Elbow arthrodesis performed primarily for stabilization. Arthrodesis is indicated when no muscle is available, and when the extremity is extremely weak, but hand function is possible. As far as the paralyzed shoulder is concerned, tendon trans-

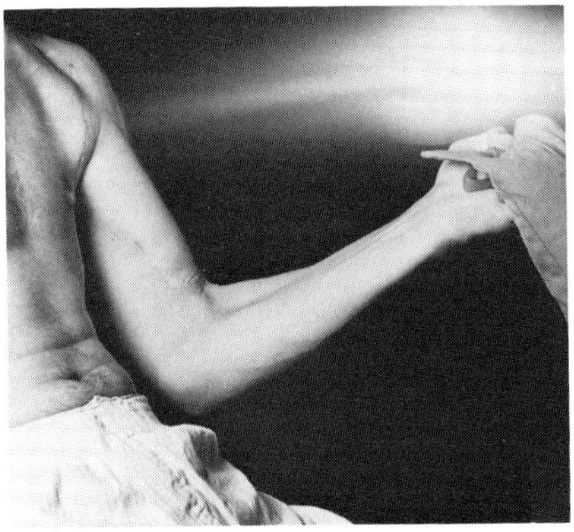

Fig. 22-7. This patient had a musculocutaneous nerve injury, with partial loss of elbow flexion. The biceps and brachialis were paralyzed except for the segment of brachialis innervated by the radial nerve. The brachioradialis was normal. The patient could flex against gravity but did not have good resistance. Furthermore, he desired to have the muscle mass replaced, as he was conscious of the loss of symmetry of the arms. The pectoralis major muscle was transferred from the anterior chest wall to the humerus and anchored into the radial tubercle, using external oblique fascia for elongation. This demonstrates the patient's ability to flex a 10 lb. weight against gravity with ease. Note the course of the pectoralis major muscle, its enlargement with flexion, and its effect on supinating the forearm. He also flexes the fingers and the wrist, in order to maintain elbow flexion.

fers to augment the weakened shoulder muscles can be performed, and strong function of the extremity is often possible. This approach is superior to an external motor, to a cable on the opposite shoulder, or, in certain instances, to an arthrodesis. I believe that tendon transfers about the shoulder should be attempted rather than resorting to arthrodesis provided, of course, that an adequate number of muscles are available.

References

1. Basmajian, J. V., and Latif, A.: Integrated actions and functions of the chief flexors of the elbow, J. Bone Joint Surg. **39A**:1106, 1957.
2. Brooks, D., and Seddon, H. J.: Pectoral transplantation for paralysis of the flexors of the elbow, J. Bone Joint Surg. **41B**:36, 1959.
3. Bunnell, S.: Restoring flexion to the paralytic elbow, J. Bone Joint Surg. **33A**:566, 1951.
4. Carroll, R. E.: Restoration of flexor power to the flail elbow by transplantation of triceps tendon, Surg. Gynecol. Obstet. **95**:685, 1952.
5. Carroll, R. E., and Gartland, J. J.: Flexorplasty of the elbow, J. Bone Joint Surg. **35A**: 706, 1953.
6. Carroll, R. E.: Use of sternocleidomastoid muscle for restoration of elbow flexion, personal communication.
7. Clark, J. M. P.: Reconstruction of biceps brachii by pectoral muscle transplantation, Br. J. Surg. **34**:180, 1946.
8. d'Aubigne, Merle, Seddon, H. J., Hendy, A. M., and Brooks, D. M.: Symposium on small reconstructive surgery of the paralyzed upper limb, Proc. R. Soc. Med. **42**:831, Section 53-66, 1949.
9. Dickson, F. D.: Fascial transplants in paralytic and other conditions, J. Bone Joint Surg. **19**:405, 1937.
10. Eyler, Don: Transfer of one half of the flexor carpi ulnaris as modification of Steindler

flexorplasty, Paper from Duke Orthopaedic and Affiliated Institutions Training Program, 1951.
11. Irwin, C. E.: Restoration of elbow flexion in patients with poliomyelitis, personal communication, 1949.
12. Kettlekamp, D. B., and Larson, C. B.: Evaluation of the Steindler flexorplasty, Paper No. 21, AAOS, January 31, 1962.
13. Mayer, L., and Greene, W.: Experiences with the Steindler flexorplasty at the elbow, J. Bone Joint Surg. **36A**:775, 1954.
14. Seddon, H. J.: Transplantation of pectoralis major for paralysis of the flexors of the elbow, Proc. R. Soc. Med. **42**:837, 1949.
15. Segat, A., Seddon, H. J., and Brooks, D. M.: Treatment of paralysis of the flexor of the elbow, J. Bone Joint Surg. **41B**:44, 1959.
16. Spira, E.: Replacement of biceps brachii by pectoralis minor transplant, J. Bone Joint Surg. **39B**:126, 1957.
17. Steindler, A.: Transplantation of tendons at elbow, AAOS, Lecture, T. 276, 1944.
18. Zancolli, E.: Transfer of latissimus dorsi muscle belly to restore paralyzed elbow flexors. Lecture presented Massachusetts General Hospital, October, 1974.

23. Operations to restore thumb opposition

a historical review

Frederick V. Minkow, M.D.

Opposition of the thumb is a basic requirement for normal use of the hand. Without the ability to oppose the thumb, the hand is weakened and dexterity is lost. The act of opposition implies motion of the tip of the thumb through a large arc. It involves many muscles and motions in all three thumb joints.

The successive position assumed by the thumb in transcribing its normal forward arc of opposition has been demonstrated by Sterling Bunnell by attaching toothpicks to the thumb. The thumb begins at the side of the hand with the thumbnail at a right angle with the palm. The thumb abducts, and after the first one third of the arc has been transversed, it pronates until it is opposite the base of the long finger with the thumbnail parallel to the palm.

The loss of opposition of the thumb is commonly caused by peripheral nerve injury, spinal cord lesions such as poliomyelitis or injury to the cord, and direct injury to muscle.

Many operations to restore thumb opposition have been described in the literature. All too often, however, the articles were brief, undocumented, without follow-up, and without definite goals. Some procedures were more successful than others; but, in general, they didn't lack for originality. Chosen for presentation are articles of classic significance and related interest that have contributed to the historical development of opponensplasty.

REVIEW OF LITERATURE

1918 to 1929

Steindler was the first to report on an operation to restore opposition of the thumb. At the 69th annual session of the American Medical Association in June, 1918, he described his procedure and gave two case reports (Fig. 23-1).[46]

Steindler split the flexor pollicis longus tendon longitudinally into two halves. The radial half of the tendon was severed at the distal end, and the tendon was carried around through a tunnel in the soft tissues to the base of the proximal phalanx. The tendon was fastened to the periosteum of the proximal phalanx

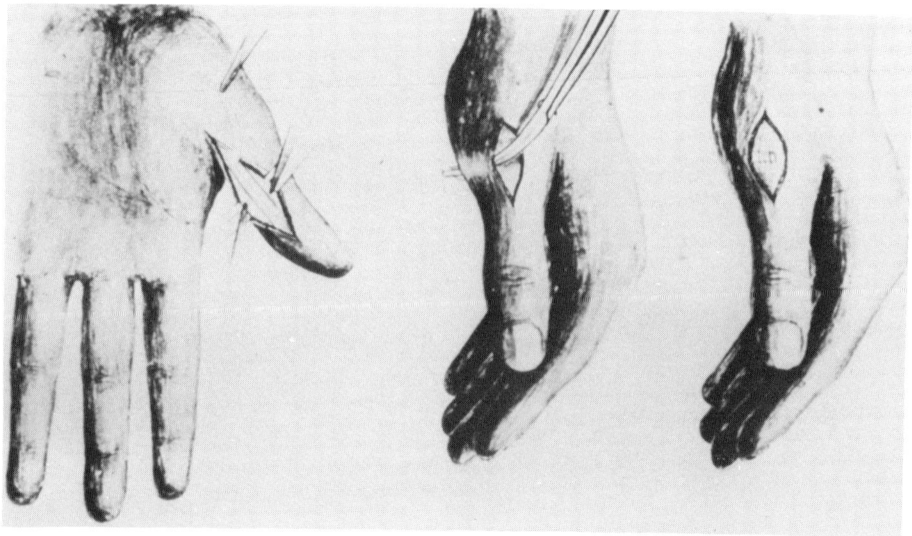

Fig. 23-1. Illustration of A. Steindler's operation, which was first described in 1918. Radial half of a split flexor pollicis longus tendon was fastened to dorsal surface of the proximal phalanx. (From Steindler, A.: Operative orthopedics, New York, 1925, Appleton-Century-Crofts, p. 94.)

well on its dorsal surface. The sheath of the flexor pollicis longus was reunited over the remaining ulnar half of the tendon.

Several operations were described in 1921 by Taylor[50] Krukenberg,[23] Ney,[33] Huber,[15] Nicolaysen,[34] Baldwin,[1] and Spitzy.[44] Cook, a military surgeon on the service of R. T. Taylor, during World War I, treated a patient who had been shot through the first web space. R. T. Taylor described Cook's procedure in which the extensor digiti minimi tendon was passed around the ulnar border of the wrist to the palmar side of the hand and inserted into the distal end of the first metacarpal.[50] More recently Schneider reported success using the extensor digiti minimi tendon transfer in ten patients.[42]

Krukenberg split the long finger sublimis tendon from the middle phalanx to the transverse carpal ligament. The radial half of the split sublimis tendon was passed around a notch in the transverse carpal ligament and sutured to the periosteum of the first metacarpal.

Ney devised a procedure for retaining the thumb in a normal position when complete intrinsic paralysis was present. The extensor pollicis brevis tendon was sectioned at the wrist and brought through a small hole in the palmar fascia. It was sutured to the palmaris longus or flexor carpi radialis tendon proximal to the transverse carpal ligament. This rerouting of the extensor pollicis brevis was subsequently incorporated into other procedures that will be mentioned later (Fig. 23-2).

In 1921, Huber[15] and Nicolaysen,[34] independently transferred the abductor

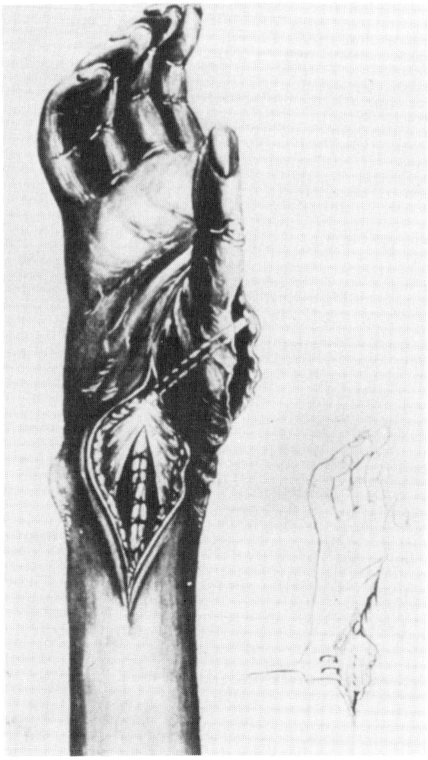

Fig. 23-2. Ney rerouted the extensor pollicis brevis tendon and attached it to palmaris longus or flexor carpi radialis proximal to the transverse carpal ligament. (From Ney, K. W.: Tendon transplant for intrinsic hand muscle paralysis, Surg. Gynecol. Obstet. 33:342, 1921.)

digiti minimi muscle on its neurovascular bundle and attached it to the first metacarpal. In 1963, Littler and Cooley[25] renewed interest in this procedure and emphasized the technical aspects of preserving the neurovascular bundle to the abductor digiti minimi.

Also in 1921, Baldwin[1] and Spitzy[44] independently performed arthrodesis of the carpal metacarpal joint of the thumb. Through a short incision, the joint was exposed and the thumb twisted into internal rotation, complete abduction, and slight flexion. The desired result was a fibrous union that allowed just enough flexion for useful movement.

Although Bunnell's classic paper on opponensplasty wasn't published until 1938,[4] he was writing about this subject as early as 1924.[5] Initially, he passed the ring sublimus tendon across the palm in the subcutaneous tissue to the outer side of the thumb. This merely adducted the thumb. Next, he combined this procedure with another in which he passed the palmaris longus subcutaneously to the outer side of the distal end of the thumb metacarpal.

Not satisfied with the combined procedure, Bunnell rerouted either the ring finger sublimis, the flexor carpi ulnaris with a free graft, or a palmaris longus around a pulley created near the pisiform. The point of insertion was the distal end of the first metacarpal. Later, the site of insertion was changed to the dorsal-ulnar aspect of the proximal phalanx of the thumb. When the thumb had assumed a flexed position due to weak thumb extensors, as in some cases of poliomyelitis, the tendon transfer was attached to the extensor pollicis longus at the metacarpophalangeal joint.

Kortzeborn, in 1924, described a static way to fix the thumb in opposition in cases of paralysis caused by polio.[22] He thought the "monkey hand" appearance of the thumb was a result of overpull by the extensor policis longus and brevis. He lengthened these tendons and fixed the thumb in opposition by excising some palmar skin and constructing a fascia lata graft across the palm.

Howell, in 1926,[14] exposed the flexor pollicis longus through a long volar incision and severed the tendon at the wrist. The distal segment of tendon was passed subcutaneously around the extensor pollicis longus and thenar eminence and was reattached to the proximal end of the flexor pollicis longus at the wrist.

Silfverskiold, in 1928, tenotomized the flexor pollicis longus at the level of the sesamoid bones.[43] The distal part of the tendon was tenodesed to the radial sesamoid to hold the interphalangeal joint in slight flexion. The proximal part of the tendon was transplanted to the radial sesamoid and the radial border of the first metacarpal.

Jahn, in 1929, transferred the extensor digitorum communis tendon of the long finger volarward around the ulnar border of the third metacarpal.[19] It was elongated with a fascia lata graft. Loss of extension of the donor finger was restored with a fascia lata graft attached to the adjacent extensor tendons.

1930 to 1939

Foerster, in 1930, inserted a 3 cm. tibial graft between the first and second metacarpals to fix the thumb in maximum opposition.[9]

Royle, in 1938, passed the ring sublimis up the sheath of the flexor pollicis longus and inserted it into the outer edge of the opponens pollicis and flexor pollicis brevis muscles (Fig. 23-3).[39, 40]

Bunnell, in 1938, published his classic article on thumb opposition in which opposition was defined and the principles of tenoplasty were given.[4] He emphasized the wide range of motors, tendons, and pulleys that could be used if one adheres to the principles of passing the tendon subcutaneously in the direction of the pisiform and inserting it on the dorsal-ulnar aspect of the base of the proximal phalanx (Fig. 23-4).

Mayer has done extensive work in the field of opponensplasty. He wrote on the subject as early as 1927,[30] and summarized his experience in 1939.[31] Mayer presented a review of his experience with the Bunnell transfer in patients with poliomyelitis. He expressed disappointment because although the patients had powerful adduction they could not oppose. He found contractures present in the carpometacarpal joints or intercarpal joints, when paralysis was present for 2

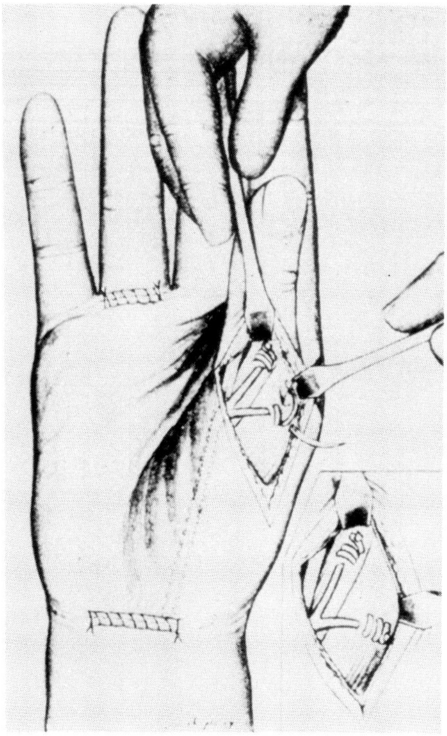

Fig. 23-3. Royle rerouted flexor digitorum sublimis tendon of the ring finger to the opponens pollicis and flexor pollicis brevis muscles. (From Royle, N. D.: Operation for paralysis of intrinsic muscles of the thumb, J.A.M.A. **111**:612, 1938.)

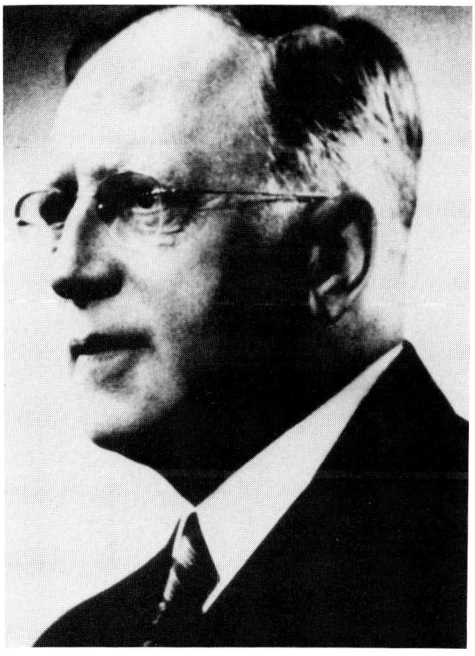

Fig. 23-4. Sterling Bunnell published his classic article on thumb opposition in 1938.

years or more. His results improved when the tight joint structures were released prior to tendon transfers, as had been advocated by Bunnell.

1942 to present

Irwin, in 1942, warned not to use a paralyzed flexor carpi ulnaris for the pulley because it would stretch out and the correct direction of pull of the transfer would be lost.[16]

Thompson, in 1942, brought the ring sublimis out in the palm, using the lower border of the transverse carpal ligaments as a pulley.[52] The sublimis was carried across the center of the thenar eminence and fixed to the distal end of the metacarpal and to the base of the proximal phalanx. Osteotomy at the base of the metacarpal could be done when and if there was an external rotation contracture of the thumb (Fig. 23-5).

Goldner and Irwin, in 1950, reemphasized the need to thoroughly evaluate the status of the thumb in poliomyelitis and the secondary changes that occur in bones, joints, and soft tissues before reconstruction is attempted.[10] They presented a classification and treatment plan based on the existing condition of the hand.

Riordan, in 1959, suggested that the tendon transplant be so directed that it reduplicated the pull of the abductor pollicis brevis.[38] The transfered tendon was sewn into the extensor pollicis longus to increase extension of the distal joint

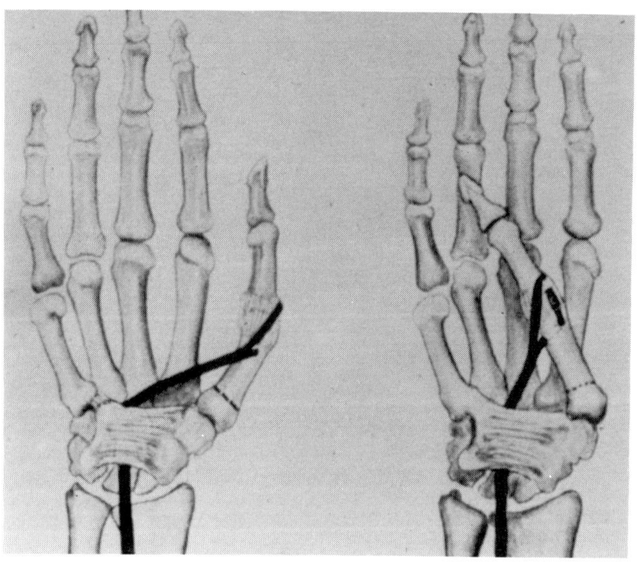

Fig. 23-5. T. C. Thompson transferred flexor digitorum sublimis of the ring finger around the lower border of the transverse carpal ligament. Osteotomy at the base of the first metacarpal could be done to correct an external rotation contracture of the thumb. (From Thompson, T. C.: Modified operation for opponens paralysis, J. Bone Joint Surg. **24**:632, 1942.)

of the thumb, and also into the abductor pollicis brevis to provide opposition and abduction.

In some situations, it is better to select a finger or wrist extensor for a motor, especially when the forearm is scarred or the flexor muscles are injured or paralyzed. Phalen and Miller[35] Henderson,[12] Zancolli,[58] and Tubiani[54] were among several authors who described operations that utilized extensor tendons for motors.

Phalen and Miller, in 1947, transferred the extensor carpi ulnaris to the rerouted extensor pollicis brevis tendon.[35] The technique of using the extensor pollicis brevis had previously been described by Ney in 1921.[33]

Henderson, in 1962, reported on his experience using any available wrist extensor tendon or brachioradialis to restore thumb opposition.[12] The muscles were elongated with either a free tendon graft or a distally attached extensor pollicis brevis tendon.

Zancolli, in 1965, transferred the extensor indicis proprius tendon around the ulnar border of the wrist.[58] In the same article he described a second procedure. The extensor pollicis brevis tendon was detached distally and brought out at the wrist. It was passed through the flexor carpi radialis sheath and fixed to the abductor pollicis brevis.

Tubiani, in 1969, modified the Zancolli procedure by rerouting the extensor pollicis brevis tendon proximally around the flexor carpi radialis before fixing it distally to the abductor pollicis brevis.[54]

DeVecchi, in 1961, described a rather simple procedure that was performed in only one patient.[7] Two incisions were made along the medial and lateral border of the thumb at the metacarpophalangeal joint. The adductor pollicis tendon was detached at its insertion and passed superficial to the sheath of the flexor pollicis longus tendon and deep to the neurovascular bundles. The tendon was sutured to the abductor pollicis brevis and opponens at the level of the metacarpophalangeal joint.

For cases of median and ulnar nerve paralysis of the thumb due to leprosy, Brand, in 1966, modified the tendon insertion to the thumb to provide stability at the metacarpophalangeal joint without it being an active mover of that joint.[2] The ring finger sublimis tendon was split with half being passed dorsal to the metacarpophalangeal joint to the adductor tendon and the other half passed to the radial side of the joint and attached to the extensor pollicis longus tendon.

Makin, in 1967, translocated the flexor pollicis longus to the radial side of the thumb through an osteotomy of the proximal phalanx without detaching the tendon.[29] The procedure avoided any tendon anastomosis and the circulatory embarrassment associated with the circumferential incision. It is a modification of the procedure described by Howell in 1926[14] and by Von Bayer in 1925.[56] Howell divided the flexor pollicis tendon at the wrist before wrapping it around the thumb. Von Bayer utilized a circumferential incision around the thumb.

Ramsellar, in 1970, emphasized the multitude of pulleys that have been used in opposition transfers and that the desired direction of pull of the transferred tendon can be altered by changing the location of the pulley.[37]

SUMMARY

Certain requirements must be met before attempting to restore opposition of the thumb. With these essentials in mind, you will be able to appreciate why some operations were more successful than others. There should be:

1. Metacarpophalangeal and interphalangeal joint stability of the thumb
2. Carpometacarpal mobility at the base of the thumb
3. A soft bed in which the tendon transfer or graft may glide
4. A muscle of sufficient power and amplitude to produce effective function
5. The proper insertion to support stability and attitude of the thumb
6. A pulley located in the correct position to provide effective pull to the thumb

The important thing to remember is that there is a multitude of motors, pulleys, and methods of insertion from which to choose, but the success of the operations depends on choosing the best procedure for each individual patient.

References

1. Baldwin, W. I.: Orthopedic surgery of the hand and wrist in bones. In Sir Robert, editor; Orthopedic surgery of injuries, Vol. 1, London, 1921, Oxford University Press, p. 277.
2. Brand, P. W.: The hand in leprosy in clinical surgery. In Pulvertaft, R. G., editor: The hand, London, 1966, Butterworth & Co. (Publishers) Ltd., p. 279.
3. Brooks, D. M.: Intermetacarpal bone graft for thenar paralysis, J. Bone Joint Surg. **31B:** 511, 1949.
4. Bunnell, S.: Opposition of the thumb, J. Bone Joint Surg. **20:**269, 1938.
5. Bunnell, S.: Reconstructive surgery of the hand, Surg. Gynecol. Obstet. **39:**259, 1924.
6. Camitz , H.: Surgical treatment of paralysis of opponens muscle of thumb, Acta Chir. Scand. **65:**77, 1929.
7. DeVecchi, J.: Opposition del pulgar fisiopathologia viva nueva operation—transplante del adductor, Boletin, de la Sociedad de Cirugia del Uruguay **32:**423, 1961.
8. Edgerton, M. T., and Brand, P. W.: "Restoration of abduction and adduction to the unstable thumb in median and ulnar paralysis, Plast. Reconstr. Surg. **36:**150, 1965.
9. Foerster, O.: Value of orthopedic fixation operations in nerve disease, Acta Chir. Scand. **67:**351, 1930.
10. Goldner, J. L., and Irwin, C. E.: An analysis of paralytic thumb deformities, J. Bone Joint Surg. **32A:**627, 1950.
11. Grunkorn, J.: Die daumenopposition, Hre Muskelphysiologische Erklarung Und Die Belandlung des OppositionsausFalls, Z. Ortho. Chir. Scand. **57:**517, 1932.
12. Henderson, E. D.: Transfer of wrist extensors and brachioradialis to restore opposition of the thumb, J. Bone Joint Surg. **44A:**513, 1962.
13. Hill, N. A.: Restoration of opposition for the paralyzed thumb, Clin. Ortho. **61:**234, 1968.
14. Howell, D. W.: A new operation for oppenens paralysis of the thumb, Lancet **1:**131, 1926.
15. Huber, E.: Hilfsoperation bei Medianuslahmung, Deutsche Ztschr, F. Chir. **126:**271, 1921.
16. Irwin, D. E.: Transplants to restore function of opposition, end results, South Med. J. **35:**257, 1942.
17. Iselin, M.: Chirurquie de la Main, ed. 2, Paris, 1955, Masson & Cie Editeurs, p. 314.
18. Jacobs, B., and Thompson, T. C.: Opposition of the thumb and its restoration, J. Bone Joint Surg. **42A:**1015, 1960.

19. Jahn, A.: akhver Ersata be. Oppositionslahmung des Daumens, Z. Orthop. Chir. **51**:100, 1929.
20. Kaplan, E.: Functional and surgical anatomy of the hand, ed. 2, Philadelphia, 1965, J. B. Lippincott, Co.
21. Kirklin, J. W., and Thomas C. G.: Opponens transplant: an analysis of the methods employed and results obtained in seventy-five cases, Surg. Gynecol. Obstet. **86**:213, 1948.
22. Kortzeborn, A.: Operativ-Behandlung der Sogenannten Affenhand, Arch. Klin, Chir. **133**: 465, 1924.
23. Krukenburg, H.: Uber Ersatz des M. Opponens Pollicis, Z. Orthop. Chir. **42**:178, 1921-1922.
24. Litter, J. W.: Tendon transfers and arthrodeses in combined median and ulnar nerve paralysis, J. Bone Joint Surg. **31A**:225, 1949.
25. Littler, J. S., and Cooley, S. G. E.: Opposition of the thumb and its restoration by abductor digiti quinti transfer, J. Bone Joint Surg. **45A**:1938, 1963.
26. Lyle, J. H. M.: The disabilities of the hands and their physiological treatment, Ann. Surg. **78**:816, 1923.
27. Lyle, J. H. M.: The operative treatment of thenar paralysis, Ann Surg. **84**:288, 1926.
28. Lyle, J. H. M.: Result of an operation for thenar paralysis of the thumb (extensor flexorplasty), Ann. Surg. **79**:933, 1924.
29. Makin, M.: Translocation of the flexor pollicis longus tendon to restore opposition, J. Bone Joint Surg. **49B**:458, 1967.
30. Mayer, L.: Loop operation for paralysis of the adductors of the thumb, Am. J. Surg. **2**:456, 1927.
31. Mayer, L.: Operative reconstruction of the paralyzed upper extremity, J. Bone Joint Surg. **21**:377, 1939.
32. Minkow, F. V. Operations to restore thumb opposition—a historical review, Sound Slide Program 357, AAOS.
33. Ney, K. W.: Tendon transplant for intrinsic hand muscle paralysis, Surg. Gynecol. Obstet. **33**:342, 1921.
34. Nicolaysen, J.: Transplantation des M. abductor Dig. V be: Fehlender Oppositions Fahigkeit des Daumens, Deutsche Z. F. Chir. **168**:133, 1922.
35. Phalen, G. S., and Miller, R. C.: The transfer of wrist extensor muscles to restore and reinforce flexion power of the fingers and opposition of the thumb, J. Bone Joint Surg. **29**:993, 1947.
36. Price, W. E.: A two-tendon transplant for low median ulnar palsy of the thumb in leprosy, Proc. R. Soc. Med. **61**:220, 1968.
37. Ramselaar, J. M.: Tendon transfers to restore opposition of the thumb, Leiden, 1970, H. E. Stenfert Kroese, B.V.
38. Riordan, D. C.: Surgery of the paralytic hand. In AAOS Instructional Course Lectures, The American Academy of Orthopedic Surgeons **16**:79, 1959.
39. Royle, N. D.: Operation for paralysis of intrinsic muscles of the thumb, J.A.M.A. **111**: 612, 1938.
40. Royle, N. D.: Operation for thenar paralysis, Med. J. Aust. **2**:155, 1936.
41. Scherb, R.: Uber den Ersatz Poliomyelitisch Gelamter Daumenmuskeln durch Sehnentransplantation und uber das fehlen Antagonistischer Bindungen an der Obersen Extermitat, Schweiz. Med. Wschr. 75.
42. Schneider, L. H.: Opponensplasty using the extensor digiti minimi, J. Bone Joint Surg. **51A**:1297, 1969.
43. Silverskiold, N.: Sehnentransplantation Methode be; Lahmung der Oppositions Fahiqkeit des Daumens, Acta Chir. Scand. **64**:296, 1928.
44. Spitzy, H.: Die Krankhaften Veranderungen der Oberen Extremitat, Verhandl. Deutsch. Orthop. Besellsch., 25th Congress, pp. 76-113, 1931.
45. Steindler, A.: Orthopedic operations on the hand, J.A.M.A. **71**:1288, 1918.
46. Steindler, A.: Orthopedic operations on the hand, Transactions of the Section on Orthopedic Surgery of the A.M.A., 69th Annual Session, Chicago, 1918, A.M.A. Press, p. 64.

47. Steindler, A.: Flexorplasty of thumb in thenar palsy, Surg. Gynecol. Obstet. **50**:1005, 1930.
48. Steindler, A.: Operative orthopedics, New York, 1925, Appleton, p. 94.
49. Steindler, A.: Tendon transplant in the upper extremity, Am. J. Surg. **44**:260, 1939.
50. Taylor, R. T.: Reconstruction of the hand, Surg. Gynecol. Obstet. **32**:237, 1921.
51. Thompson, C. F.: Fusion of metacarpals of thumb and index finger to maintain functional position of thumb, J. Bone Joint Surg. **24**:907, 1942.
52. Thompson, T. C.: Modified operation for opponens paralysis, J. Bone Joint Surg. **24**:632, 1942.
53. Troxell, E. L.: The thumb of man, Sci. Monthly **43**:148, 1936.
54. Tubiani, R.: Anatomic and physiologic bases for the surgical treatment of paralysis of the hand, J. Bone Joint Surg. **51A**:613, 1969.
55. Tubiani, R.: Paliative treatment of paralytic deformities of the thumb, Ortho. Clin. North Am. **4**:4, 1141, 1973.
56. Von Baeyer: Bewegungslehre und Orthopadie, Z. Orthop. Chir. **46**:24, 1925.
57. Williams, H. W. G.: The leprosy thumb, Br. J. Plast. Surg. **19**:136, 1966.
58. Zancolli, E.: Tendon transfers after ischemic contracture of the forearm, Am. J. Surg. **109**:356, 1965.

24. Thumb disabilities in rheumatoid arthritis: classification and treatment

Alfred B. Swanson, M.D., F.A.C.S.
Genevieve deGroot Swanson, M.D.

Any study of reconstructive surgery of the thumb must consider the entire ray—its balanced musculotendinous system and the position, mobility, and stability of its joints. Arthritic and posttraumatic disabilities often seriously interfere with the normal functional adaptations of the thumb. Fortunately, however, most of these disabilities respond well to reconstructive measures of arthroplasty, fusion, capsulodesis, tendon transfers, or other procedures.[1, 5, 14, 16]

In thumb disabilities the joints may be primarily affected, or they may be secondarily affected as a result of imbalances of other joints of the articular chain, as in the boutonniere and swan-neck deformities. Treatment therefore requires a knowledge of the functional anatomy of the thumb and the pathogenesis of the deformity presented.

ANATOMY

The thumb of man is unique in the animal kingdom. Its functional interaction with the fingers for both strength and precision gives man the greatest prehensile ability of all animals. The thumb is relatively strong as compared with the digits to which it opposes. All three joints of the thumb are important in functional adaptations, and each one is designed for a specific purpose in the articular chain.[6, 14]

Interphalangeal joint

The interphalangeal joint of the thumb is essentially the same as the distal interphalangeal joint of the fingers. It is a ginglymus or hinge joint, which moves in one axis only—flexion-extension—and is strongly reinforced by its capsule, collateral ligaments, and volar plate. The flexor pollicis longus muscle flexes this joint to an average of 80°. The extensor pollicis longus tendon and the winglike insertion of the lateral and medial intrinsic muscles into a dorsal hood provide active extension and hyperextension to an average of 5° to 10°; however, passive hyperextension can measure 30° to 40°. The arrangement of this extensor apparatus is similar to that in the fingers.

Flexion of the distal joint of the thumb is important in pinch activities (especially to the ulnar fingers), in grasp activities to hold objects in the palm, and in the manipulation of small objects to position them against the other digits. Adequate flexion and extension of this joint are also very important to the positioning of the sensitive palmar surface of the thumb for fine sensory appreciation.

Metacarpophalangeal joint

The metacarpophalangeal joint of the thumb is a condyloid articulation like the metacarpophalangeal joint of the fingers; however, it also has some of the characteristics of the ginglymus joint. The thumb metacarpophalangeal joint moves in two separate axes: flexion-extension and abduction-adduction. However, the laxity of the capsular ligaments also allows a considerable degree of rotation.

The head of the first metacarpal has a biconvex surface corresponding to the shallow biconcave surface of the base of the proximal phalanx. The collateral ligaments are especially strong and allow approximately 10° of radial or ulnar deviation. The musculotendinous units that cross the joint provide a strong stabilizing system. The intrinsic muscles have insertions into the proximal phalanx, the volar plate, and the extensor hood to help stabilize the joint during prehensile movements. The fibrocartilaginous volar plate contains two sesamoid bones into which the flexor pollicis brevis and the oblique head of the adductor pollicis are inserted. Active or passive extension of this joint is usually less than 10° under normal circumstances. Greater values of extension can be considered abnormal and may signal an important disability. Flexion varies from 30° to 100° in normal individuals, with an average of 75°. Strong active flexion forces can be applied across this joint in prehensile activities and are important in the flexion-adduction position in which the thumb is placed across the palm.

Carpometacarpal joint of thumb

The carpometacarpal joint makes possible the wide circumduction motion of the normal thumb and has great functional importance in activities involving grasp and pinch. It is a saddle joint in which the convexity of one surface fits into the concavity of the other to allow movement in two separate planes: adduction-radial abduction and retroposition-palmar abduction. The capsuloligamentous system around the joint is relatively loose and allows some actual motion in a third axis of movement: rotation. The articular surfaces are kept in apposition by muscle tone and the capsular ligaments, the most important being the anterior oblique (deep ulnar) ligament, which anchors the volar beak of the thumb metacarpal to the deep intercarpal ligaments. The loss of this ligament in either traumatic or arthritic disabilities allows radial subluxation of the metacarpal to occur. It is important to reconstruct this ligament in many arthritic cases associated with

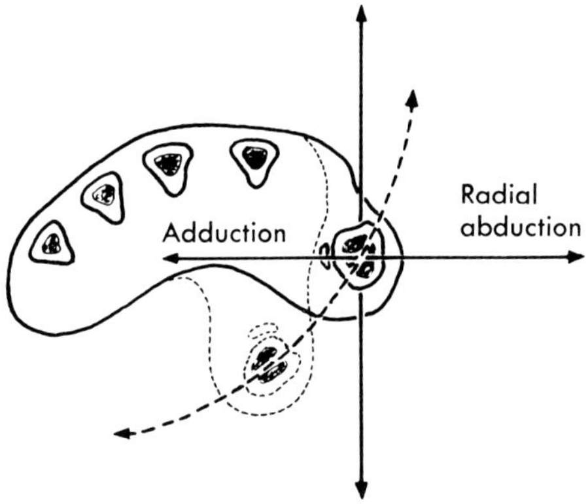

Fig. 24-1. Positional movements of the thumb are adduction, radial abduction, palmar abduction or anteposition, and retroposition. Opposition (dotted line) is accomplished by movements of axial rotation, abduction, and flexion of all three joints of the thumb, resulting in rotation of the thumb in position to present its palmar pad to the pad of any finger. (Redrawn from Tubiana, R.: Surg. Clin. North Am. **48**:967, 1968.)

subluxation. The stability of the carpometacarpal joint also depends on the tone of the musculotendinous units that surround it.

The positional movements of the thumb can be arbitrarily divided into (1) adduction, which moves the thumb toward the index finger on the palmar plane; (2) radial abduction, which is the opposite of adduction and brings the thumb away from the index finger on the palmar plane; (3) palmar abduction, which can also be described as anteposition and moves the thumb away from the palm in a plane perpendicular to the palmar plane; (4) retroposition, which moves the thumb in a plane perpendicular to the palmar plane and in a direction posterior to this plane; and (5) opposition, which is characterized by the ability to carry the thumb away from the palm and to achieve rotation of the thumb ray to present the palmar pad of the distal phalanx of the thumb to the pad of any of the fingers.[21]

Opposition is an essential feature of normal prehension (Fig. 24-1). The actual rotation is accomplished by a circumduction movement that is a geometrical result of the two movements of abduction and the flexion of all three joints of the thumb. The muscles, acting during opposition, also provide a motion of pronation that occurs at the carpometacarpal and metacarpophalangeal joints. The average rotation obtained in normal opposition ranges between 90° and 120°. Passive rotation of the thumb ray is possible between 60° and 80°, and is greater at the metacarpophalangeal joint than at the carpometacarpal joint. However, the range of active rotation is less than half the range of passive rotation. The remainder of the apparent rotation occurs through the abduction and flexion components of the circumduction movement.

CLASSIFICATION AND PATHOMECHANICS OF DISABILITIES

A long standing experience in the evaluation of the rheumatoid arthritic thumb has led us to attempt to classify its disabilities.[8, 9]

I. Postural deformities
   A. Longitudinal collapse deformities
      1. Boutonniere (primary MP joint disturbance)
      2. Swan-neck (primary CM joint disturbance)
      3. Other
   B. Fixed positional deformities
      1. Adducted retropositioned thumb
      2. Other
II. Unstable, stiff, or painful joints
   A. Interphalangeal joint
   B. Metacarpophalangeal joint
   C. Carpometacarpal joint
III. Tendon disabilities (contracture, displacement, rupture)
   A. Flexor pollicis longus
   B. Extensor pollicis longus
   C. Extensor pollicis brevis
   D. Abductor pollicis longus
   E. Intrinsics

The joints of the thumb may be impaired from osteoarthritis, rheumatoid arthritis, or posttraumatic arthritis. A sound understanding of the mechanism of deformities is important to select the proper treatment.[11, 14, 20]

The boutonniere deformity

The boutonniere deformity is the most common collapse deformity of the thumb in rheumatoid arthritis. It is found in 57% of the rheumatoid hands and is caused primarily by an arthritic involvement of the metacarpophalangeal joint.[2, 3] Initially, the joint capsule and extensor apparatus around the metacarpophalangeal joint are stretched out by a synovitis process. The extensor pollicis longus tendon and adductor expansion are displaced ulnarward. The lateral thenar expansions are displaced radially. The attachment of the extensor pollicis brevis tendon to the base of the proximal phalanx is lengthened and becomes ineffective. The ability to extend the metacarpophalangeal joint is decreased and results in a flexion deformity of the proximal phalanx. The extensor pollicis longus tendon and the extensor insertions of the intrinsic muscles apply all their power to the distal phalanx and secondarily produce hyperextension of the interphalangeal joint. Pinch movements further aggravate the deformity and a vicious circle is established: the more the flexion of the metacarpophalangeal joint, the greater the tendency for the interphalangeal joint to hyperextend and the thumb ray to collapse. In time, as contractures develop, the deformity becomes fixed. Destructive articular changes compound the deformity and disorganization, and subluxation of the joint may occur.

The swan-neck deformity

The swan-neck deformity of the thumb is usually initiated by destructive changes at the carpometacarpal joint. This deformity is present in 9% of the rheumatoid thumbs; it is by far more common in osteoarthritic thumbs. When restriction of motion occurs at the base of the thumb, compensatory movements occur at the distal joint to provide thumb function. Instability and deformity of the swan-neck type may result from these compensatory changes. Similarly, when the normal sliding motion of the trapeziometacarpal joint during abduction becomes painful, the patient avoids abduction and an increasing adduction contracture develops. If there is an effusion in the joint, further loosening of the capsule occurs permitting a radial proximal subluxation of the metacarpal. As a result the normal movements required in pinch become increasingly painful and the distal joints are used to compensate for the lack of movement at the base of the thumb. The result is hyperextension of the interphalangeal joint, but more frequently hyperextension of the metacarpophalangeal joint and further adduction of the first metacarpal. A vicious circle is therefore established. The more the adduction contracture of the metacarpal, the greater the tendency for the metacarpophalangeal joint to hyperextend and the thumb ray to collapse. Occasionally, severe erosive changes in the carpometacarpal joint and absorption of the trapezium occur. This decompresses the joint and the severity of the deformity is decreased.

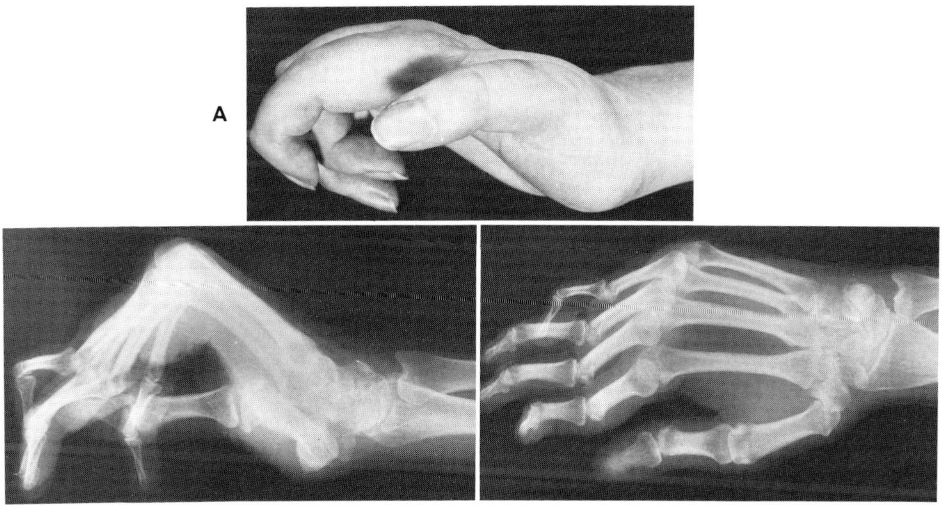

A

B

C

Fig. 24-2. A, The adducted retroposition is a fixed positional deformity of the postural deformity category. It is caused by a radial palmar dislocation of the metacarpal base off the trapezium. A contracture of the extensor pollicis longus further aggravates the adducted, retropositioned, and externally rotated position, which precludes opposition movement of the thumb for normal functional pinch and grasp activities. **B,** The lateral radiographic view of the hand demonstrating the dislocation of the first metacarpal base off the trapezium in the radiopalmar direction. **C,** The antero-posterior radiograph of this hand showing the dislocation at the basal joint of the thumb and the externally rotated thumb ray.

The adducted retropositioned thumb

A deformity occasionally seen in the rheumatoid hand is one in which the thumb metacarpal is retropositioned, adducted, and externally rotated (Fig. 24-2). This is seen in less than 5% of the patients with rheumatoid arthritis; it has been seen most frequently in the young patient with rheumatoid arthritis, in which cases it presents difficult treatment problems. It appears that the deformity is initiated by a synovitis at the carpometacarpal joint. Awkward positioning of the thumb on a flat board during acute illness can result in a permanent deformity. The ability of the extensor pollicis longus muscle to adduct and externally rotate the metacarpal is predominant. Palmar and radial subluxation of the metacarpal off the trapezium occurs. Consequently, the patient has difficulty abducting the metacarpal and may develop an abduction deformity of the metacarpophalangeal joint by stretching the ulnar collateral ligament in grasp activities.

Unstable, stiff, or painful joints

Instability of the interphalangeal, metacarpophalangeal, or carpometacarpal joint may occur as isolated deformities in rheumatoid arthritis, resulting from synovial invasion and erosive changes of the bone. These deformities are accentuated by the forces applied during pinch. Joint instability may be seen in association with other deformities such as the instability of the interphalangeal joint present in the late stages of the boutonniere deformity. In rheumatoid thumbs not presenting a collapse deformity, instability is seen in 35% of the metacarpophalangeal joints and in 7% of the interphalangeal joints.

Tendon disabilities

Tendon disabilities in the rheumatoid thumb may be related to muscle contracture, tendon displacement, adhesions, or ruptures, similar to what is seen in the other digits of the rheumatoid hand.

The extensor pollicis longus tendon is the most commonly ruptured tendon in the rheumatoid thumb. Its most frequent site of disruption is within the third extensor compartment in the area of Lister's tubercule. The tendon may suddenly give way or may gradually thin out and lengthen by several centimeters as the attempted healing process occurs. The etiology of ruptured tendons include invasion of the synovial tissue into the tendon substance especially at points of pulley constriction. The additional erosive effect of rough bone on the tendon takes its toll. The sudden ruptures of the extensor pollicis tendon result in a sudden drop of the metacarpophalangeal joint of the thumb and some loss of extensor power at the distal phalanx. The deformity may be confused with the classical boutonniere deformity, which is also an extrinsic minus problem. The hyperextension of the distal joint is, however, not as prominent; the lack of extension of the metacarpophalangeal joint is usually associated with less flexion contracture and, most importantly, the long extensor tendon cannot be prominently palpated on the back of the hand in forced extension and retroposition positions of the thumb.

Rupture of the flexor pollicis longus is not rare and must be thought of in any hyperextended interphalangeal deformity of the thumb. This rupture may occur suddenly with the patient's awareness or may be a gradual process of loss of flexion of the distal joint. Ruptures of the flexor pollicis longus frequently occur at the radial aspect of the flexor canal. Erosive and subluxating changes in the trapezium and scaphoid bones may present an abrading surface over which the tendon must slide. Ruptures of this tendon may also occur at the entrance of the digital flexor canal, similar to that occurring in the other flexor canals. In this situation, the hypertrophied synovial covering around the tendon abuts against the relatively rigid opening of the fibro-osseous canal as the tendon glides. The synovium bunches up proximal to the pulley and acts as a block to further tendon movement. The increased fluid pressure in the synovium finally forces the synovium into the tendon substance, which eventually loses its blood supply and becomes necrotic. Careful examination of active flexion will help differentiate the hyperextended interphalangeal thumb joint of the boutonniere deformity from that of the ruptured flexor pollicis longus.

Ruptures of the abductor pollicis longus and extensor pollicis brevis are rare. Disability of the intrinsics usually results from their displacement and secondary contracture caused by synovial invasion and stretching of the dorsal hood of the metacarpophalangeal joint of the thumb. The intrinsic attachment to the dorsal hood is consequently displaced palmarly and this results in a distortion of its normal function.

SURGICAL TREATMENT

The most frequently used methods in our clinic for surgical treatment of thumb disabilities include: flexible implant resection arthroplasty for the carpometacarpal, metacarpophalangeal, and interphalangeal joints; capsulodesis or fusion of the metacarpophalangeal joint; and hemitenodesis or fusion of the interphalangeal joint.

The basal joints

A study of the roentgenograms of patients selected for reconstructive surgery of the thumb demonstrated that the arthritic changes most frequently occur at the trapeziometacarpal joint but that the trapezioscaphoid, trapeziotrapezoid, and trapezium–second metacarpal joints are also involved in a significant number of cases. The trapezium was the center of the arthritic process in all cases of osteoarthritis and of traumatic arthritis.[10] Patients with rheumatoid arthritis may have a similar localized involvement of the basal thumb joints. They may also have severe absorptive changes of the trapezium and base of the metacarpal, which produces a result not unlike a resection arthroplasty. If the joint is reasonably stable, mobile, and pain-free, no surgery is indicated. However, some patients have a dislocation of the metacarpal off the trapezium in addition to severe erosive and absorptive bone changes and ligamentous loosening at the base of the thumb. It is important to realign the thumb ray but the destructive changes are too great to allow an implant arthroplasty or other stabilizing procedures. In these cases, we have resected the base of the metacarpal and partially resected the carpus so that the base of the metacarpal can be reduced in position. The metacarpal is held in a position of function with a temporary Kirschner wire fixation. A pain-free, reasonably stable fibrous ankylosis results. This has allowed us to perform other procedures necessary at the metacarpophalangeal and interphalangeal joints such as fusion or arthroplasty.

That the arthritic process most frequently involves more than the trapeziometacarpal joint is significant since it suggests that total excision of the trapezium will be necessary in most cases to eliminate all arthritic pain. Fusion procedures of the trapeziometacarpal joint does not remove the disease problem in the other three joints.

Trapezium implant resection arthroplasty

Trapezium implant resection arthroplasty can be used in selective cases of rheumatoid arthritis in which adequate bone stock is present. This procedure has been described for the osteoarthritic thumb disabilities in great detail; certain technical considerations are of great importance to obtain good results.[10, 11, 14, 15, 17]

Indications. Trapezium implant resection arthroplasty is indicated in the presence of the following conditions whether the disability is due to degenerative, posttraumatic, or rheumatoid arthritis:

1. Localized pain and palpable crepitation during circumduction movements with axial compression of the thumb (grind test)
2. Decreased motion, pinch, and grip strength
3. Radiologic evidence of arthritic changes of the trapeziometacarpal, trapezioscaphoid, trapeziotrapezoid, and trapezium–second metacarpal joints, singly or in combination
4. Unstable, stiff, or painful distal joints of the thumb or swan-neck collapse deformity

Surgical procedure (Fig. 24-3). A 5 cm. to 7 cm. incision is made over the radial aspect of the thumb and wrist (Fig. 24-3, *A*). This incision is centered over the trapezium, parallel to the extensor pollicis brevis. It is preferred because of the excellent exposure provided to identify the branches of the superficial radial nerve and the trapezium. This incision can be extended distally to expose the metacarpophalangeal joint and proximally to inspect the first dorsal compartment, the flexor carpi radialis tendon, or the trapezioscaphoid joint. The branches of the superficial radial nerve are identified, mobilized, and carefully retracted. The base of the first metacarpal and the trapeziometacarpal joint are first identified. The capsule is incised longitudinally and reflected by sharp dissection from the base of the metacarpal and trapezium. It is very im-

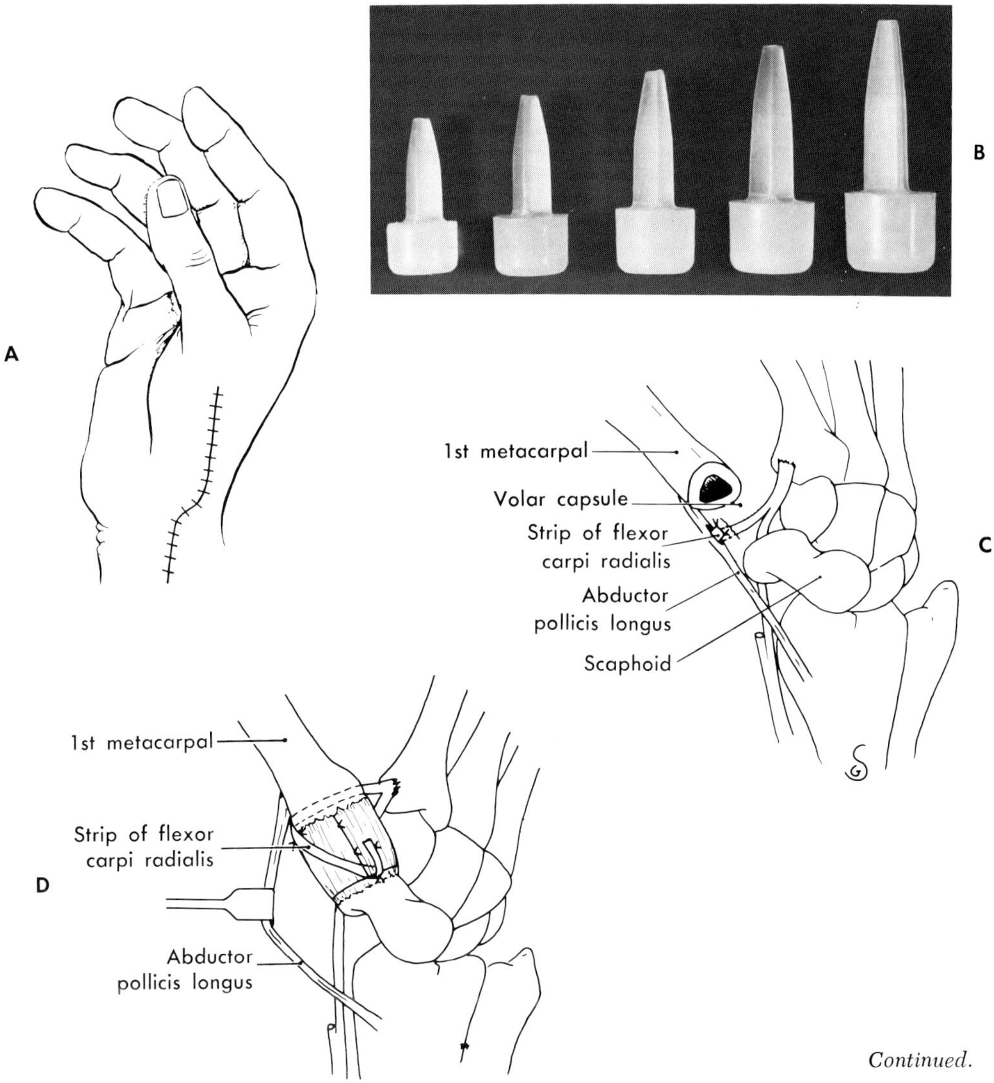

Continued.

Fig. 24-3. Trapezium implant resection arthroplasty technique. **A,** The longitudinal incision is placed over the short extensor tendon and has a short transverse and palmarward arm to then continue proximally in a longitudinal direction. This incision allows excellent exposure of the nerves, vessels, tendons, and joint structures important to the procedure. **B,** Intramedullary stemmed silicone rubber implant improves the results of excision arthroplasty of the trapezium by acting as a space filler and preserving the joint space relationships. This implant is available in five sizes. **C,** This illustration demonstrates a method of reinforcement of the volar capsule with a strip of flexor carpi radialis tendon. This technique may be used when there is evidence of inadequate volar capsular support for the implant following removal of the trapezium bone. **D,** A method utilizing a 7 cm. strip of the flexor carpi radialis tendon to reconstruct an ulnar check ligament. The tendon strip is dissected proximally in the wrist, passed into the area of the trapezium resection through the fibro-osseous canal and dissected to the base of the second metacarpal; the strip is then passed on the volar aspect of the base of the first metacarpal and secured over the dorsal capsule. Displacing the first metacarpal towards the second metacarpal and securely suturing the tendon strip to the capsular structures provides a firm ulnar check ligament to stabilize the first metacarpal and its implant.

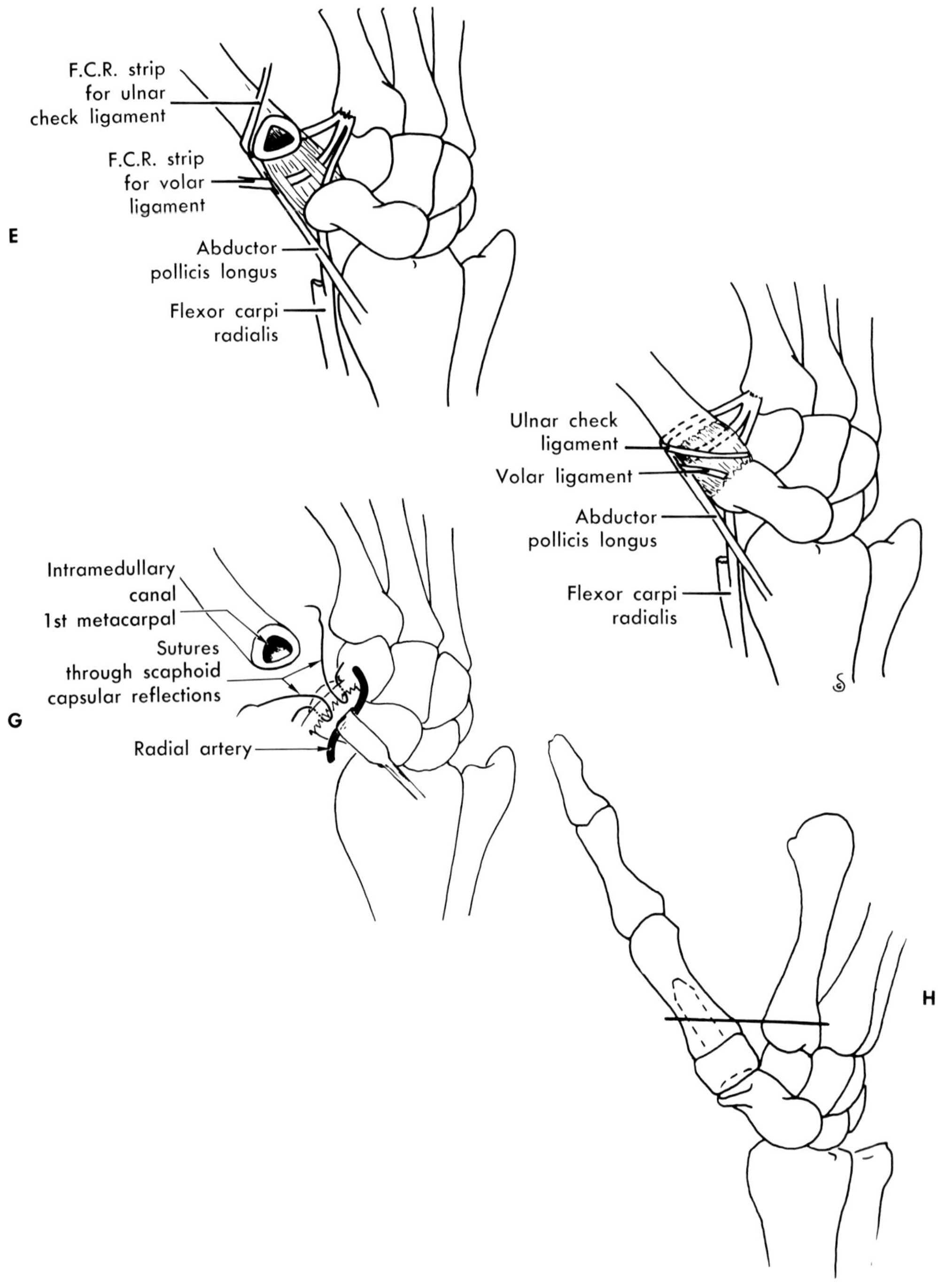

Fig. 24-3, cont'd. For legend see opposite page.

portant to preserve the capsule to provide substance for a strong closure at the end of the procedure. The overlying branch of the radial artery is carefully dissected off the trapezium. A small articular branch may be tied off to facilitate this mobilization. Careful retraction of the artery is important during the entire procedure. The dissection is then continued around to the palmar surface of the trapezium, carefully freeing the attachment of the transverse carpal ligament on the trapezium. It is important to stay close to the bone during this dissection to avoid injury to the artery, tendons, or capsule.

The entire trapezium is removed including its medial portion by a piecemeal method sectioning the bone into two or three pieces with an osteotome and then removing the fragments with a bone biting rongeur. During this step, it is essential to avoid injury to branches of the radial artery, the flexor carpi radialis tendon, and the joint capsule of the trapezium, especially the volar portion. Any osteophytes or irregularities on the distal end of the scaphoid are trimmed.

The base of the metacarpal is squared off with a rongeur leaving most of the cortical and subchondral bone intact. A hole is then made in the base of the metacarpal to open up the intramedullary canal using a drill, small curettes, or a broach. The base of the metacarpal may be elevated into the wound by using a small, sharp two prong retractor. The canal should not be opened any more than necessary to receive the stem of the implant easily. A set of test implants is used to determine the proper implant size that fits easily into the space left by resection of the trapezium, and allows full thumb circumduction yet maintains stability. The concave base of the implant should seat properly over the scaphoid bone (Fig. 24-3, *B*).

Using instruments and a no-touch technique, the stem of the implant is inserted into the intramedullary canal of the metacarpal. It is important that

---

Fig. 24-3, cont'd. E and **F,** These illustrations show how the two preceding techniques, **C** and **D,** can be combined using a double tendon slip from the flexor carpi radialis to form both a volar ligament support and an ulnar check ligament. The residual length of the strip can be used to reinforce the dorsal capsule. **G,** This illustration emphasizes the importance of proper exposure and retraction of the radial artery over the scaphoid bone to allow sutures to be placed in the capsular reflection of the scaphoid bone. These sutures are very important in providing dorsal capsular stability of the implant on closure. **H,** Kirschner wire fixation between the first and second metacarpals with the thumb positioned midway between palmar and radial abduction is of extreme importance in assuring ideal position of the implant during the capsular ligamentous healing stage. A 0.045 in. Kirschner wire can be drilled through the cortex of the first and second metacarpals while holding the thumb in the abducted position and also maintaining the implant over the scaphoid. This wire can be passed more easily using power equipment; however, this can also be done efficiently with a hand drill. The wire can be cut under the skin and is extracted when the plaster cast is removed 6 weeks later. The wire may also be passed through the head of the implant into the trapezoid bone. It is left protruding 1 cm. out of the skin. It should be removed through a window in the cast in 2 weeks.

the collar of the implant be in intimate contact with the base of the metacarpal throughout its circumference to avoid wobbling. The thumb is then held in abduction to place the implant well into the recess left by the removal of the trapezium.

At the end of the surgical procedure, it is important to thoroughly secure the implant in place by reconstruction of the carefully preserved capsuloligamentous structures. Before inserting the implant, the volar capsule and ligaments should be inspected in the depths of the wound for inadvertent tears during removal of the trapezium. This can be verified by forceful manipulation of the metacarpal with the implant in position. If present, these tears should be sutured with 3-0 Dacron on a PR-2 needle to provide a firm supporting capsule on the volar surface of the implant. A strip of the flexor carpi radialis tendon can also be used for reinforcement of the volar capsule (Fig. 24-3, *C*).

If there are only mild or moderate destructive changes around the trapezium, the normal capsuloligamentous structures suffice to maintain the implant in position. The dorsal radial capsular structures are brought together tightly over the implant and are carefully sutured with 2-0 or 3-0 Dacron or other nonabsorbable suture material using multiple interrupted sutures and inverted knot technique.

A careful closure of the dorsal capsule must include firm suturing over the scaphoid bone. The radial artery in this area is carefully retracted proximally for exposure. If necessary, a small drill hole through the dorsoradial surface of the scaphoid may be made to receive 2-0 Dacron sutures for firm fixation of the capsule.

If the capsule is loose, it should be imbricated. If it is thinned out, it should be reinforced using local tendons such as the abductor pollicis longus, the flexor carpi radialis, and the extensor carpi radialis longus.

Ulnar check ligament reconstruction with flexor carpi radialis. A slip of the flexor carpi radialis tendon may be used to reconstruct an ulnar oblique ligament between the first and second metacarpals (Fig. 24-3, *D*). This is especially important in patients who have had subluxation of the metacarpal off the trapezium with stretching out of this ligament.[3, 10] It is also important in patients who will be expected to do heavy work. Strong pinch forces require stability of the base of the metacarpal to prevent subluxation and a simple capsular repair may not be adequate. The flexor carpi radialis is exposed either by extending the initial longitudinal incision in a palmar proximal direction or through a separate incision. A slip 6 cm. to 7 cm. in length and one third to one half the width of the flexor carpi radialis tendon is prepared leaving its distal insertion at the base of the second metacarpal intact. The slip is dissected proximally and passed through the carpal tunnel of the flexor carpi radialis to be withdrawn into the area left by the resected trapezium. The flexor slip is then further dissected longitudinally from the main flexor carpi radialis tendon as it crosses the depths of the wound and attaches to the base of the second metacarpal. A small hemostat is then used to develop a tunnel under the capsule and to bring the tendon slip around the base of the metacarpal between the capsule and the bone. We now prefer to bring this slip around the radial aspect because it improves the pronation position of the first metacarpal. The tendon slip is then pulled tight to provide a check ligament between the base of the second metacarpal and the first metacarpal. The slip is then sutured to the capsule, placed underneath the insertion of the abductor pollicis longus tendon, and overlapped and sutured across the dorsal capsule to further reinforce this area on closure. The insertion of the abductor pollicis longus tendon is usually advanced distally on the metacarpal as the closure is completed to improve its abduction force. The flexor carpi radialis tendon slip can be split in half to be used for reconstruction of both the volar capsule and the ulnar check ligament (Fig. 24-3, *E-G*). We prefer this procedure now because it provides capsular reinforcement circumferentially around the implant as well as giving material for the ulnar check ligament reconstruction. The weak points of the capsule that must be carefully checked before the procedure is completed include capsular reflection at the scaphoid bone and the radiopalmar and ulnar-dorsal areas.

The first dorsal compartment is routinely inspected and released longitudinally to improve the moment force of the abductor pollicis longus and the extensor pollicis brevis, as well as to relieve the frequently associated tendinitis in the area.

The postoperative fixation must maintain the correct position for 6 weeks until a strong capsule has formed around the implant.[7, 12] We routinely place a 0.045 Kirschner wire between the first and second metacarpals to maintain the position of the trapezium implant during the healing phase (Fig. 24-3, *H*). The wire is inserted before final closure of the capsule so that the position of the implant can be observed. The wire is drilled through the base of the first metacarpal approximately 1 cm. from the base and directed towards the base of the second metacarpal. The wire may go through the stem of the implant; however, it usually is possible to insert the wire through the cortex of the first metacarpal. Care must be taken to avoid injury to the radial artery. Fixation should hold the thumb securely in the recommended palmar abducted position. The firmly sutured and reinforced capsule and the postoperative wire fixation have prevented the complication of subluxation of the implant.

Temporary fixation of the implant to the base of the first metacarpal may be important in some unstable cases. The implant and first metacarpal base may also be transfixed to the trapezoid or scaphoid bones with a small Kirschner wire. Any trapezium implant fixation must be temporary; otherwise the implant can be torn or there may be localized bone absorption tendencies. The wire is usually left extruding from the skin about 1 cm. When the wire is placed through the head of the implant into the trapezoid bone for temporary fixation, it is removed through a window in the cast in about 2 weeks.

Special considerations. Adduction of the first metacarpal is frequently an associated problem in arthritic disabilities of the basal joints of the thumb. If severe and untreated, it will imbalance the thumb and seriously affect the result of resection arthroplasties of the trapezium. If the angle of abduction between the first and second metacarpals does not reach at least 45° or more, the origin of the adductor pollicis muscle must be released from the third metacarpal through a separate palmar incision. Once sufficient abduction has been achieved, proper seating of the implant on the scaphoid should be established. A Kirschner wire can be passed through the first and second metacarpals for temporary fixation in severe cases.

Hyperextension deformity of the metacarpophalangeal joint contributes to the adduction tendency of the metacarpal and prevents proper abduction of the metacarpal and seating of the implant. If the metacarpophalangeal joint hyperextends less than 10°, no treatment is necessary except to apply the postoperative cast so that the metacarpal is abducted and not the proximal phalanx. If the metacarpophalangeal joint hyperextends from 10° to 20°, a Kirschner wire is placed obliquely across the joint while it is held in 10° of flexion. The wire is extracted when the cast is removed 4 weeks to 6 weeks after surgery. This fixation facilitates maintenance of abduction of the metacarpal during the healing phase. If hyperextension of the metacarpophalangeal joint is greater than 20°, stabilization is an absolute necessity either by palmar capsulodesis or fusion. In patients who have a 30° to 40° flexion of the metacarpophalangeal joint of the thumb, a capsulodesis is the operation of choice to save the available flexion. These procedures should be performed at the same time as the implant is inserted. If the swan-neck deformity is severe with no flexion available at the

A

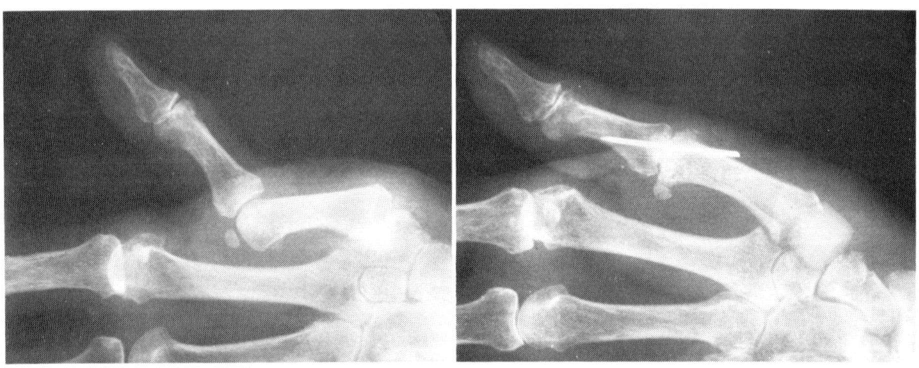

B

Fig. 24-4. A, The preoperative roentgenogram shows a thumb in a 69-year-old woman with the swan-neck deformity secondary to severe arthritis involving the trapeziometacarpal joint. The base of the metacarpal is subluxated radially and adduction contracture of the metacarpal and a hyperextension deformity of the metacarpophalangeal joint has resulted. **B,** The postoperative roentgenogram demonstrates an implant resection arthroplasty of the trapeziometacarpal joint. The patient has also had proximal release of the adductor muscle and arthrodesis of the metacarpophalangeal joint. The patient has had an excellent functional and cosmetic result from her problem.

metacarpophalangeal joint, fusion of this joint and temporary fixation of the distal joint in extension is performed (Fig. 24-4).

A boutonniere deformity of the thumb is usually not associated with arthritis of the basal joints of the type that would require implant arthroplasty. However, when this situation does occur, fusion of the metacarpophalangeal joint and release of the extensor pollicis longus at the distal joint may be performed at the same time as the implant procedure.

Postoperative care. The hand and forearm are placed in a voluminous conforming dressing with a roll of cotton or Dacron batting between the first and second metacarpals to maintain 40° to 60° of palmar abduction. A plaster splint is incorporated in the dressing. A scaphoid type cast is applied after 3 to 4 days, taking care to place the abduction pressure on the metacarpal and the phalanges to avoid later pain and deformity of the metacarpophalangeal joint. The cast is removed after 6 weeks, and abduction and opposition movements of the thumb are encouraged. If there is a tendency for adduction contracture, a roll of soft material such as sheet wadding or a cylinder of wood or plastic of 4 cm. to 5 cm. in diameter is given to the patient to hold across the palm and the thumb web space. Full unguarded movements are usually possible in 6 to 10 weeks.

The metacarpophalangeal joint

Treatment possibilities for disabilities of the metacarpophalangeal joint of the thumb include flexible implant resection arthroplasty, capsulodesis, and arthrodesis.

Implant resection arthroplasty. Implant resection arthroplasty of the metacarpophalangeal joint of the thumb has been carried out successfully in our clinic for the last 9 years.[11, 13, 14, 18, 19] It is indicated for severely destroyed metacarpophalangeal joints with associated stiffness of the distal or basal joints and in boutonniere deformities in which the metacarpophalangeal joint is destroyed and the distal joint requires fusion. This procedure has provided adequate stability and the increased movement of flexion has been important especially for fine coordinated movements (Fig. 24-5).

The metacarpophalangeal joint is approached through a dorsal, longitudinal, obliquely directed incision. This can also be made in continuation with the incision for reconstruction of the basal joints of the thumb. The dorsal veins are preserved and the extensor hood is exposed by blunt dissection.

A careful reconstruction of the extensor mechanism is essential for good results. The extensor pollicis longus tendon is released from the wing-like expansions of the intrinsic muscles on each side and retracted. The intrinsic expansions are then dissected free on each side of the joint including the insertion of the extensor pollicis brevis, which is released from the base of the proximal phalanx.

The neck of the metacarpal is exposed subperiosteally and transected with

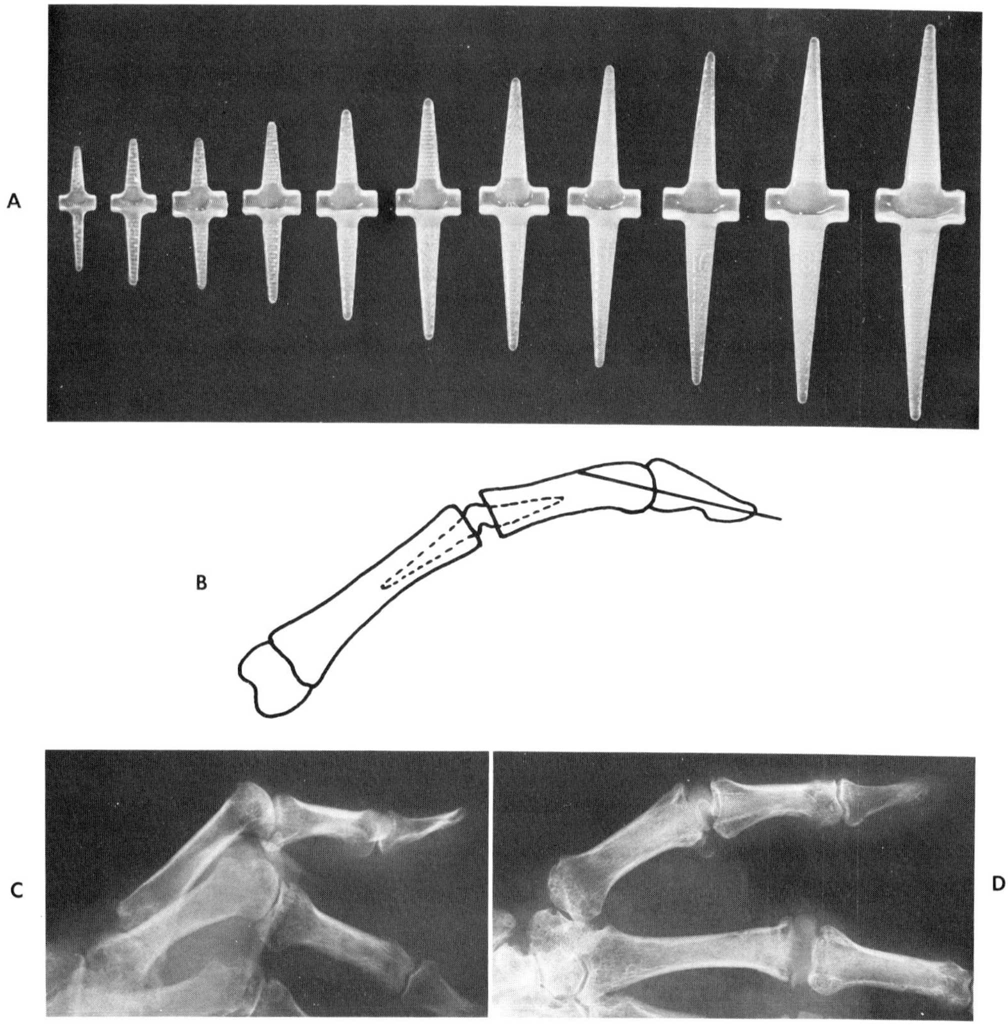

Fig. 24-5. **A**, The intramedullary stemmed silicone rubber implants for the finger joints are available in 11 anatomical sizes. Implant sizes 4 through 9 are usually used for reconstruction of the metacarpophalangeal joint. **B**, The head of the metacarpal is resected and the intramedullary canals are prepared to receive the stems of the implant. The implant midsection must fit snugly against the collar of resected bone. All flexion contractures must be released. If the distal joint is destroyed, fusion in the appropriate position is indicated; otherwise, the joint is temporarily pinned in 10° of flexion with a small Kirschner wire to encourage motion of flexion and extension at the level of the metacarpophalangeal joint during the rehabilitation phase. **C**, Preoperative radiogram showing a severe boutonniere deformity with subluxation of the metacarpophalangeal joint in a patient with rheumatoid arthritis, who also had involvement of the metacarpophalangeal joints of the fingers. **D**, Postoperative radiogram showing the flexible implant in position in the metacarpophalangeal joint of the thumb. Implant arthroplasty of metacarpophalangeal joints 2 through 5 was also carried out. The patient had an excellent result with adequate stability and good flexion/extension of the thumb metacarpophalangeal joint.

an air drill, motor saw, or bone cutting forceps leaving part of the flair of the metaphysis. Care should be taken to avoid splintering the bone. The head of the metacarpal is then grasped and removed en masse with the attached synovial tissue. The collateral ligaments and capsular attachments are left intact. All capsuloligamentous structures must be carefully preserved during the procedure. Synovectomy of the joint is completed, using a pituitary rongeur.

If there is a severe contracture of the metacarpophalangeal joint, the collateral and accessory collateral ligaments and palmar plate may be incised. All flexion contractures must be released.

No bone resection of the base of the proximal phalanx is usually performed except for marginal osteophytes that might interfere with the implant. Occasionally in patients with osteoporosis and longstanding dislocation, the base of the proximal phalanx will be severely deformed and shaping of the base may be necessary.

The intramedullary canal of the metacarpal is prepared with a curette or broach. We prefer an air drill with a special burr that has a smooth leader point to prevent perforation of the lateral cortex of the metacarpal. Care should be taken to avoid excessive reaming of the canal, especially in patients with thin bones. Test implants are used to select the proper implant size. The stem of the implant should fit well down into the canal so that the transverse mid-section of the implant abuts against the smoothened bone end. The largest size possible should be selected. Sizes 4 through 9 are usually used. A rectangular hole is then made in the base of the proximal phalanx and the intramedullary canal is reamed to receive the distal stem of the implant.

An adequate extensor mechanism must be restored. A small area of cortical bone is removed from the base of the proximal phalanx and a small drill hole is placed through the bone for later fixation of the extensor pollicis brevis tendon.

The wound is irrigated with saline to remove debris and the implant is inserted using blunt instruments and a no-touch technique. With the joint in extension, the phalanx and the metacarpal should not impinge on the implant. If there is impingement, either the soft tissue release or bone resection has been inadequate. Reshaping of the implant must be avoided because it might create mechanical weakness. Shortening of the end of the stem is permissible.

Once the implant is in place, the extensor pollicis brevis tendon is sutured through the drill hole to the bony depression at the base of the proximal phalanx with 3-0 Dacron taking care to properly adjust the tension. The extensor expansions of the medial and lateral intrinsic muscles are brought over the area and sutured to each other with 3-0 Dacron. This improves the extension power of the proximal phalanx and the stability of the joint. The extensor pollicis longus is then advanced distally and maintained over the center of the phalanx with a few Dacron sutures. Closure of the skin is completed and a small drain is inserted subcutaneously.

The usual conforming dressing is applied for 3 to 5 days. A padded aluminum splint may then be taped on the thumb metacarpophalangeal joint in 0° of extension. This is worn for 3 to 4 weeks. Contrary to implant arthroplasty of the fingers, the goal of implant arthroplasty of the MP joint of the thumb is primarily stability with some amount of useful flexion movements. No special exercises are prescribed after splint removal except normal functional adaptations. Forceful activities should be avoided for 6 to 8 weeks.

Mild to moderate boutonniere deformity of less than 10° fixed flexion contracture of the metacarpophalangeal joint can be treated by preserving the joint surfaces and using the same tendon reconstruction technique as for the implant arthroplasty. The metacarpophalangeal joint is fixed in 0° of extension with a Kirschner wire for a period of 4 weeks. If the distal joint is destroyed, implant arthroplasty or fusion in the appropriate position is indicated. If the distal joint is adequate but presents a hyperextension deformity with contracture of the extensor pollicis longus tendon, it is lengthened or simply transected distally to decrease the extensor power at the distal joint. The distal joint is then pinned in 10° of flexion with a small Kirschner wire for a period of 4 to 6 weeks until the tendons have healed.

Occasionally, a flexible hyperextension deformity of the interphalangeal joint occurs that seems to be related to a palmar plate and collateral ligament relaxation. The patient may be able to actively flex the joint, but on strong pinch, severe hyperextension occurs that results in considerable disability A flexor tenodesis procedure can prevent hyperextension and still allow flexion; this procedure may be used instead of arthrodesis of the distal joint especially if lateral stability is present and the joint surfaces are intact (Fig. 24-6).

Capsulodesis for swan-neck deformity. If hyperextension of the metacarpophalangeal joint is present to more than 20° and flexion of the joint is possible

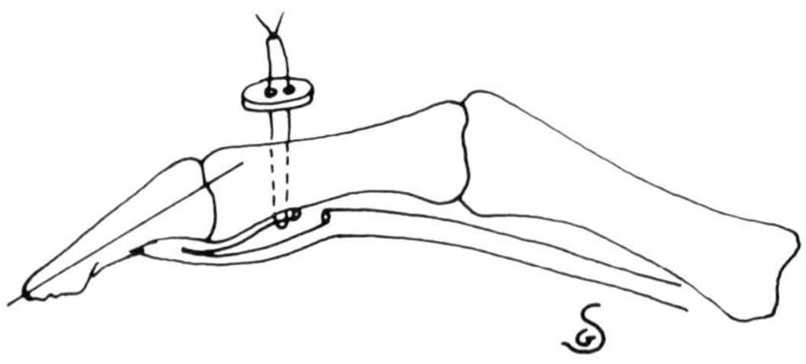

Fig. 24-6. A flexor tenodesis of the thumb interphalangeal joint can be carried out for certain flexible hyperextension deformities of this joint. A slip of the flexor pollicis longus is prepared, leaving its distal attachment to the distal phalanx intact. The periosteum is stripped from the volar aspect of the neck of the proximal phalanx; two small drill holes are made through the bone in a vertical direction and converted with a curette to form a small cavity to receive the tendon slip. The flexor slip is secured in position, using a pull-out type suture exiting dorsally over a button to obtain 10° to 15° flexion of the interphalangeal joint. A small Kirschner wire is placed across the joint to maintain the desired degree of flexion. The pull-out wire is removed in 3 weeks and the Kirschner wire in 6 weeks.

to only 30 to 40°, the joint being otherwise stable with good articular surfaces, a palmar capsulodesis procedure is indicated (Fig. 24-7). The palmar aspect of the joint is exposed through a lateral incision. The proximal membranous insertion of the palmar plate is incised. The sesamoid bones and their tendinous attachments are left intact. The periosteum is stripped from the volar aspect of the neck of the metacarpal and two small drill holes, made through the bone in a vertical direction, are converted with a curette to form a cavity to receive the palmar plate flap. The dorsal aspect of the palmar plate is scarified and pulled up into the bony depression with a pull-out type suture exiting dorsally over a button. The suture is placed through the palmar flap as to obtain 10° to 15° of flexion of the metacarpophalangeal joint. A small Kirschner wire is placed obliquely across the joint to maintain the desired degree of flexion. The pull-out suture is removed in 3 weeks and the Kirschner wire in 6 weeks. This procedure has worked well in correction of hyperextension deformity if attention is paid to obtain a firm union between the palmar plate and the bone.

Arthrodesis. A fusion of the metacarpophalangeal joint of the thumb is indicated in cases of severe joint destruction by rheumatoid arthritis provided there is adequate mobility at the distal and basal joints. Fusion of the metacarpophalangeal joint to simplify the articular chain system of the thumb ray by subtracting a joint can also be of great importance in balancing a severe collapse deformity of either the boutonniere or the swan-neck type when the distal and basal joints are adequate.

The joint is exposed through a longitudinal dorsal incision and the extensor hood is longitudinally incised through the middle. The head of the metacarpal is shaped convexly to fit the concavity formed at the base of the proximal phalanx. A longitudinal wire is placed in a retrograde fashion through the entire

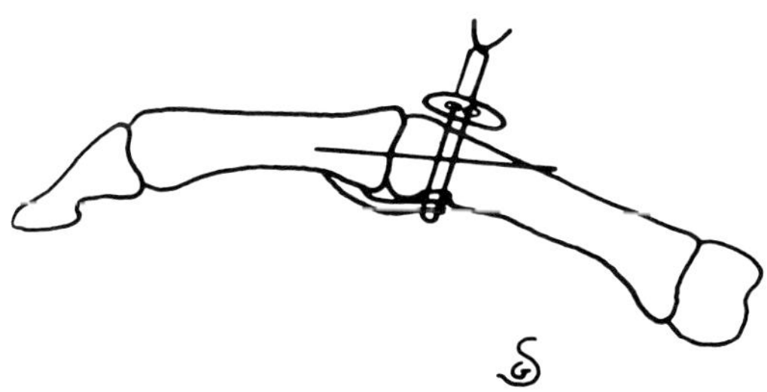

Fig. 24-7. Capsulodesis of the metacarpophalangeal joint of the thumb: the palmar aspect of the joint is exposed through a lateral incision. The proximal membranous insertions of the palmar plate are incised. The tendinous attachments on the sesamoid bones are left intact. The periosteum is stripped from the volar aspect of the neck of the metacarpal. Two small drill holes are made vertical to the bone and converted into a cavity with a small curette. The dorsal aspect of the palmar plate is roughened and fixed in the bony depression with a pull-out wire suture exiting dorsally over a button. The tension of the palmar plate flap must be such as to obtain 10° to 15° of flexion of the metacarpophalangeal joint. The desired degree of flexion of the joint is maintained with a Kirschner wire left in place for 6 weeks. The pull-out wire is removed after 3 weeks.

A

B

C

D

E

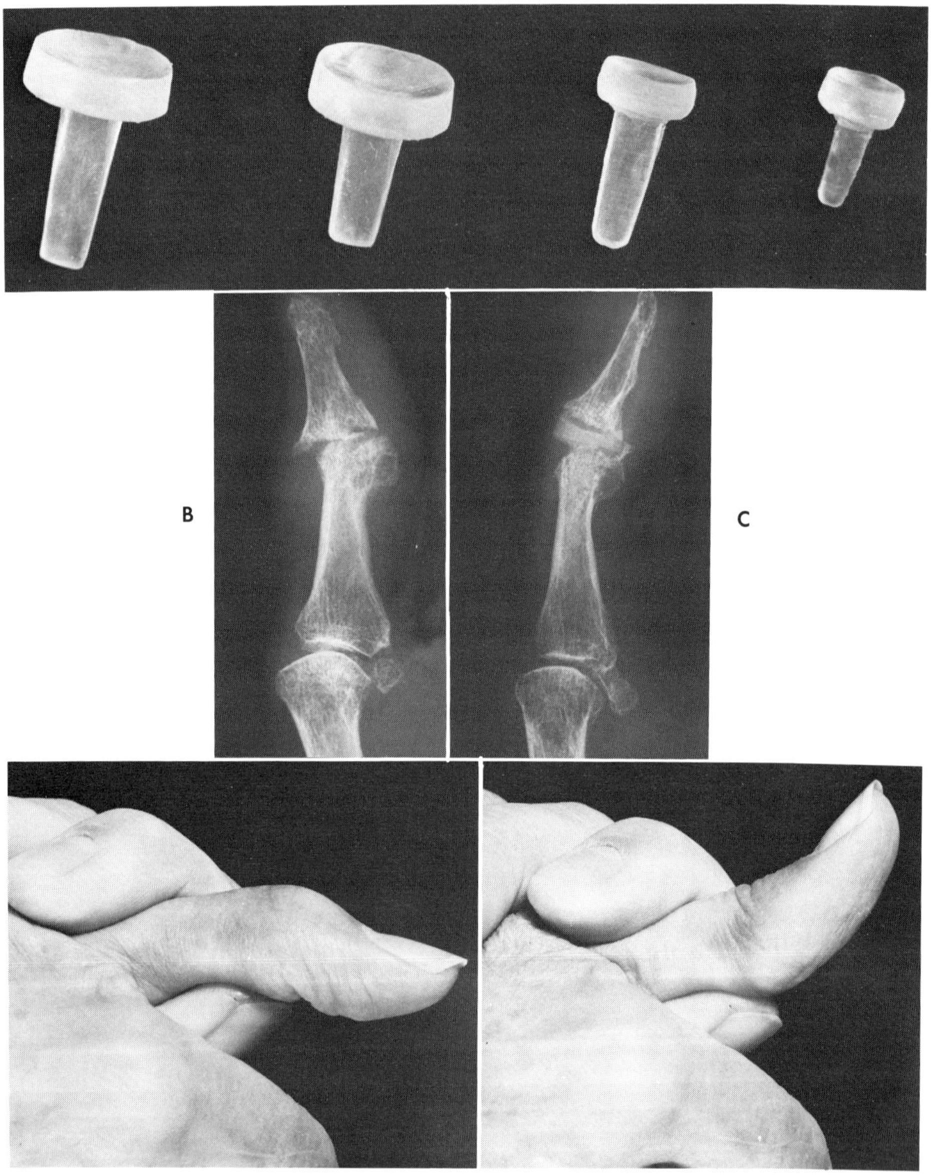

Fig. 24-8. **A,** Flexible intramedullary stemmed spacer used for implant arthroplasty of the thumb interphalangeal joint. **B,** Preoperative radiogram showing severe destruction of the thumb distal joint in a patient with rheumatoid arthritis. **C,** Postoperative radiogram showing the implant in position with its stem in the proximal phalanx. **D** and **E,** The range of active flexion/extension obtained in this case. The patient was very pleased with the result. This amount of movement has been very useful to perform certain finely coordinated hand activities.

thumb ray and is bent in place by flexing the joint to the desired position. The fusion must be performed with the thumb in a functional position of 10° of flexion, 5° of abduction, and slight pronation as required. A few fragments of cancellous bone can be inserted as a graft between the bone ends. A small Kirschner wire is introduced obliquely across the joint to further stabilize it and the bone ends are firmly compressed together. The wire is sectioned subcutaneously and removed after 6 to 8 weeks or left in place indefinitely. The longitudinal wire is removed without difficulties after 6 weeks. This procedure is usually successful because good bone contact and fixation are easily obtained in this joint.

The interphalangeal joint

In rheumatoid arthritis, severe erosive changes of the interphalangeal joint result in angulation deformity and subluxation as seen in 35% of the cases. Arthrodesis of this joint is indicated and, occasionally, bone grafting will be necessary when severe bone absorption is present. A single, relatively large (0.062) intramedullary wire and a .035 cross pin to further assure the fixation are used. It is important to obtain good bone-to-bone contact and to maintain the fixation until firm healing can be demonstrated radiologically, usually 6 to 10 weeks after surgery.

In a small number of cases presenting moderate erosive changes with secondary ligamentous instability and pain, implant resection arthroplasty of the interphalangeal joint of the thumb has been performed using a single stemmed silicone implant (Fig. 24-8). This procedure is similar to the great toe implant arthroplasty. In this case the stem is inserted in the distal aspect of the proximal phalanx and the implant acts as an articular spacer. We have used a lateral approach, releasing the radial collateral ligament, and dislocating the joint to expose the articular surfaces that are trimmed. The intramedullary canal of the proximal phalanx is prepared to receive the implant stem. The collateral ligament is resutured to the proximal phalanx. Care should be taken to avoid the small sensory branches of the radial nerve in this dissection. The joint is splinted in neutral position for approximately 3 weeks with a small aluminum splint. This procedure, when indicated, has the advantage of preserving some flexion of the interphalangeal joint that can be important in certain prehensile activities especially when the other joints are disabled.

SUMMARY

In any reconstructive procedure, the thumb ray must be evaluated as a functional unit in relation to functional adaptations of the entire hand. The prognosis of treatment of thumb disabilities has been greatly improved by a sound knowledge of the pathomechanics of deformities, proper techniques for reconstruction of the fine tendon balance, and development of the flexible implant resection arthroplasty method. The indications and important surgical steps of the most frequently used methods for reconstruction of the joints of the thumb are presented.

References

1. Boyes, J. H.: Bunnell's surgery of the hand, ed. 5, Philadelphia, 1970, J. B. Lippincott Co.
2. Clayton, M. L.: Surgery of the thumb in rheumatoid arthritis, J. Bone Joint Surg. **44A:** 1376, 1962.
3. Eiken, O.: Prosthetic replacement of the trapezium in surgery of the hand, Scand. J. Plast. Reconstr. Surg. **5:**131, 1971.
4. Entin, M. A.: Surgical treatment of rheumatoid arthritis, Surg. Clin. North Am. **44:**1081, 1964.
5. Flatt, A. E.: The care of the rheumatoid hand, ed. 3, St. Louis, 1974, The C. V. Mosby Co.
6. Kaplan, E. B.: Functional and surgical anatomy of the hand, ed. 2, Philadelphia, 1965, J. B. Lippincott Co.
7. Madden, J. W., and Peacock, E. E., Jr.: Studies on the biology of collagen during wound healing; dynamic metabolism of scar collagen and remodeling of dermal wounds, Ann. Surg. **174:**511, 1971.
8. Nalebuff, E. A.: Diagnosis, classification, and management of rheumatoid thumb deformities, Bull. Hosp. Joint Dis. **29:**119, 1968.
9. Ratliff, A. H. C.: Deformities of the thumb in rheumatoid arthritis, J. Bone Joint Surg. **54A:**557, 1972.
10. Swanson, A. B.: Disabling arthritis at the base of the thumb—treatment by resection of the trapezium and flexible (silicone) implant arthroplasty, J. Bone Joint Surg. **54A:**456, 1972.
11. Swanson, A. B.: Disabilities of the thumb joints and their surgical treatment, including flexible implant arthroplasty. In AAOS Instructional Course Lectures, Vol. 22, St. Louis, 1973, The C. V. Mosby Co.
12. Swanson, A. B.: Finger joint replacement by silicone rubber implants and the concept of implant fixation on encapsulation, Ann. Rheum. Dis. (supp.) **28:**47-55, 1969.
13. Swanson, A. B.: Flexible implant arthroplasty for arthritic finger joints—rationale, technique, and results of treatment, J. Bone Joint Surg. **54A:**435, 1972.
14. Swanson, A. B.: Flexible implant resection arthroplasty in the hand and extremities, St. Louis, 1973, The C. V. Mosby Co.
15. Swanson, A. B.: A flexible implant for replacement of arthritic or destroyed joints in the hand, N. Y. Univ. Inter-Clin. Inform. Bull. **6:**16-19, 1966.
16. Swanson, A. B.: The need for early treatment of the rheumatoid hand, J. Mich. State Med. Soc. **60:**348, 1961.
17. Swanson, A. B.: Silicone rubber implants for replacement of arthritic or destroyed joints in the hand, Surg. Clin. North Am. **48:**1113-1127, 1968.
18. Swanson, A. B.: Surgery of established rheumatoid deformities in the hand. In Cruess, R. L., and Mitchell, N., editors: Surgery of rheumatoid arthritis, Philadelphia, 1971, J. B. Lippincott Co.
19. Swanson, A. B., Meester, W. D., Swanson, G. deG., Rangaswamy, M. B., and Schut, G. E.: Durability of silicone rubber implants—an in vivo study, Orthop. Clin. Am. **4:** 1097-1112, 1973.
20. Swanson, A. B., and Swanson, G. deG.: Pathogenesis and pathomechanics of rheumatoid deformities in the hand and wrist, Orthop. Clin. North Am. **4:**1039-1056, 1973.
21. Tubiana, R., and Valentin, P.: Opposition of the thumb, Surg. Clin. North Am. **48:**967, 1968.

25. The recognition and treatment of tendon ruptures in the rheumatoid hand

Edward A. Nalebuff, M.D.

Tendon ruptures are common complications of rheumatoid arthritis. The cause and location of ruptures vary. Attrition ruptures of the extensor tendons occur most frequently and are usually seen either at the distal end of the ulna[12, 13] or at Lister's tubercle, where the extensor pollicis longus tendon turns radialward to the thumb. Attrition ruptures of the flexor tendons occur on the volar aspect of the wrist at the carpal navicular.[4] Tendon ruptures may also be caused by direct tendon invasion by rheumatoid tenosynovitis. A third factor leading to tendon ruptures is a diminished blood supply secondary to increased pressure under either the dorsal retinaculum, the transverse carpal ligament, or the digital pulleys. Although the correct diagnosis of tendon rupture is usually not difficult, it requires both an observant patient and an informed physician. There is usually a sudden loss of digital extension or flexion. The ruptures are usually painless and result from trivial activities. Patients with rheumatoid arthritis, who become accustomed to frequent variations and limitations of hand function, are apt to delay seeking medical attention unless the functional loss following a tendon rupture is obvious or significant.

Isolated ruptures of the extensor digiti quinti or extensor pollicis longus may cause only limited functional loss and may go unrecognized or be overshadowed by more significant deformities. The factors leading to a single tendon rupture, unless corrected, are often responsible for additional ruptures with more significant functional loss. Following a rupture of the extensor of the small finger, the next finger to be involved is the ring digit. The progress of multiple tendon ruptures is usually in a radial direction affecting the index finger's tendon last. In our experience, patients with multiple extensor tendon ruptures, especially those that occur in rapid sequence, are the result of attrition against the bony spicule on the ulnar aspect of the wrist. When a patient describes a sudden loss of finger extension, usually in the small digit, followed by subsequent loss of extension of the ring and middle digits, the diagnosis of multiple extensor tendon ruptures is most likely correct.

What are the conditions that simulate multiple tendon ruptures? There are three other situations encountered in rheumatoid arthritis that can mimic tendon rupture and should be ruled out before proceeding to surgery to restore extensor power to the digits. The most common condition is metacarpophalangeal (MP) joint dislocations with the fingers fixed in a flexed and ulnar deviated

A B C D E F

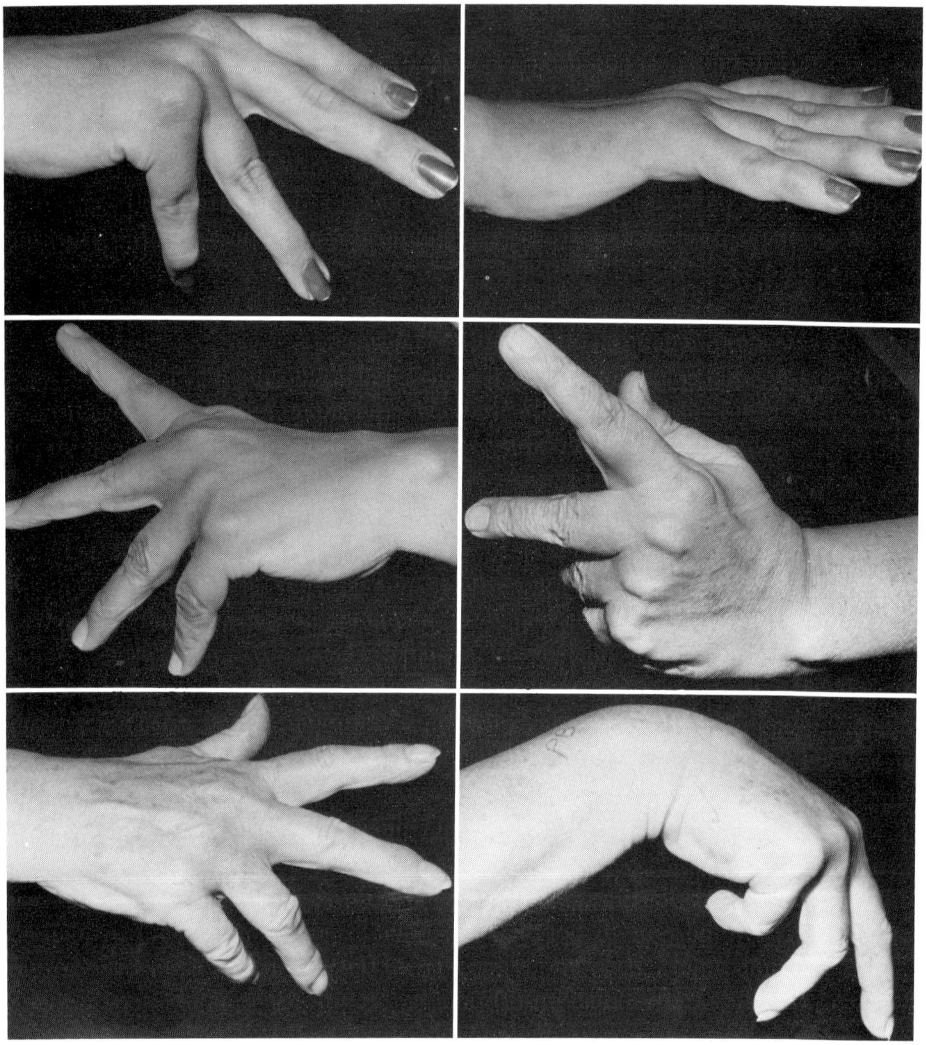

Fig. 25-1. Factors to consider in diagnosis of extensor tendon ruptures. **A** and **B**, Example of a patient with lack of active finger extension secondary to subluxation of the extensor tendons into the intermetacarpal valleys. This patient has the ability to maintain extension of the fingers, once the deformity has been corrected passively. **C** and **D**, An example of a patient with posterior interosseous nerve paralysis. This patient was incorrectly diagnosed as having multiple tendon ruptures. The radial deviation of the wrist should have been a significant clue to the correct diagnosis. **D** and **E**, The lack of tenodesis effect with extensor tendon rupture. The patient does not show any extension of the digits as the wrist is flexed.

position. This typical posture of advanced MP joint disease can mimic tendon rupture. However, the lack of passive MP joint extension and the presence of visible extensor tendons on the back of the hand should make the differentiation between MP joint dislocations and tendon ruptures easy. The second condition that must be ruled out is displacement of the extensor tendons into the valleys between the metacarpal heads. When this occurs, the extensor force is lost, as the tendon is volar to the arc of motion of the joint. The posture of the fingers on attempted active extension simulates that of multiple extensor tendon ruptures or dislocated MP joints. The differentiation, however, can be made between subluxation of the tendons and the joints by the presence of passive metacarpophalangeal joint extension. In fact, once the fingers are passively extended, these patients can usually actively maintain this extension (Fig. 25-1, *A*, *B*). The treatment for subluxation of the tendons is their relocation over the MP joints with or without MP arthroplasty, depending upon the status of the joints.

The least common entity that may be misdiagnosed as multiple extensor tendon ruptures is a paralysis secondary to posterior interosseous nerve compression. There are, however, subtle differences that should prevent misdiagnosis. In addition to the lack of active finger extension, patients with posterior interosseous nerve compression usually demonstrate some radial deviation of the wrist due to weakness of the extensor carpi ulnaris (Fig. 25-1, *C*, *D*). One should check for soft tissue fullness about the elbow in these patients. An excellent diagnostic test is to note finger extension, as the wrist is flexed. A positive tenodesis effect is noted in the paralytic condition. With tendon ruptures, flexion of the wrist has no effect on digital extension (Fig. 25-1, *E*, *F*). In addition, patients with multiple extensor ruptures usually have dorsal tenosynovitis or a prominent distal ulna to explain the ruptures, while those patients with posterior interosseous nerve compression usually have a negative examination about the wrist.

On the flexor side of the hand and wrist, the most common tendon to rupture is the flexor pollicis longus. Patients with this type of rupture lose their ability to actively flex the distal joint of the thumb. The diagnosis of a flexor pollicis longus rupture is not difficult, unless there is a previous hyperextension deformity or stiffness of the distal joint. An isolated rupture of a flexor digitorum profundus tendon causes a lack of distal joint flexion. A patient with this rupture can flex the involved finger well into the palm but without terminal joint flexion. A condition that mimics deep flexor tendon ruptures and, in fact, is a precursor to it, is a rheumatoid nodule in the intact tendon within the digital sheath. The nodule restricts profundus excursion, and, as the digit is flexed by the superficial flexor, the terminal joint loses its power. The situation can be correctly diagnosed as follow: Is there flexor power of the terminal phalanx with the digit held in extension? With the tendon nodule, power is present but disappears as the finger is actively flexed. Palpation of the volar aspect of the digit often reveals the source of difficulty. Patients with either a rupture of or a nodule within the flexor digitorum profundus demonstrate a discrepancy between active and passive flexion of the finger. The differentiation between the two diagnoses is made by the presence or absence of the terminal power with the digits held in extension. It should be added, however, that a hidden rupture of the deep flexor can mimic a flexor tendon nodule. If the deep flexor has ruptured in the palm and has reunited to the adjacent tendons in a lengthened position, the patient will have some active distal interphalangeal (DIP) flexor control with the finger extended but will lose it upon digital flexion. The correct diagnosis of tendon rupture may then be made by noting an alteration in digital posture with the involved finger maintaining a more extended position in relationship to the adjacent digits.

Isolated ruptures of a superficial flexor tendon can also occur and may lead to undiscernible functional loss. Testing for sublimis function should be part of the examination of the rheumatoid hand. The examiner holds the other fingers in extension (to block profundus action) and tests each finger for proximal interphalangeal (PIP) joint flexion. The presence of PIP joint flexion with a flail distal joint confirms the presence of an intact and functioning superficial flexor.

Rupture of both flexor tendons leads to such an obvious functional loss that the diagnosis is relatively easy. The patient lacks interphalangeal joint motion and flexes only at the MP joint. Of course, the examiner should confirm the presence of good passive motion before concluding that both tendons are ruptured. Even after recognizing that flexor tendon ruptures have occurred, one is still faced with the difficult task of determining at what site the ruptures have occurred. These ruptures can occur at the wrist, the palm, and within the digit. Palpation for fullness or lack of it within the digit can aid in diagnosing the level of tendon rupture. However, in the final analysis, one often has to investigate surgically before the exact site of rupture may be determined.

TREATMENT

Rupture of the extensor pollicis longus

Rupture of the extensor pollicis longus (EPL) is common in rheumatoid arthritis. The functional loss varies depending upon the functional capacity of the extensor pollicis brevis. One might think that a spontaneous rupture of the extensor pollicis longus would lead to a droop or a lack of extension of the distal joint of the thumb. This can occur, but more commonly the patient maintains the ability to extend the terminal joint in spite of the rupture. This function is shared with the intrinsic muscles of the thumb, which can maintain almost normal posture of the distal joint making the functional loss less significant. More commonly, the patient with an EPL rupture loses extension of the MP joint, as the extensor pollicis brevis is not strong enough to extend the joint alone (Fig. 25-2, *A*, *B*). In some cases with an EPL rupture, no de-

A B C D E F

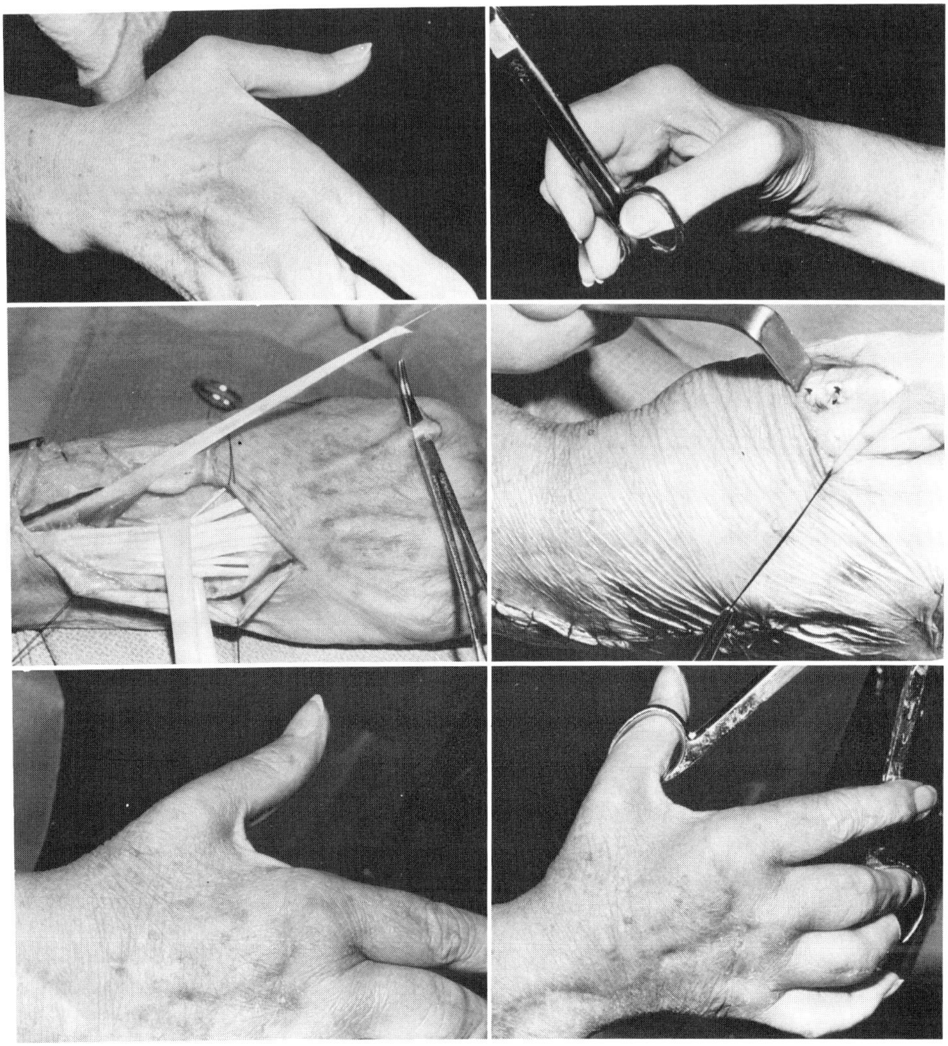

Fig. 25-2. The diagnosis and treatment of extensor pollicis longus tendon rupture. **A,** The typical posture of an extensor pollicis longus rupture with lack of metacarpophalangeal joint extension. The functional loss using scissors is demonstrated in **B. C,** The technique of extensor indicis proprius transfer. **D,** The interweaving of the transfer into the extensor mechanism over the metacarpophalangeal joints. **E** and **F,** The postoperative improvement in thumb posture and the improved functional capability.

formity occurs in either joint level. The diagnosis is often missed, unless specific examination for the tendon is made by asking the patient to bring the thumb backward with the palm resting on a flat surface. If a diagnosis of EPL rupture is made and the functional loss and deformity is significant, EPL function should be restored. Various options are available including *end-to-end repair, tendon graft,* or *tendon transfer.* Although a tendon rupture can occasionally be repaired if explored shortly after rupture, this is an exception. One should not expect to be able to achieve end-to-end repair. Although tendon grafts through areas of diseased rheumatoid tissue tend to become adherent and have not been recommended in treating extensor tendon ruptures in rheumatoid arthritis,[2] they can function well for this particular rupture. The powerful flexion and wide excursion of the thumb overcome the adhesions that occur.

However, to be effective, one requires a proximal motor that is not contracted. For this reason, tendon transfers are preferred in treating the EPL rupture. The two tendons most commonly used are the extensor indicis proprius or the extensor carpi radialis longus.[3] We prefer the extensor indicis proprius for several reasons (Fig. 25-2, *C*). It can be taken from the index at the MP joint level without interferring with the index finger function. In our experience, the patient does not lose independent extension of the index as a result of this transfer. We prefer not to weaken radial wrist extension, which is very important in maintaining proper wrist alignment. In performing the EIP transfer the tendon is identified at the MP joint level. It is the most ulnar of the two tendons at this level. It is withdrawn at the wrist through a second incision and passed subcutaneously to the thumb. Until a few years ago, we would make an end-to-end or weaving anastomosis of the transfer with the distal stump of the EPL. This was always the most tedious part of the procedure. The judging of proper tension is the hardest part, because once the tendon is sutured, it is quite difficult to readjust the tension. At the present time, we pass the tendon directly to the MP joint level and interweave the transfer into the extensor mechanism (Fig. 25-2, *D*). A temporary stitch is used to judge tension. With the correct tension, the thumb will stay in extension with the wrist flexed. With the wrist extended, one should be able to bring the thumb to the small digit. The interweaving of the transfer through the extensor mechanism makes a very strong anastomosis and gives us confidence about starting motion after 4 or 5 weeks of immobiization. The results of a properly performed tendon transfer to restore extensor pollicis longus function are usually excellent (Fig. 25-2, *E*, *F*).

Rupture of the digital extensors

Single tendon ruptures can involve any finger, but, most commonly, the small digit is affected. The patient will demonstrate a droop at the MP joint level. The amount of limited extension depends upon whether or not both the extensor digiti quinti and the comminus tendon from the ring finger are ruptured. With an isolated EDQ rupture, the finger may droop only 30° or 40°. One can confirm that the extensor digitorum comminus is supplying some extensor power to the small finger by holding the index, middle, and ring fingers in MP flexion and asking the patient to extend the small digit. The increased deformity represents the contribution to extension provided by the EDC. Because of the danger of additional ruptures that complicate the treatment, patients in whom a diagnosis of a single rupture has been made are best advised to have early surgery. Surgical treatment of an isolated rupture of any finger extensor is relatively easy and the functional result is usually excellent. The treatment we prefer is *adjacent anastomosis*. As noted previously, end-to-end repair is seldom feasible. The proper approach is to carry out a dorsal tenosynovectomy, remove any bony spicules from the distal end of the ulna (or resect it) to eliminate the cause of rupture. We replace the distal ulna with the Swanson ulnar head prosthesis. This preserves ulnar length and provides a smooth surface beneath the extensor tendons. The dorsal retinaculum should then be placed deep to the extensor tendons. These steps should be carried out prior to restoring power to the involved digit by adjacent anastomosis. For an isolated rupture of the middle or ring finger, adjacent anastomosis is especially easy. A side-to-side suture is performed using a nonabsorbable material. Tension is determined by restoring the proper sequence posture to the fingers. The use of intravenous regional anesthesia simplifies the task of judging proper tension. After the tendon suture has been completed, the tourniquet may be released when one is ready for skin closure. Within minutes, muscle control is restored. The patient is then asked to flex and extend the fingers. If there is a lag in extension, it can be corrected at this time. Infiltration of the skin with a local anesthetic permits skin closure. The slight inconvenience of this step is a small price to pay in order to be certain of the proper tension.

Multiple ruptures of the extensor tendon

As additional tendons rupture, the surgical treatment becomes more complicated. With double ruptures of the third and fourth fingers, it is still possible to use adjacent anastomosis; the fourth finger tendon is sutured to the fifth and the third finger tendon to the second. However, double ruptures more frequently involve the ring and small digits. One can carry out adjacent anastomoses in some of these patients (Fig. 25-3), although there may be difficulty with the small digit. The distal stump may be so short that it will not reach the adjacent finger without excessive abduction of the small digits necessitating a more direct restoration of extensor power to the small finger. We usually turn to our old friend, the extensor indicis proprius, to act as a tendon transfer. It is not necessary to divide the tendon as far distally as when it is utilized for thumb tendon rupture. Other tendon transfers have been advocated, such as the extensor carpi ulnaris to restore power in this situation.[11] However, the wrist extensor tendon is very important for maintaining wrist alignment and power. We feel it is best left in its normal position. In addition, it does not have the same excursion as the digital extensor. Therefore, there will usually be a lack of either full flexion or extension following this particular transfer.

As additional extensor tendons rupture, the difficulty in restoring extension multiplies. With three or four extensor tendons gone, one can no longer combine the adjacent anastomosis with extensor indicis proprius transfer to supply enough power for four fingers. One must look elsewhere for power; a strong motor that is expendable and has the necessary length to reach the distal tendons just proximal to the MP joints is needed. For the past few years we have handled this problem

A B C D

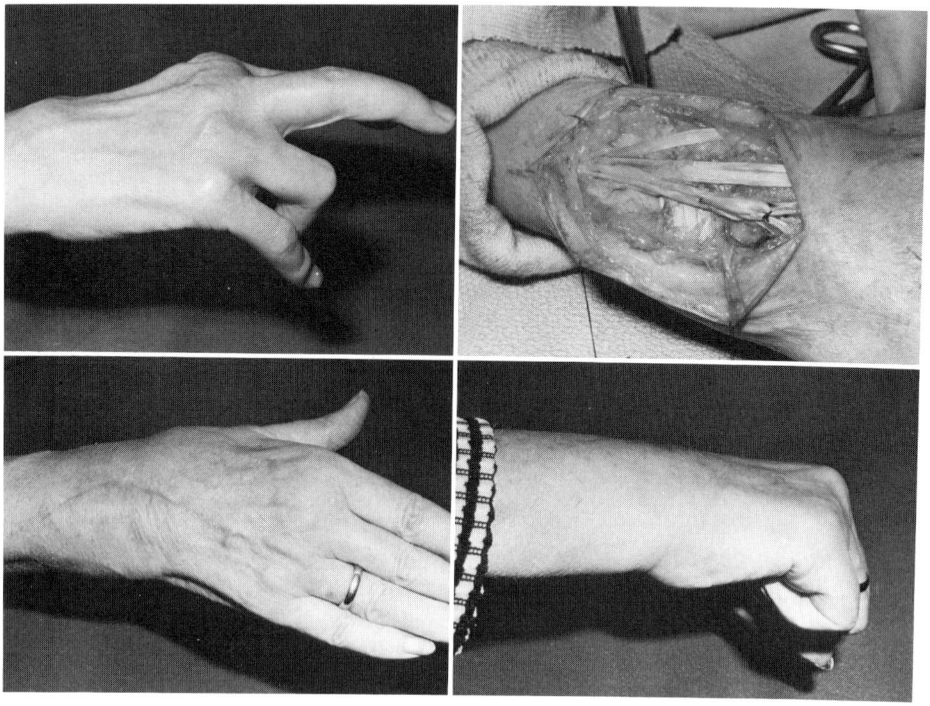

Fig. 25-3. An example of double extensor tendon rupture treated by adjacent anastomoses. **A,** Clinical appearance of the patient with lack of metacarpophalangeal extension of the ring and small digits. **B,** The condition at surgery following tenosynovectomy, dorsal retinaculum relocation, and adjacent anastomoses. **C** and **D,** Patient's postoperative extension and flexion ability.

with one or more of the flexor digitorum sublimis tendons. This transfer was first advocated by Boyes for a radial nerve palsy. He showed that patients learned quickly to use the former finger flexor as an extensor. In his technique, he brought the transferred tendon through a wide opening in the interosseous membrane to achieve a direct route to the site of anastomosis. For the past 5 years, we have modified this approach. We utilize the third sublimus muscle as the motor and bring its tendons subcutaneously around the radial aspect of the forearm. This direction of pull was chosen to eliminate the risk of pulling the digits into increased ulnar deviation. The transfer is carried out through three incisions. A small transverse incision within the palm is made, and the tendon divided after applying traction. This will given enough length to reach the MP joints. A second incision is made on the volar aspect of the forearm. It should be placed ulnarward to the midline, so that the final transfer will pass deep to unscarred tissue. The third incision is on the dorsal aspect of the hand, where the anastomosis is made. The transfer is sutured to the ring and small fingers' extensors. We ordinarily suture the mid finger tendon to the adajcent index. With quadruple tendon ruptures, two superficial flexor tendons are utilized. One to restore extension of

A

B

C

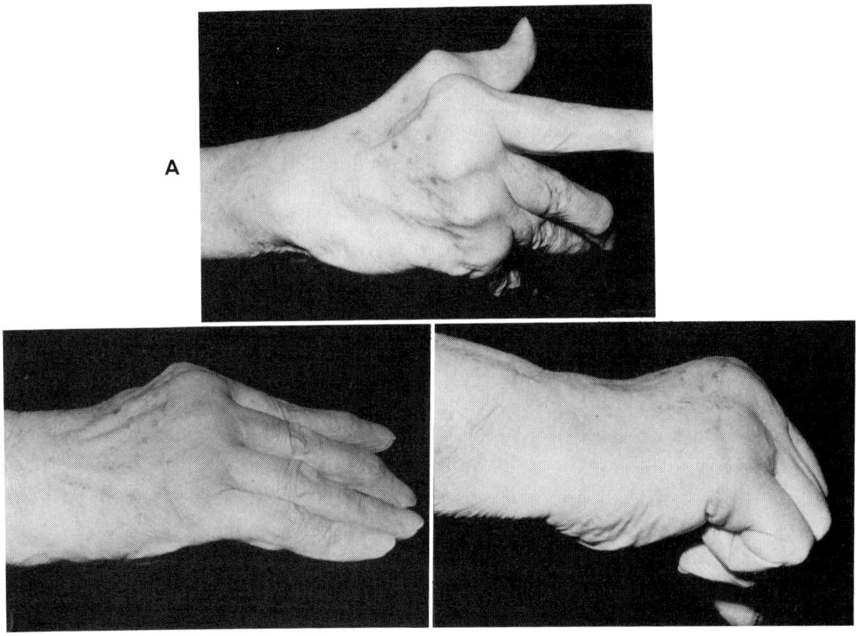

Fig. 25-4. Example of multiple extensor tendon ruptures in a patient who has dislocations of the metacarpophalangeal joints requiring arthroplasty. **A,** Preoperative appearance demonstrating functional loss and deformity. **B** and **C,** Postoperative extension following combined metacarpophalangeal joint arthroplasty and tendon transfer. **C,** Postoperative flexion achieved.

the index and mid fingers and the other to the small and ring digits. The judgment of tension is again critical. The transfer should be tight enough to have a tenodesis effect. In other words, without any muscle contraction we like to see the other fingers extend with the wrist flexed. We try to adjust the transfer so that there is enough slack with the wrist in extension to allow almost full flexion of the digits. There is some tendency to stretch out the transfer because of the remaining strong flexors. This transfer definitely does not always work as a tenodesis. We have utilized the flexor digitorum sublimis (FDS) transfer in patients in whom wrist fusion has been performed, and they are still able to achieve satisfactory extension of the digits. It would be appropriate at this time to state that in patients with fused wrists one also has the opportunity to utilize the wrist motors to restore the finger extension. As noted before, the excursion of these muscles is limited, but these powerful muscles are idle with the fused wrist and can be used to activate the digits without taking away any power of finger flexion. We have used both the wrist extensors and flexors to restore finger extension, when there is an associated or planned wrist fusion. When utilizing the wrist flexors, there is not enough length to reach the ruptured tendon ends and a tendon graft is needed. If one is performing a wrist fusion and plans to do tendon transfer for multple tendon ruptures at a later date, a Hunter rod can be placed in position at the time of the wrist fusion. This makes the second stage tendon graft procedure easier and minimizes the risk of postoperative adhesions.

Before leaving the subject of extensor tendon ruptures, I would like to comment upon the not infrequent situation of multiple extensor tendon ruptures with associated MP joint disease. What should you do with a patient who requires both MP joint arthroplasty as well as restoration of digital extension (Fig. 25-4)? One thing is definite. Do not try to restore digital extension by transfer before restoring joint motion. Unless the MP joints can be extended passively, any transfer is bound to become adherent. One can restore function to these patients in two steps. Initially, an MP arthroplasty can be done. Postoperatively, one relies upon dynamic splinting to substitute for the absent tendons. At a second stage, appropriate transfers are done to supply active extensor power. With experience, it is possible to combine MP joint arthroplasty with a tendon transfer in one operative procedure. The arthroplasty is done in routine fashion and then a flexor digitorum sublimis is brought around the forearm and sutured to the extensor mechanism at the arthroplasty site. The postoperative management of patients with combined arthroplasty and tendon transfers is geared to protecting the tendon transfer. Active motion, therefore, should be delayed for 3 weeks. One should not expect to regain full motion in these cases. Certainly, the results of a combined procedure will quite naturally fall short when compared with an arthroplasty with normal tendons or a tendon transfer with normal joints.

TREATMENT OF FLEXOR TENDON RUPTURES

Rupture of the flexor pollicis longus

The most common flexor tendon to rupture in rheumatoid arthritis is the flexor pollicis longus. It is usually secondary to attrition at the carpal navicular. The functional loss is variable. If the patient has a good interphalangeal joint with passive motion, the loss is readily apparent. If the MP joint is badly involved with rheumatoid disease or fused, the loss of any terminal joint function is substantial. One must chose either to provide terminal joint stability by fusion or to attempt to restore active motion. If a decision is made to fuse the distal joint to provide a stable pinch, one has not eliminated the need to explore the volar aspect of the wrist. The bony spicule that has disrupted the flexor pollicis longus will next affect the tendons of the index finger. We have seen the sequence of FDL rupture followed by FDP (index) rupture and FDS rupture before treatment was instituted (Fig. 25-5).

In treating these ruptures, the volar aspect of the wrist is exposed through a curved incision along the thenar crease extending proximally. The bony spicule should be removed surgically and covered by adjacent soft tissues. Attention should then be directed toward restoring tendon function. The choice of treatment includes a bridge graft, a full tendon graft, or tendon transfer. If the tendon ends can be identified at the wrist, we prefer to insert a short bridge graft (Fig. 25-6). If the distal tendon stump cannot be brought into the wrist incision, we will use the full length graft as utilized following a laceration. Another alternative is to transfer the superficial flexor divided in the distal palm and passed through

A B C D

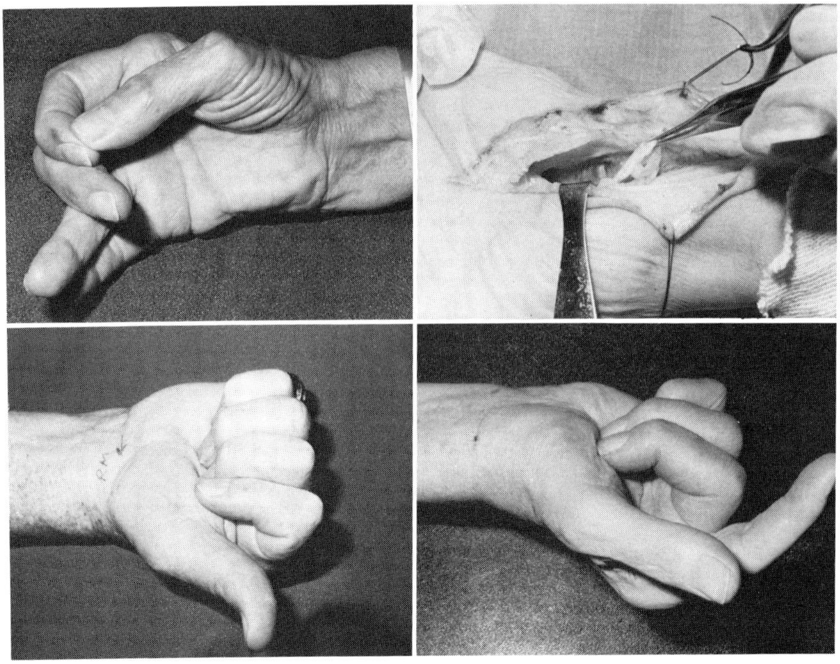

Fig. 25-5. The dangers of attrition rupture on the flexor aspect of the wrist. **A,** Patient who has rupture of the flexor pollicis longus treated with terminal joint fusion. However, exploration of the volar aspect of the wrist was carried out to remove bony spicule that might have caused additional ruptures. **B,** The typical pathology with a bony spicule of the carpal navicular. **C,** The clinical appearance of a patient who has ruptured both the flexor pollicis longus and the deep flexor of the index finger secondary to attrition rupture at the wrist. **D,** The posture of a patient who has ruptured both flexors of the index finger as well as the long flexor of the thumb due to the same pathology.

the digital sheath and sutured distally through the terminal phalanx of the thumb with a pull-out wire.

Rupture of the flexor digitorum profundus

Rupture of one or more of the deep flexors is not uncommonly encountered. If these patients maintain superficial flexor function both in range of motion and in strength, the functional loss is minimal. The treatment should match the functional loss. If the distal stump becomes adherent, the patient may only lose active flexion but maintain enough terminal stability to preclude the need for surgical stabilization. Probably the most important factor determining the course of treatment is the level of tendon rupture. These ruptures can occur within the digits, palm, or at the wrist. The easiest location to restore function is in the palm. Ruptures in this area are actually less obvious, as the ruptured tendon adheres to the common mass of deep flexors. This confuses the diagnosis, in that terminal joint flexion is possible with the digit extended, but is lost as the finger is flexed (passively or actively). One could readily confuse this with a flexor

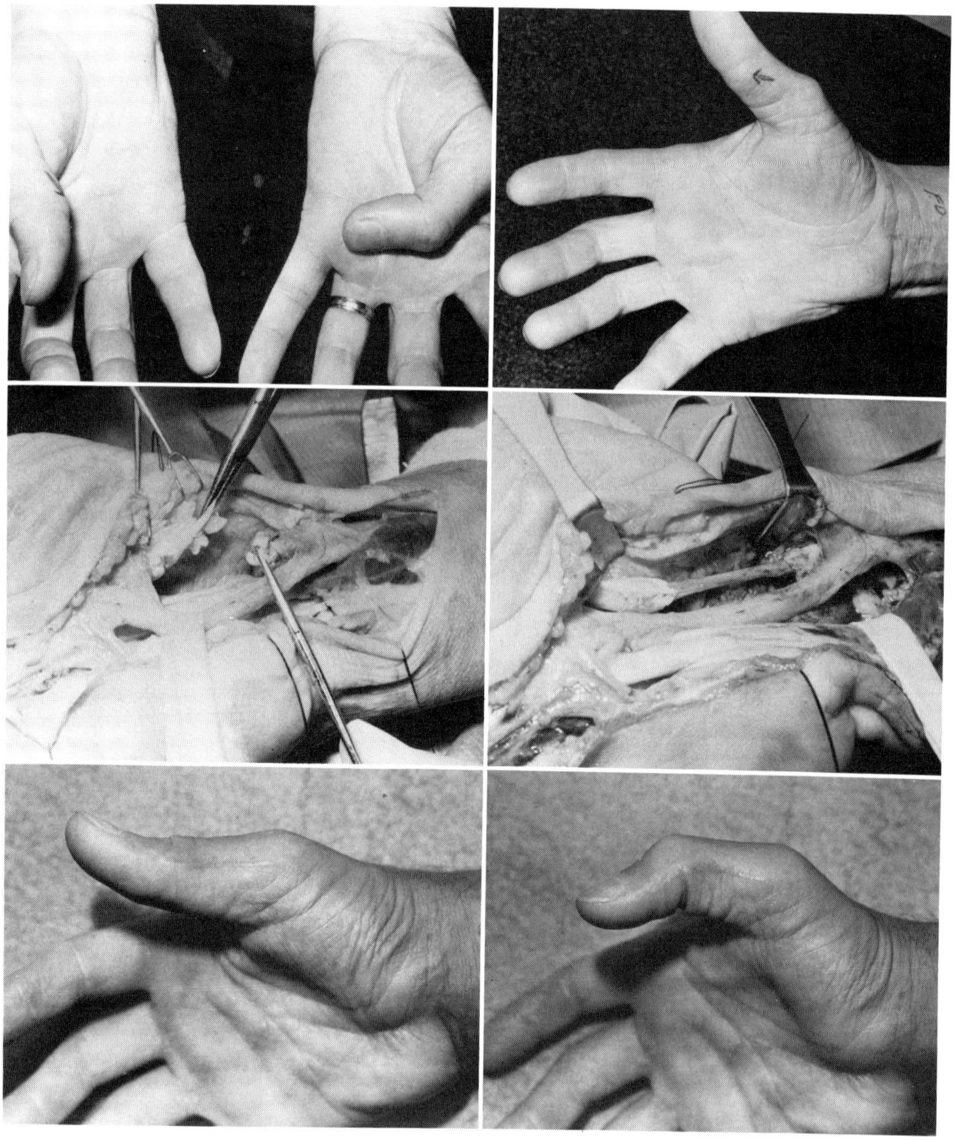

Fig. 25-6. An example of flexor pollicis longus rupture treated with a bridge graft. **A,** The lack of terminal joint flexion preoperatively. **B,** The flexor tendon nodule can be palpated distally, which confused the diagnosis as far as location of the tendon rupture. **C,** The true pathology at the wrist. **D,** The insertion of short bridge graft. **E** and **F,** Postoperative functional return.

tendon nodule that blocks active excursion of the profundus. Clues to the proper diagnosis include the lack of a palpable nodule and an alteration of the resting digital posture. The finger assumes a more extended position than the adjacent digits. Ruptures at the palm and wrist levels are best treated by adjacent anastomoses to the neighboring intact muscle. However, within the digit this is not possible, and one should carry out surgery only to remove any diseased synovium from the intact superficial flexor, which is now vital to the digit's function. We

A B C D

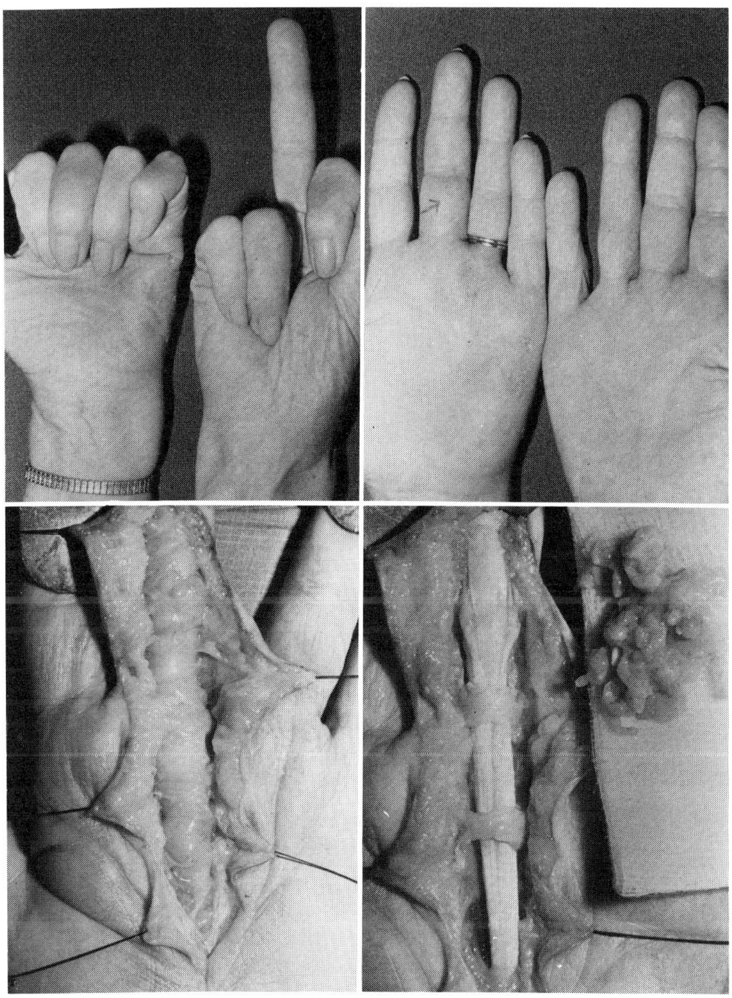

Fig. 25-7. Flexor tendon rupture within no-man's-land and the importance of flexor tenosynovectomy as a prophylactic treatment. **A,** Lack of active flexion of the left middle finger, as the result of rupture of both flexor tendons. **B,** Location of palpable flexor tendon nodule in the opposite middle digit. **C,** The appearance of flexor tendon sheath of right middle finger at time of prophylactic tenosynovectomy. **D,** The amount of diseased synovium removed in an attempt to preserve flexor tendon function.

prefer to stabilize the terminal joint in these patients rather than to consider a flexor tendon graft through an intact sublimis.

Rupture of the flexor digitorum sublimis

Loss of the flexor digitorum sublimis function within the digit causes no obvious functional loss. In fact, in patients with extensive flexor tenosynovitis involving both tendons we will occasionally sacrifice the superficial flexor in order

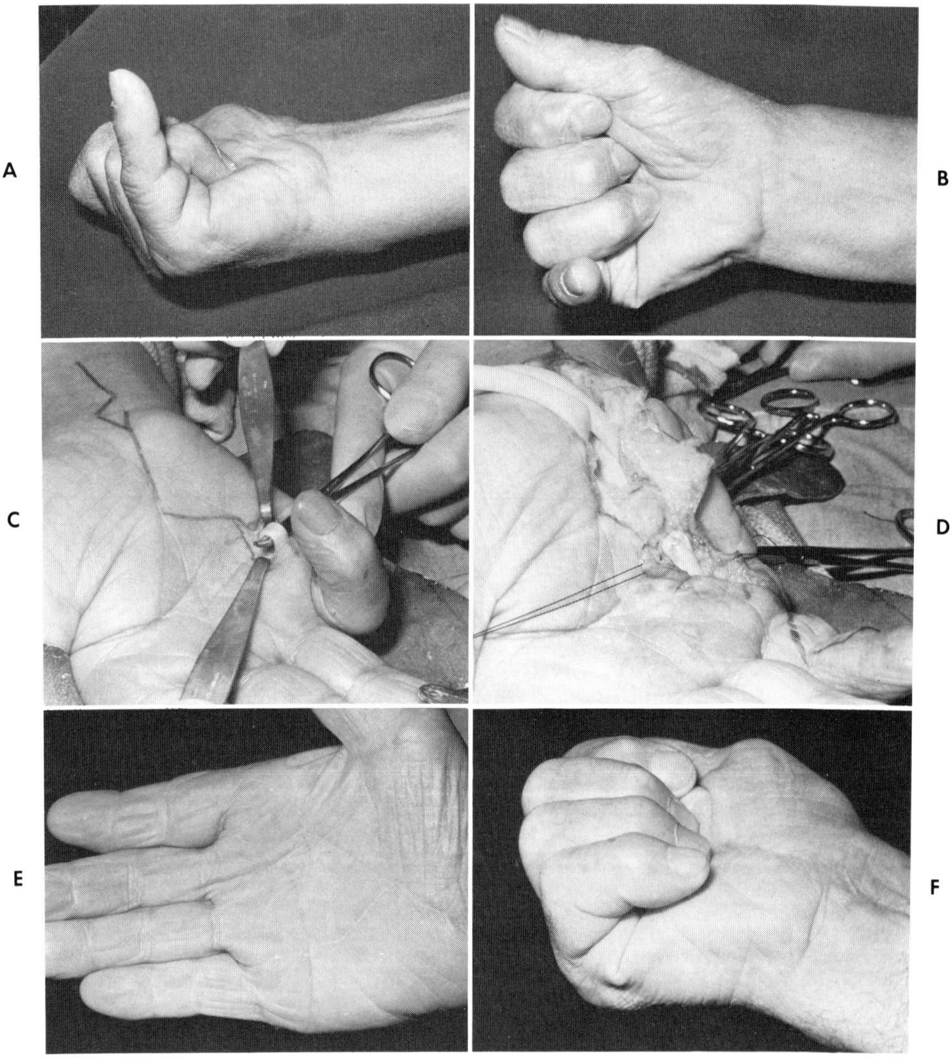

Fig. 25-8. An example of flexor tendon rupture within the palm treated by adjacent anastomosis. **A** and **B**, The functional loss preoperatively. **C**, Incision at the base of the digit to determine the site of tendon rupture. **D**, The rupture within the mid palm. **E** and **F**, Postoperative functional result following adjacent anastomosis.

to restore proper deep flexor function. A true diagnosis may only be made by careful examination. Again, treatment should not jeopardize existing function. Adjacent anastomosis within the palm or the wrist is feasible.

Rupture of both digital flexors

With loss of both digital flexors the functional loss becomes obvious and significant. The finger sticks out from the other fingers, and, like its traumatic counterpart, "gets in the way." Restoration of digtal flexion is our goal, although it is not always possible to achieve. For this reason, it is far better to look for the nodular tenosynovitis and to carry out a prophylactic tenosynovectomy before the actual rupture has occurred (Fig. 25-7). Important factors determining treatment as well as the result are: (1) the level of tendon rupture, (2) the status of the adjacent fingers, and (3) the status of the digital joints of the involved finger. If the ruptures have occurred at the wrist, one can restore the function by adjacent anastamosis or by a short bridge graft for the profundus with the suture lines above and below the carpal tunnel area. If the rupture is in the palm, one can use either adjacent anastomoses of the profundus (Fig. 25-8) or a transfer of a superficial flexor to the distal profundus.

Within the digit in no-man's-land one is faced with the same problem encountered in laceration at this level, except the situation is worse. The disease is not as localized, and the dissection needed for exposure leaves a very poor bed for a tendon graft. In addition, the adjacent joints may have restricted and painful motion. In our experience, free flexor tendon grafts have not been followed by particularly good results in patients with rheumatoid arthritis. For this reason, we have treated these patients with a two stage approach, inserting an artificial tendon rod as a preliminary to the insertion of a tendon graft. This technique is essentially the same as in traumatic cases and need not be expanded here.

Finally, there are patients in whom, because of advanced age, poor status of the interphalangeal joints, or just generalized disease, the wisest choice of action with both flexor tendons ruptured within the digital sheath is to fuse both interphalangeal joints in a functional position. In this way, we can restore satisfactory function to the digit and eliminate pain with one simple operation. This approach rightfully is at the bottom of our therapeutic list but should be given serious consideration as the proper way to handle this complicated problem in selected cases.

CONCLUSION

In conclusion, tendon ruptures, both extensor and flexor, are frequently encountered in rheumatoid arthritis patients. The associated joint deformities may obscure the diagnosis but should not fool the informed examiner. Once the diagnosis has been made, treatment should be instituted, as additional ruptures are likely to occur. The use of adjacent anastomoses, transfers, or joint fusions, has made it possible to restore significant function to these patients.

References

1. Boyes, J. H.: Tendon transfers for radial palsy, Bull. Hosp. Joint Dis. **21**:97-105, 1960.
2. Flatt, A. E.: The care of the rheumatoid hand, St. Louis, 1963, The C. V. Mosby Co.
3. Goldner, J. L.: Tendon transfer in rheumatoid arthritis, Orthop. Clin. North Am. **5**(2): 425-444, April, 1974.
4. Mannerfelt, L., and Norman, O.: Attrition ruptures of flexor tendons in rheumatoid arthritis caused by bony spurs in the carpal tunnel, J. Bone Joint Surg. **51B**(2):270-277, May, 1969.
5. Millender, L. H., and Nalebuff, E. A., et al.: Dorsal tenosynovectomy and tendon transfer in the rheumatoid hand, J. Bone Joint Surg. **56A**(3):601-610, April, 1974.
6. Millender, L. H., Nalebuff, E. A., and Holdsworth, D. A.: Posterior interosseous nerve syndrome secondary to rheumatoid arthritis, J. Bone Joint Surg. **55**(4):753-757, June, 1973.
7. Nalebuff, E. A.: Surgical treatment of rheumatoid tenosynovitis in the hand, Surg. Clin. North Am. **49**:799-809, 1969.
8. Nalebuff, E. A.: Surgical treatment of tendon rupture in the rheumatoid hand, Surg. Clin. North Am. **49**:811-822, 1969.
9. Nalebuff, E. A., and Patel, M. R.: Flexor digitorum sublimus transfer for multiple extensor tendon ruptures in rheumatoid arthritis, Plast. Reconstr. Surg. **52**:530-533, 1973.
10. Nalebuff, E. A., and Potter, T. A.: Rheumatoid involvement of tendons and tendon sheaths in the hand, Clin. Orthop. **59**:147-159, 1968.
11. Straub, L. R., and Wilson, E. H., Jr.: Spontaneous rupture of extensor tendons in the hand associated with rheumatoid arthritis, J. Bone Joint Surg. **38A**:1208-1217, Dec., 1956.
12. Vaughan-Jackson, O. J.: Attrition ruptures of tendons in the rheumatoid hand. In Proceedings of the Joint Meeting of the Orthopaedic Associations of the English Speaking World, J. Bone Joint Surg. **40A**:1431, Dec., 1958.
13. Vaughan-Jackson, O. J.: Rupture of extensor tendons by attrition at the inferior radio-ulnar joint, Report of two cases, J. Bone Joint Surg. **30B**:528-530, Aug., 1948.

26. Staged flexor tendon reconstruction: current status

James M. Hunter, M.D.
Lawrence H. Schneider, M.D.

In 1971 one of us (J. M. H.) presented more than 10 years of experience of a technique in which severely damaged flexor tendon systems were rebuilt around a silicone-Dacron reinforced gliding implant.[5] The implant, fixed only at its distal end, was left free at its proximal extremity in the distal forearm and a passive exercise program was instituted to recondition the finger prior to the second stage. At that time, the implant was replaced 3 months postoperative with a long tendon graft that was carried out with as little disturbance as possible to the newly-formed sheath, created in response to the rubber implant.

This work was based on the earlier studies with artificial tendons.[1, 8, 9] The concept of a flexible silicone rubber rod that could serve as a template on which a new sheath would be created with minimal reaction was introduced later.[2] This would thereby organize a severely scarred area, one in which standard one-stage tendon grafting would most certainly fail, and grade such a finger up to where tendon grafting would have a reasonable prospect for success. The flexible rod allowed joint exercise and seemed to promote the formation of a superior sheath system. The tendon implant described in the 1971 article was constructed of silicone rubber in a new shape and a Dacron woven tape was added within the rubber to give body to the implant, enhancing its gliding in the passive motion program, and also supplying better hold for the necessary distal sutures.

In the 4 years that have elapsed since that publication we have continued to employ the staged tendon technique. If anything, indications have broadened, partially because of natural enthusiasm for the method and mainly because of disappointment with the results of standard tendon grafting. While the main source of case material is in the area of failed flexor tendon surgery or in crushing injuries in which the flexor system has been destroyed, we also use the technique in occasional extensor tendon reconstructions and opponensplasties performed under suboptimal conditions. Another rare indication has been in grafting the profundus in cases in which the sublimis is intact.

The use of this tool is not without its problems and painstaking attention to all minor technical details is necessary if success is to be achieved.

We will enumerate the various technical pitfalls and problems along the course of the staged flexor tendon reconstruction. For details of the technique the reader is referred to the literature.[3-5]

PATIENT SELECTION

This critical decision must take many factors into account. Does the patient understand the complexity of the problem and the nature of the two-stage procedure? Will the patient be able to cooperate in a difficult postoperative therapy program? Is the finger itself salvageable? The surgeon must ask whether it is justifiable to subject a severely damaged finger to two more surgical assaults, and in some cases we must offer arthrodesis or even ablation as a better reconstructive alternative. While it is true that joints can be released, nerves repaired, and scar tissue excised at Stage I, most of these hands should be subjected to a preoperative softening period in which various physical therapy techniques are applied in an effort to regain maximum passive range of motion and soft tissue healing. This period also allows us to get to better know the patient, his attitudes, abilities, and willingness to work. After this preliminary period, the final decision on what direction to take can be made. It is probable that those patients with fingers that have severe vascular impairment will at best have very limited gain and should be rejected as candidates for the staged reconstruction.

STAGE I

Technical details are followed scrupuously as in the article.[5] At Stage I the implant must be firmly attached distally to the profundus stump and adjacent fibrous tissues. The wire suture is reinforced with at least two nonabsorbable sutures. The surgeon must be certain that the added sutures catch the Dacron tape as they will cut out if they are only holding the rubber alone. Preservation of as much sheath material as possible is stressed as long as it doesn't bind the implant and prevent passive gliding. Do not hesitate to reconstruct the needed pulleys at this stage. If there is any question of bowstringing of the implant or ineffective passive gliding and buckling, then pulleys should be built using sublimis tendon remnants as free grafts fixed firmly to the periosteum, original pulley, or even through bone when no soft tissue is available. The importance and location of the various pulley levels is discussed in Chapter 9.

Synovitis, the most common problem seen with Stage I is usually associated with either loosening of the distal juncture or buckling of the implant due to tight or absent pulleys. Attention to the above technical details has markedly reduced our incidence of this problem.

Another cause of buckling of the implant is the short cul-de-sac at the proximal end of the artificial tendon. To insure adequate room within the new sheath it is stressed that the wrist be placed in 40° of flexion, at the close of Stage I, to ensure a long proximal extension of the sheath. This position is maintained for 3 weeks. If this is not done, later passive exercises will abut the proximal end of the implant against the closed tube causing buckling in the hand and later synovitis.

Availability of the implant in sterile packaging is a new development that has, we believe, led to a reduced incidence of synovitis attributable to surface contaminants and particulate matter. At this time we have available in the operating room one implant in each size that is reused only for estimation of the correct implant size. In this way the bulk of the procedure can be carried out and only when all is ready is the actual implant broken out of its wrapper and immediately inserted. This cuts down on the handling and contamination of the implant.

When synovitis does intervene we still return these patients to a resting splint and cut down on their exercises. If the problem persists, then an early Stage II procedure is recommended. Repeat cultures have failed to reveal bacterial or fungal growth when fluid from these inflammed sheaths is removed by aspiration or surgery. In the few infections seen after Stage I it is apparent that synovial irritation and subsequent skin breakdown allow for bacterial contamination of the sheath. The breakdown usually occurred in the finger with the sheath being seeded secondarily. We have treated these with antibiotic irrigations and have accomplished a successful Stage II graft with antibiotic coverage. The only other choice, which is the more conservative one, is removal of the implant and, after adequate healing, re-evaluation for a repeat Stage I.

STAGE II

The problems associated with the Stage II procedure, as with any tendon grafting procedure, could be avoided to a great degree by careful attention to the technical details involved in creating a strong proximal and distal graft juncture. The sheath is removed in the forearm allowing free mobility of the proximal juncture. We have performed some of these procedures under local anesthesia[6] in an effort to better understand the dynamics of the situation and also to learn how to best adjust tension on the graft.

The procurement of satisfactory tendon graft material can provide another obstacle for the surgeon. When the plantaris is present and of adequate size it is the preferred source. Present in over 80% of patients, it is, at times, of insufficient girth to be used. Rather than use a flimsy graft that doesn't hold sutures, our second choice is one of the long toe extensors. Because of interconnections between the toe extensors, it usually requires more extensive surgery for its removal.

Handling of the graft material with great care and generally applying the rules of good tendon surgery will help reduce the formation of adhesions seen after Stage II. When this problem occurs and is unresponsive to hand therapy measures, tenolysis will occasionally be necessary (see Chapter 18). When tendon adhesions prevent adequate gliding, it is seen at lysis that these occur chiefly at the proximal juncture in the forearm and it is gratifying to see that on release at this level the graft can be salvaged. The quality of the graft itself within the created tendon sheath is often excellent, appearing much the way it looked when placed 6 months earlier. These lysis procedures are performed under local anesthesia for a more complete understanding of the problem.[6]

The importance of patient input after Stage II cannot be overemphasized. We have found that the best way to interest and activate patients is through an effective hand therapy program administered by trained therapists in close communication with the surgeon. The use of wood blocks, web straps, and dynamic splints along with an active motion program, which gradually increases the forces applied through the tendon graft, is the keynote of the postcasting period. The application of a work-directed therapy program in the later stages of recovery has also been helpful.

For the future, effort is being directed toward the development of an active artificial tendon, one that can be implanted at one stage with sturdy proximal and distal attachments that can withstand the forces applied with active use. This is a formidible challenge. A method is needed in which inorganic material can be bonded to the living tissue: at the terminal end fixation on the distal phalanx, or at the proximal end attachment to the motor tendon unit that allows motion. This bonding problem is being attacked through the use of woven synthetic fabric tapes that allow for tissue ingrowth, thereby fixing the artificial tendon to the tissues. Titanium rings have been used for the distal insertion. At present the active tendon is feasible and has been subjected to limited clinical trial. This active tendon will probably have to be replaced by a standard tendon graft at some later time but the flexor system created will be a dynamic one. The prospects for a permanent artificial tendon, which can withstand the tremendous forces placed on normal tendon, are not at this time within the realm of our present technology.

References

1. Biesalski, K., and Mayer, L.: Die Physiologische Sehnenverp Flanzung; Berlin, 1916, Springer.
2. Carroll, R. E., and Bassett, A. L.: Formation of tendon sheath by silicone rod implants. Proceedings of The American Society for Surgery of the Hand, J. Bone Joint Surg. **45A:** 884-885, 1963.
3. Hunter, J. M.: Artificial tendons; early development and application, Am. J. Surg. **109:** 325-338, 1965.
4. Hunter, J. M.: Artificial tendons; their development and application. Proceedings of The American Society for Surgery of the Hand, J. Bone Joint Surg. **47A:**631-632, 1965.
5. Hunter, J. M., and Salisbury, R. E.: Flexor tendon reconstruction in severely damaged hands, J. Bone Joint Surg. **53A:**829-858, 1971.
6. Hunter, J. M., Schneider, L. H., Dumont, J., and Erickson, J. C.: A dynamic approach to problems of hand function, Clin. Orthop. **104:**112-115, 1974.
7. Hunter, J. M., Subin, D., Minkow, F., and Konikoff, J.: Sheath formation in response to limited active gliding implants (animals), J. Biomed. Mater. Res. Symposium, No. 5, Part 1: 163-173, 1974.
8. Mayer, L., and Ransohoff, N.: Reconstruction of the digital tendon sheath, a contribution to the physiological method of repair of damaged finger tendons, J. Bone Joint Surg. **18:** 607-616, 1936.
9. Milgram, J. E.: Transplantation of tendons through preformed gliding channels, Bull. Hosp. Joint Dis. **21:**250, 1960.

27. The active gliding tendon prosthesis: progress

James M. Hunter, M.D.
Scott H. Jaeger, M.D.

The passive gliding tendon implant has been shown to be clinically effective in reconstructive tendon surgery.[3, 5, 6] When a smooth silicone tendon implant glides passively, in a short period of time, it produces a pseudosynovial sheath that can accept and nourish a free tendon graft.[7, 8] This concept represents an advancement in the field of reconstructive hand surgery. However, in practice, it has its limitations. Since gliding of the implant is necessary for the production of the sheath, a supervised program of hand therapy consisting of manual range of motion and active finger trapping is required to generate the necessary passive gliding of the implant. In addition, the total treatment plan requires at least two, and occasionally three, operative procedures: the first stage for implantation of the implant, a second stage for replacement with the free tendon graft, and occasionally, tenolysis.

The ultimate solution to these limitations would be to develop an active gliding tendon prosthesis. Then, only one procedure would be required, and once the prosthesis is secure, the patient's own muscular activity could provide the necessary excursion to produce the pseudosheath and maintain supple finger joints. In instances where Stage II tendon replacement is indicated, young patients, heavy laborers, tendon grafting at a later date becomes simplified as the soft tissue gliding planes are already present (Fig. 27-1).

The idea of an active gliding tendon prosthesis is not new as evidenced by several unsuccessful attempts at its development since the early 1900s.[2, 9-11] In the past, the obstacles have been in two major areas: (1) the materials and design of the prosthesis shaft and (2) attachment of the prosthesis distally to bone and proximally to muscle (Fig. 27-1). In this article, we will discuss the present status and what is currently being done to solve the problems in the development of an active gliding tendon prosthesis.

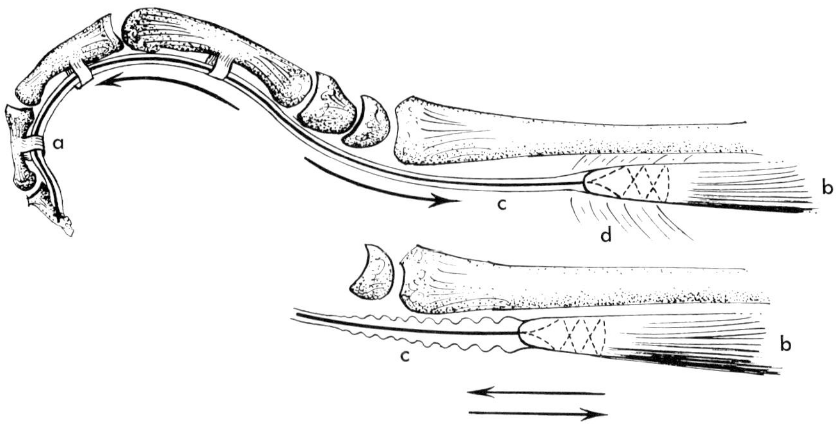

Fig. 27-1. Side view of an active gliding tendon prosthesis. *a,* Distal juncture to bone. *b,* Muscle. *c,* Soft tissue gliding plane, in which sheath is mobile and pleats allow excursion of motor tendon. *d,* Proximal juncture to musculotendinous junction. Soft tissue planes must organize to permit movement of sheath *(c)* juncture to tendon and implant *(d)* as one unit.

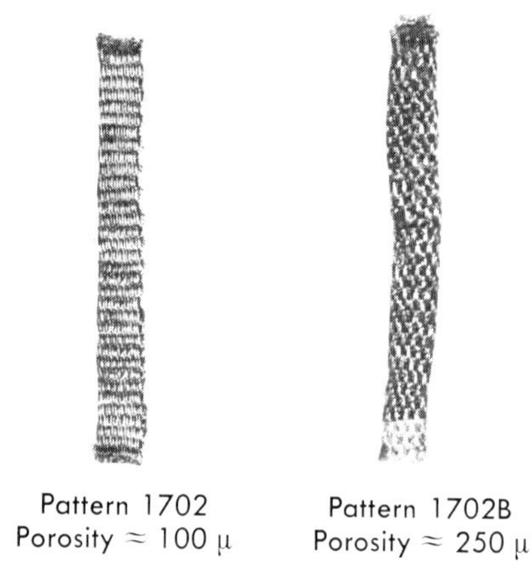

Fig. 27-2. Samples of stainless steel fibrile woven into 5 mm. wide tapes—useful core material and site for tissue ingrowth.

THE TENDON PROSTHESIS SHAFT

One of the key requirements of the shaft of an active gliding tendon prosthesis is that it closely conform to the physical characteristics of a normal flexor tendon, that is, tensile strength, flexibility, and resistance to elongation. At the same time, it must have the properties required of all biologic implants, that is, biocompatibility, resistance to biodegradation, and favorable wear characteristics.

The passive gliding implant is a good prototype for an active tendon. It has a woven dacron core and a molded cover of silicone rubber. This passive implant fulfills all of the above requirements except tensile strength. It cannot sustain repeated tensile loads of 25 kg. without failure. Therefore, the silicone rubber coating is acceptable, but the woven core must be strengthened to increase the tensile strength of the prosthesis. Three core materials have promising qualities for this purpose. Through a special industrial process, 31 6 L stainless steel can be pulled similar to wool to produce a yarn that can be woven into a ribbon of high tensile strength (Fig. 27-2). However, the current process leaves traces of heavy metals such as copper that may accelerate biodegradation of the implant. Hopefully, this problem is only temporary. However, other less reactive metals may be substituted in the weaving process. Titanium wire is being studied currently with regard to tensile strength and resistance to flexion fatigue for this purpose. The third material being studied is a new synthetic fiber, Kevlar (Du Pont Fiber B). The fiber can be woven into a ribbon that has excellent tensile strength, flexibility, and resistance to elongation and flexion fatigue. Studies are now in progress to determine the biocompatibility of Kevlar.

Therefore, the problem of the prosthesis shaft is approaching solution and it is not a significant obstacle in the realization of an active gliding tendon prosthesis.

THE JUNCTURE INTERFACE

Each year, implants are playing a larger role in a wide variety of surgical procedures. In the majority of instances, the primary problem is securing the implant. In the case of the tendon prosthesis, the problem is particularly perplexing because the juncture must resist tensile stresses of significant magnitude. Static and cyclic compressive forces are well tolerated, but little is known of the reaction to dynamic tensile forces.

In order for a tendon prosthesis to function, two junctures must be operative: (1) a distal junction between the prosthesis and bone and (2) a proximal junction between the prosthesis and the tendon stump, musculotendinous junction, or muscle (Fig. 27-1). Two types of attachment are required at each end. A short-term, temporary junction is necessary that offers immediate fixation and allows early range of motion and function for gliding and development of the complete sheath system. For full function, a long-term durable junction is necessary that can accept the responsibility for the tensile stresses slowly over a period of time.

The short-term distal and proximal junctions have few demands placed on them and they can be achieved by available suture techniques. Distally, the tendon prosthesis core can be wired down to the periosteum through drill holes in the bone or by a wire pull-out suture. Proximally, the core can be sutured either to the tendon stump or the musculotendinous junction where the connective tissue is strong enough to provide purchase for the sutures. These techniques will provide the low level tensile strength to allow minimally loaded excursion of the tendon prosthesis in the early postoperative period. The resultant excursion allows generation of the new sheath and maintains the integrity of digit motion.

The long-term junctures or interfaces are a much more perplexing problem

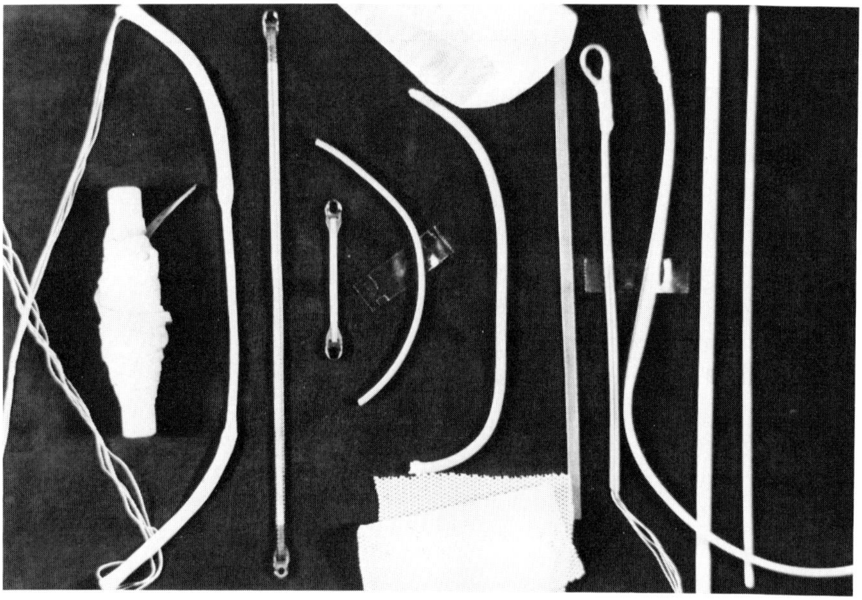

Fig. 27-3. Prototype active gliding tendon prostheses demonstrating loop concepts. Left, Chinese finger trap of polyester fiber discarded because of excessive tissue reactions.

toward which the major thrust of present research is being directed. These junctures must be permanent and must withstand repeated tensile stresses in excess of 50 kg. However, the bulk of the juncture cannot exceed the limitations offered by the area available in the distal phalanx and the proximity of the distal interphalangeal joint, nor can the bulk interfere with the gliding necessary in the volar compartment of the forearm or palm.

The solution to the problem of the long-term junctures may lie in one or a combination of two types of interfaces. One type has a relatively small interface surface area, but the nature of the interface is such that its ability to resist tensile stress per unit surface area is large. An example of this in the distal attachment is where a metal eyelet endpiece is secured to the tendon prosthesis core (Fig. 27-3). This eyelet can be secured to the bone with either a screw or a heavy wire suture. Here the surface area of the endpiece interface to bone is small, but because of the strength of the materials, good tensile strength of the juncture is achieved. The major drawback is that with the tensile stress focused to one small area, fatigue may cause failure of the attachment.

Attachment of the implant eyelet to tendon can be applied proximally through the use of hard and soft loops. The tendon prosthesis core can be attached back on itself, producing a soft loop, or an endpiece of metal in the shape of a hard loop can be affixed to the core. Through these loops, the tendon stump can be passed, woven, and sutured to produce an interlocking loop. The interface surface area is small, but once the tendon heals to itself, the attachment is quite secure.

A B C D

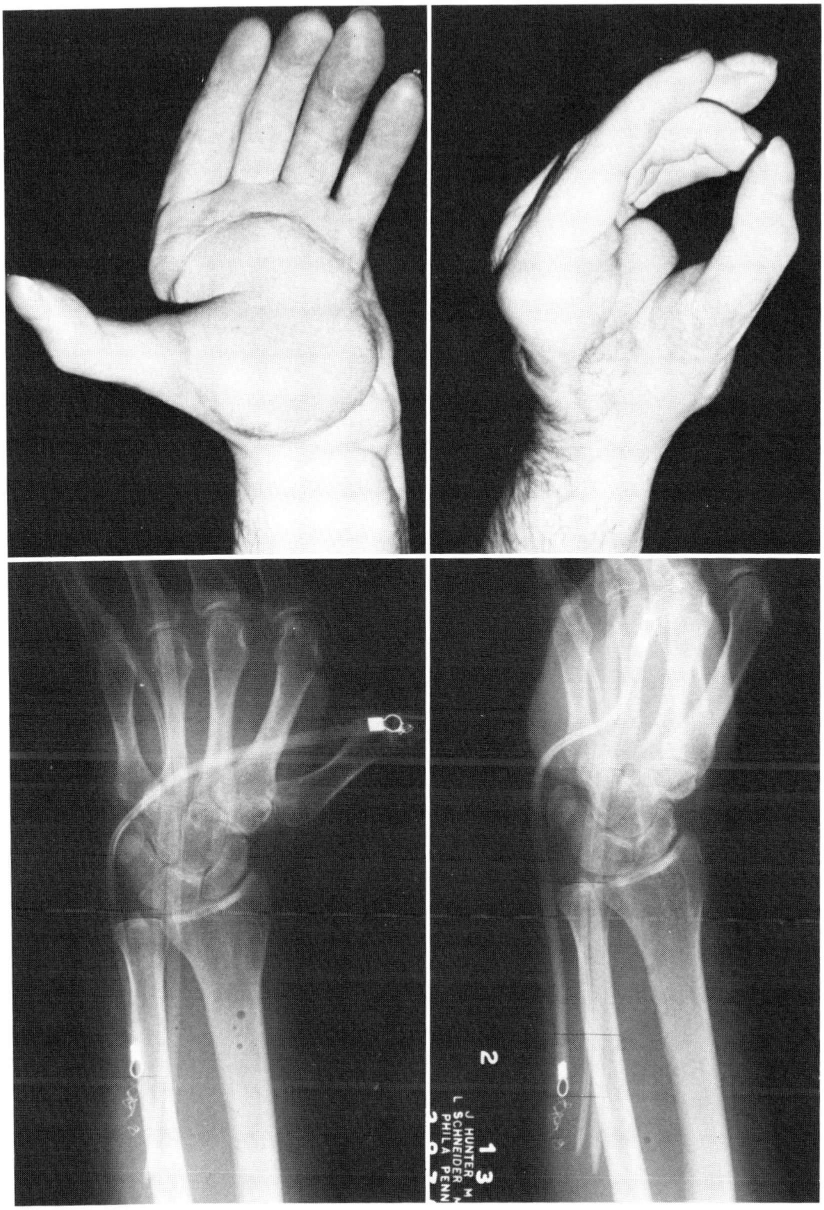

Fig. 27-4. A and B, Opponensplasty using active gliding tendon prosthesis—loop type. Motor tendon is flexor sublimis of long finger. **A,** Thumb extended. **B,** Thumb in apposition. **C and D,** Radiograph of patient shown in **A** and **B** demonstrating active excursion of the tendon prosthesis, approximately 2.5 to 3 cm. **C,** Thumb extended. **D,** Thumb in apposition.

This technique is attractive because it is simple and it is easy to achieve proper tension of the flexor system by adjusting the amount of tendon that is passed through the loop of the tendon prosthesis. This concept has been used with initial short-term success in both human and animal subjects (Fig. 27-4). Theoretically, the problem of all the tensile stresses being focused to the small surface area of the interface still remains, and the long-term utility of the technique has yet to be realized.

The other concept involving the long-term attachment of the active gliding tendon prosthesis deals with an interface that has a large surface area and therefore little tensile stress is applied per unit surface area. This concept utilizes tissue ingrowth and it is based on the fact that when a biocompatible material with the appropriate pore size is implanted in tissue, the tissue will infiltrate into the tissue and remain viable.[1] Since the optimal pore size is approximately 250 microns, the available surface area for the interface is enormous. Therefore, the tensile stress per unit surface area is quite small despite the fact that the total tensile stress applied to the interface is quite large.

The importance of the dispersion of tensile stresses on the durability of the juncture is realized when the character of the tissue interface is considered. Any time a foreign material is placed in tissue, a tissue reaction is produced that is determined by the nature and the shape of the implant. The best possible result is a thin layer of nonreactive fibrocytes that act as an interface between the normal tissue, be it bone, muscle, or tendon, and the implant. The more reactive the implant, the thicker the interface, and a thick, soft interface offers little secure fixation. The tissue reaction is also dependent on the amount of motion that occurs between the implant and the tissue. The fibrocytes of the interface tend to become reactive in response to undue motion and stress. Therefore if the stress is distributed over a large surface area, the reaction that decreases the efficiency of the interface will be less apt to occur.

The tissue ingrowth concept can be well applied as a technique for the long-term distal juncture. Distally, the prosthesis must be attached to bone, which offers an excellent site for ingrowth. Secure bone ingrowth will occur in sintered titanium[1] and, in this laboratory, bone ingrowth into 31 6 L stainless steel woven ribbon and wire mesh has been performed with early good results. If the metal has the appropriate pore size, is well impacted, and toggle is not allowed to occur, tensile strengths of up to 50 kg. per square centimeter of surface area can be obtained at 12 weeks (Fig. 27-5). Therefore, bone ingrowth into selected porous metals gives adequate tensile strength as the distal juncture to bone. The present thrust of study in this laboratory is to design suitable endpieces of sintered titanium for attachment of the tendon prosthesis using the bone ingrowth concept.

The tissue ingrowth concept may also be applied to the proximal juncture to tendon and muscle but its use here is more complicated. Whenever two materials are interwoven and stressed, in order to maintain the continuity of the bond, the

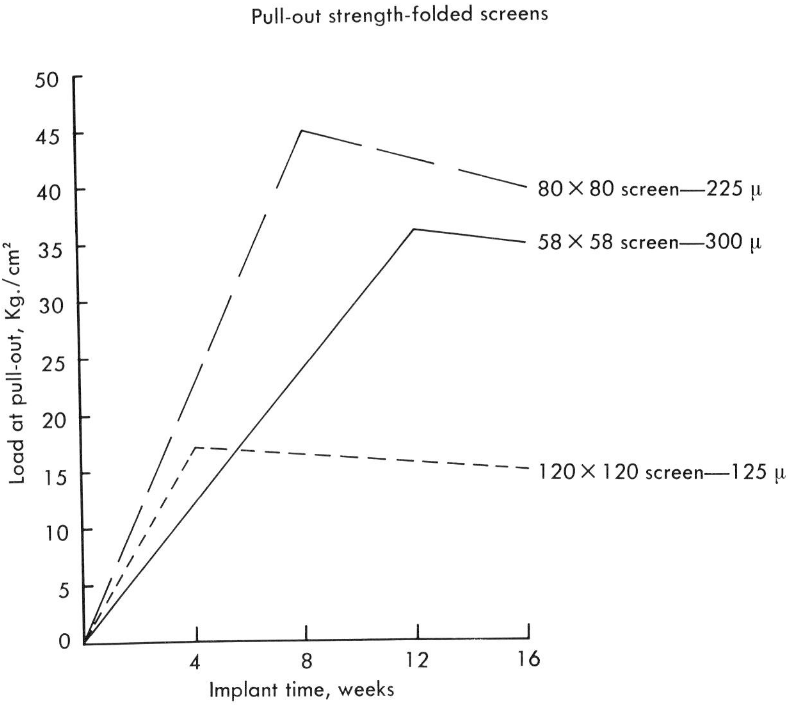

Fig. 27-5. Tensile strength of bone ingrowth into 316 L stainless steel wire mesh. Load strength decreases after 12 weeks, apparently caused by continuing tissue reactivity to stainless steel.

two materials must react similarly to the stress applied. In other words, the Young's modulus of the materials must be closely matched. This is fairly simple with regard to bone because it has a high modulus and is easily matched to the materials available for ingrowth. Soft tissue is an entirely different case because its modulus is quite low, and it is difficult to match it with a material that is strong. Essentially all the materials that are strong enough to be used in the proximal attachment have a high modulus; therefore, it is necessary to develop a method to use these materials despite the difference in modulus.

This laboratory is studying two possible solutions to the problem of modulus matching. The first concept deals with the theory that if the high modulus material is composed of many small interlocking pieces, the essential overall modulus of the implant can, in effect, match the modulus of the soft tissue. This is believed to be possible because strain can therefore occur in response to stress by motion at the junctions of the interlocking components of the high modulus material. The second concept deals with the use of a modulus buffer. A material of intermediate modulus is interposed between the high modulus metal and the low modulus soft tissue. No results are available yet, but publications are forthcoming that will deal more deeply with these concepts.

The last problem in the use of an active gliding tendon prosthesis is how to adjust the tension of the entire flexor system when the prosthesis is implanted. As previously stated, in the loop system, the problem is solved easily by varying the amount of tendon passed through the loop. In the tissue ingrowth system in which specific endpieces are necessary, the problem is more perplexing. The solution lies in the use of an adjustable adhesive connection or a universal joint that can connect the appropriate length tendon prosthesis shaft to the implanted endpieces. A variety of lengths could be available to provide the correct tension.

CONCLUSION

No prosthesis can be expected to afford complete and normal function to an affected part. This is also true of the active gliding tendon prosthesis. However, this fact should not detract from the zeal necessary to accomplish its development. Given the appropriate indications, the tendon prosthesis can be an important addition to the armamentarium of reconstructive hand surgery. None of the obstacles to its development seem insurmountable; and, through the combined effort of surgeons, engineers, and manufacturers, the active gliding tendon prosthesis can become a reality.

References

1. Galante, J., Rostoker, W., Lueck, R., and Ray, R. D.: Sintered fiber metal composites as a basis for attachment of implants to bone, J. Bone Joint Surg. **53A**(1):101-114, January, 1971.
2. Grau, H. R.: The artificial tendon: an experimental study, Plast. Reconstr. Surg. **22**: 562-566, 1958.
3. Hunter, J. M.: Artificial tendons; early development and application, Am. J. Surg. **109**: 325-338, 1965.
4. Hunter, J. M., Salem, A. W., Steindel, C. R., and Salisbury, R. E.: The use of gliding artificial tendon implants to form new tendon beds, In Proceedings of The American Society for Surgery of the Hand, J. Bone Joint Surg. **51A**:790, June, 1969.
5. Hunter, J. M., and Salisbury, R. E.: Flexor-tendon reconstruction in severely damaged hands, J. Bone Joint Surg. **53A**:829-858, July, 1971.
6. Hunter, J. M., and Salisbury, R. E.: Use of gliding artificial implants to produce tendon sheaths; techniques and results in children, Plast. Reconstr. Surg. **45**:564-572, 1970.
7. Hunter, J. M., Steindel, C., Salisbury, R. E., and Hughes, D.: Study of early sheath development using static nongliding implants, J. Biomed. Mater. Res. Symposium, No. 5 (Part 1):155-162, 1974.
8. Hunter, J. M., Subin, D., Minkow, F., and Konikoff, J.: Sheath formation in response to limited active gliding implants (animals), J. Biomed. Mater. Res. Symposium, No. 5 (Part 1):163-173, 1974.
9. Lange, F.: Ueber Periostale Sehnenverpflanzungen bei Lahmungen, Munchener Med. Wochnschr. **47**:486-490, 1900.
10. Sakata, Y.: Experimental study on the combined use of arterial tissues with nylon thread in artificial tendon formation, J. Japanese Orthop. Ass. **36**:1021, 1962.
11. Sarkin, T. L.: The plastic replacement of severed flexor tendons of the fingers, Br. J. Surg. **44**:232-240, 1956.

28. Physical therapy and the staged tendon graft: preoperative and postoperative management

Evelyn Mackin, L.P.T.

Hands are very important and, for me, the two-stage tendon reconstruction surgery is very special. The cases of salvage hands are the real challenge. All patients accepted for the two-stage tendon surgery are begun on a program to mobilize stiff joints and improve the preoperative condition of the hand.

For example, an automobile mechanic sustained a crush injury to his left little finger, lacerating the profundus and sublimis tendons. Both tendons were repaired. When he came to us 3 months after the injury, he was unable to flex the little finger, and his grasp was impaired. He was unable to hold tools and therefore unable to work. As a candidate for the two-stage tendon repair, he was started on a program of whirlpool, massage, and exercise to improve the range of motion and general condition of the hand. I use lanolin and cocoa butter, preferably lanolin. I like the tackiness of the lanolin, which is more effective with massage for loosening adhesions, as well as softening the skin. Since this patient could not actively flex the little finger, he was told to trap the injured finger with his normal right ring finger. With this method of trapping (Fig. 28-1), he was able to passively flex the finger and thereby increase its pliability. A soft pliable hand with maximum passive range of motion is the goal prior to Stage I.

I sometimes find that some patients are unable to trap their injured finger with the adjacent finger. They do not seem to have the dexterity. If this is the case, we give them a Velcro trapper (Fig. 28-2). The injured finger and the adjacent normal finger are strapped together to simulate active flexion. Whenever the ring finger is used, the little finger must also come into play. The patient may also use the trapper when doing work that requires sustained grip as part of the daily activities. This way, the injured finger is incorporated to useful function. I received the trapper idea from Janice Maynard, O.T.R., at the Union Memorial Hospital in Baltimore.

Soft tissue and joint contractures must be corrected before Stage I. Passive

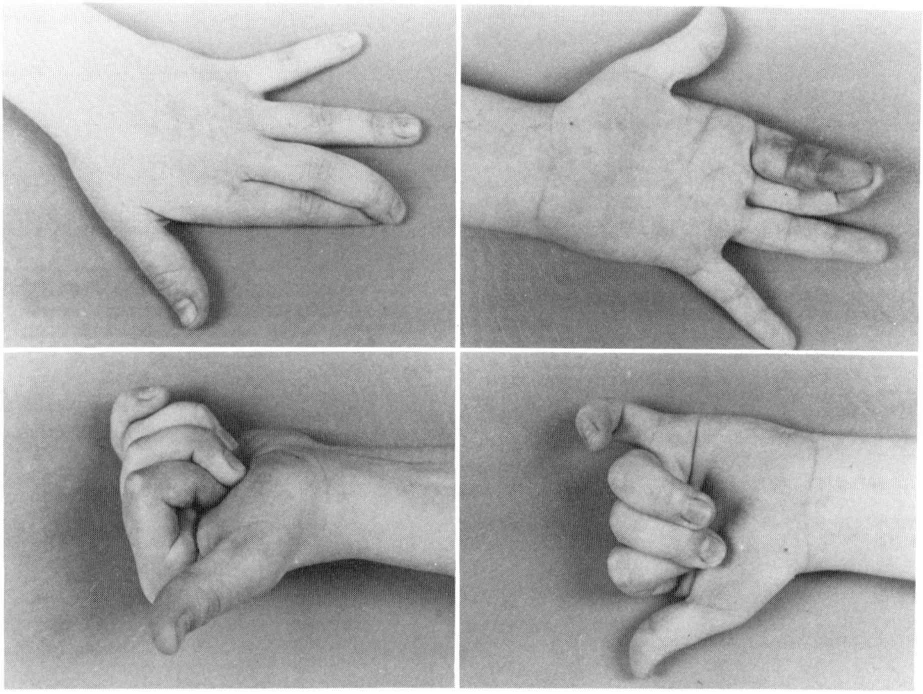

Fig. 28-1. Patient trapping injured index finger with adjacent normal long finger thereby increasing the range of motion and pliability of the index finger.

A

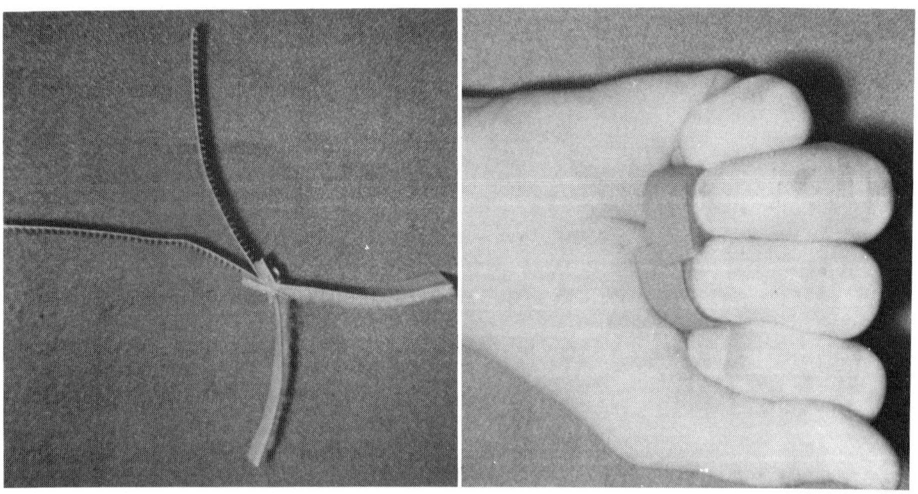

B

Fig. 28-2. Velcro trapper incorporates the injured finger to useful function. **A,** Velcro trapper. **B,** Injured finger and adjacent normal finger are strapped together to simulate active flexion.

A

B

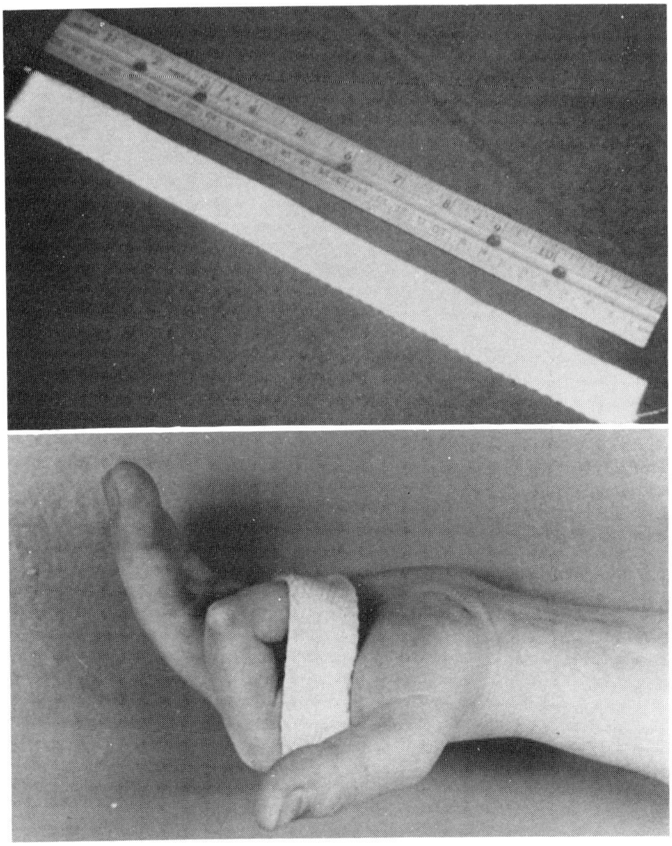

Fig. 28-3. Use of simple web strap to improve range of motion. A, Web strap made of 1″ lamp wick and small buckle. B, Patient wearing web strap over the distal interphalangeal and behind the metacarpophalangeal joints. It is the long steady stretch that corrects soft tissue and joint contractures.

stretching is necessary, which is accomplished by using a web strap (Fig. 28-3). It is made of a 1″ lamp wick and a small buckle. The strap is worn over the distal interphalangeal (DIP) or proximal interphalangeal (PIP) joint, depending on which joint is to be stretched, and behind the metacarpophalangeal (MP) joint. The time it is worn is gradually increased from 15 minutes 3 times daily to 2 hours 3 times daily. It can be worn longer. The most gain in flexion comes from wearing the strap comfortably for long periods of time. It is the long, steady stretch that improves the range of motion and it is especially helpful if the patient wears it during the night while sleeping. It doesn't have to be worn as tightly at night—only to maintain the gain made during the day. We impress on the patient that if the strap causes any pain or discomfort, it should be removed. A special thanks to Commander Theodore DuPuy of the Philadelphia Naval Hospital who suggested the lamp wick instead of a stiffer webbing. This particular patient was able to wear the web strap and made immediate improvement.

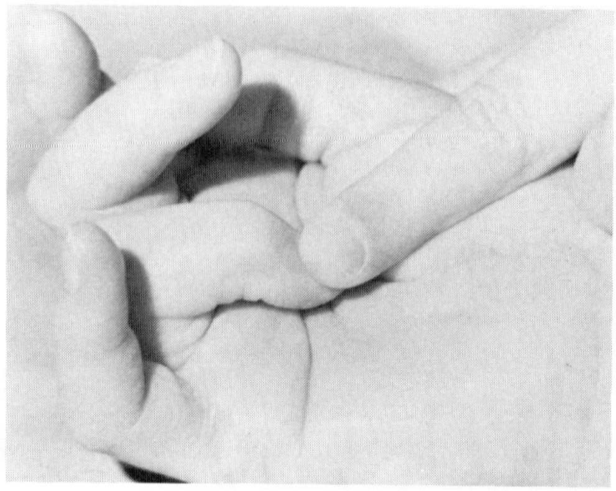

Fig. 28-4. Patient demonstrating passive potential—limit of flexion. This patient's ability to passively flex finger to distal palmar crease gives the surgeon a prediction of the future range of active motion following Stage II surgery.

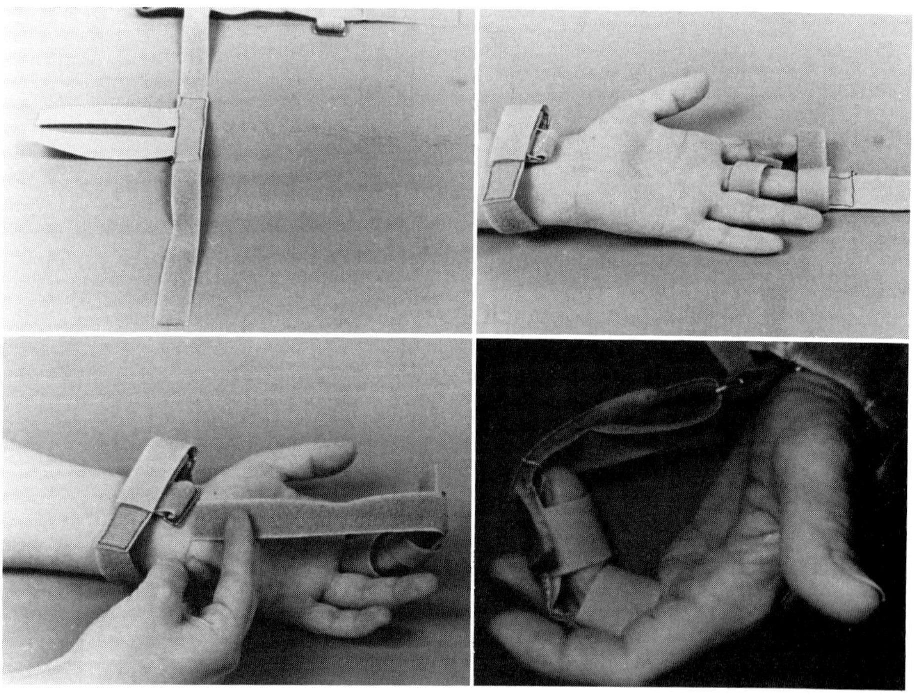

Fig. 28-5. Use of more complex web strap to improve passive range of motion when patient does not have enough flexion of finger to permit the wearing of type illustrated in Fig. 28-3.

However, many patients do not have enough passive flexion at the DIP and PIP joints to use the simple web strap and it is necessary to use one of a different construction. A patient without any PIP or DIP flexion can be started on a more involved type of passive flexion strap, and when the passive flexion improves sufficiently, the simpler web strap can be used to increase the passive potential. We try to have the patient's passive potential at the distal palmar crease prior to (Fig. 28-4) Stage II grafting so we know what to expect in active motion following Stage II. This more flexible passive flexion strap (Fig. 28-5) was introduced to me by Major Roger Salisbury, Chief of Surgical Studies, U. S. Army Institute of Surgical Research. This strap is very good when the PIP and DIP joints are limited. It is comfortable and the patient can sleep in this at night. Measurements are taken and recorded. Measuring the distance of the finger pulp from the distal palmar crease gives the surgeon a standard by which to evaluate the result of the surgery. If a patient's passive potential, for example, is ½ inch, when the preoperative Stage II is reached and the passive potential is realized following Stage II surgery, we consider it a good result.

A dorsal splint was applied to the patient's hand following Stage I surgery (Fig. 28-6). A week following surgery, the patient was fitted with a wristlet, and a hook and rubber band was applied to his finger. The hook was attached to his finger nail with quick-set Cyanoacrylate glue (Fig. 28-7). First, the fingernail is cleaned with nail polish remover, the nail is roughened a bit, and a very small dot of glue is applied to the fingernail. The hook is put on and another dot of glue is applied. With the hook and rubber band, the patient is able to exercise the finger. The patient is able to extend the finger with the antagonistic muscle and the rubber band pulls the finger back into flexion (Fig. 28-8). This is being studied following Stage I because we want to be sure that the patient extends and flexes the finger. It is important to have mobile joints and a viable gliding system before Stage II. This system may also be used after primary flexor tendon

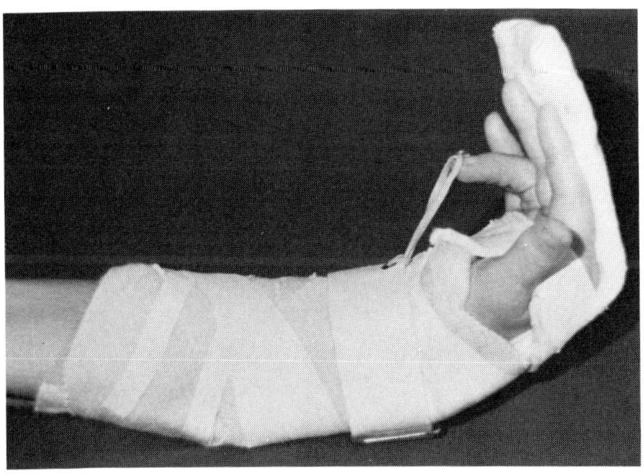

Fig. 28-6. Dorsal splint applied to patient's hand following Stage I surgery.

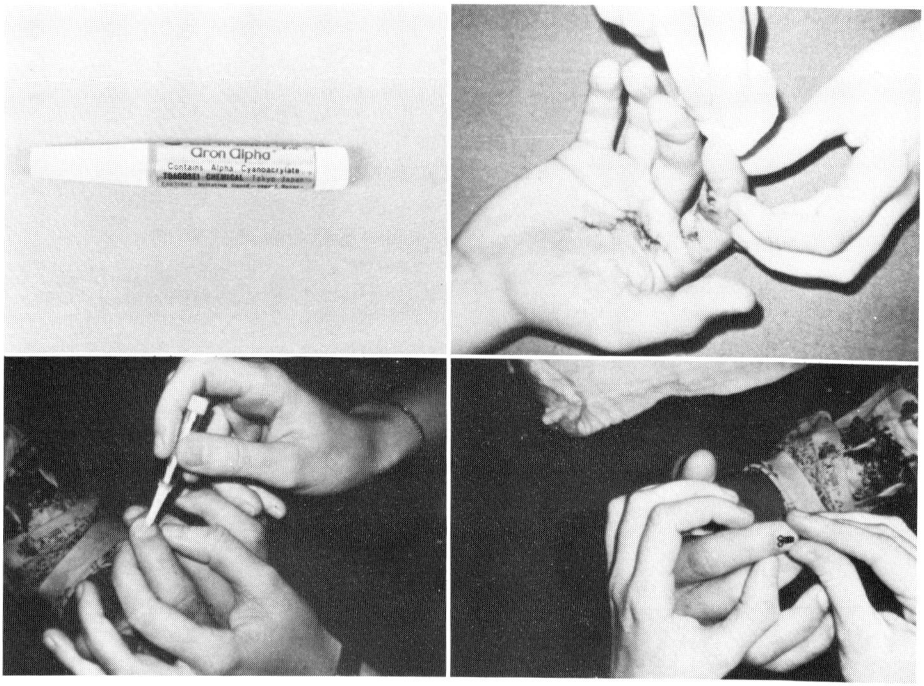

A B C D

Fig. 28-7. Use of hook on finger nail to permit the patient to exercise the finger. **A,** Quick-set glue. **B,** Finger nail is cleaned with nail polish remover. **C,** Small amount of glue is applied to finger nail. **D,** Hook applied to finger nail.

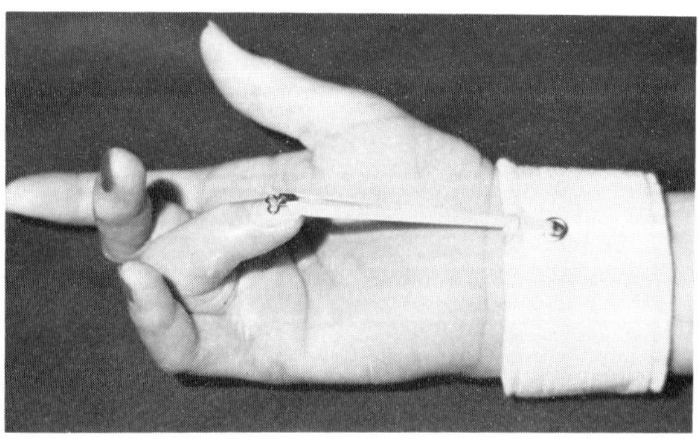

Fig. 28-8. Patient flexing finger following Stage I surgery with the use of the hook and rubber band. This method of carefully controlled passive exercising under the supervision of the hand therapist improves the mobility of the joints and gliding of the implant.

repair and in treatment of stiff interphalangeal (IP) joints. The patient is carefully checked periodically by the doctor during the 3 months between Stage I and Stage II. This patient had no evidence of reaction. He learned trapping and was training the joints appropriately. He had a Boyes' grade classification of 5, which means that he had multiple problems—joint changes, scarring of the tendon bed, and joint stiffness. He had had prior surgery. Many patients with a Boyes' preoperative classification of 5, however, are upgraded by the time they are ready for Stage II through carefully supervised therapy.

Following Stage II, another carefully fitted dorsal splint was applied to the patient's hand. It is most important that the dorsal splint be fitted properly, with the wrist and MP joints in flexion. Minimal flexion of the grafted finger is permitted while the padded dorsal splint prevents sudden forceful extension. Three weeks following the Stage II surgery, I work with the patient explaining how we want to block the PIP and MP joints with the finger to start gentle tendon pull-through. I explain to the patient the function of the tendon and its action, and guarded active motion is instituted. This retraining is so important when patients haven't used their hand for a while.

Four weeks postoperative Stage II, the button pull-out suture is ready to be removed. The surgeon tests for tendon pull-through. The protective dorsal splint is discarded at this time and the patient is ready to begin a more active exercise program with the Bunnell wood block. Now that the patient is able to actively flex the grafted finger, he is given a sponge to squeeze in the water, which provides some gentle resistive exercise. Whirlpool is an excellent preliminary to massage and exercise. Stubborn fingers that have shown contractures and stiffness prior to Stage I may require some softening again with lanolin massage. Training with the Bunnell wood block is begun 4 weeks postoperative. The wood block is ¼ inch thick and about the size of a cigarette pack (Fig. 28-9). It provides a means of training full active power ranges of the distal and proximal joints of the finger. Patients are carefully instructed in the use of the wood block when exercising. They are told to keep the MP joint firmly against the block when exercising the PIP joint. These little blocks are an excellent project for the occupational therapy department because they give patients a chance to use a sustained grip while they sand the blocks smooth around the edges. Good results from the two-stage procedure require careful attention to training and supervision. Training is always directed first to flexion of the DIP joint, then of the PIP joint, and then to flexing into the distal palmar crease. Splinting may be required intermittently. The Capener splint (Fig 28-10), which was recommended by Mr. Guy Pulvertaft, is a good splint to use during the early weeks of Stage II because, in addition to passively extending the patient's finger, it also flexes the finger.

A 23-year-old volunteer fireman, who was also a mechanic, was injured in a fireworks factory explosion. He suffered a traumatic amputation of the index, long, and ring fingers. He was treated initially with debridement and closure.

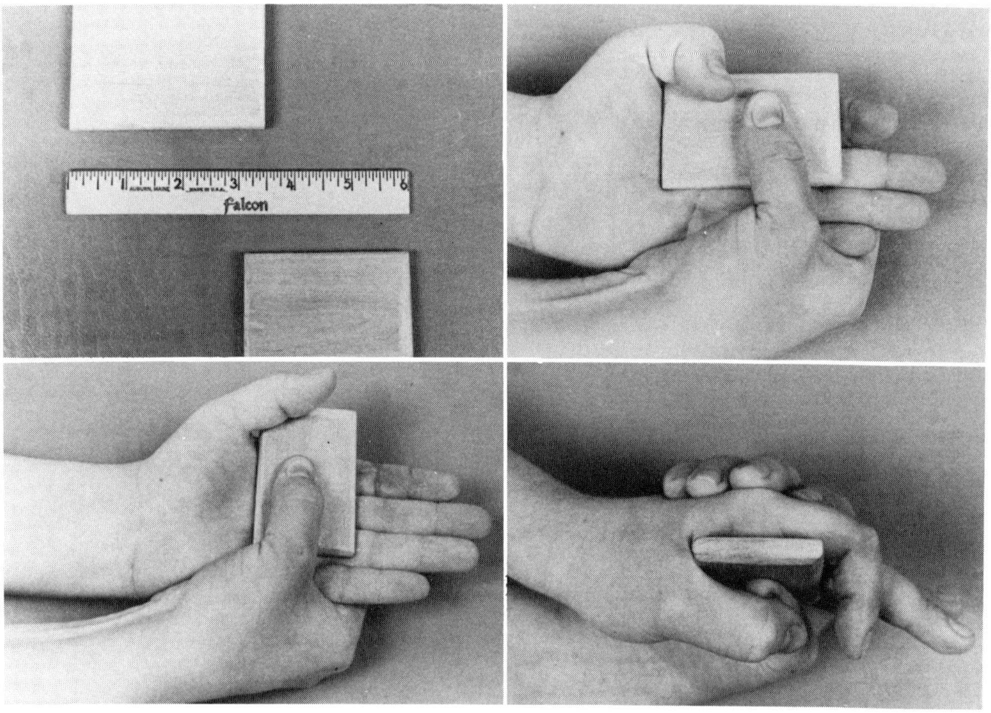

Fig. 28-9. Use of the Bunnell wood block provides the means of training full active power ranges of the distal and proximal joints of the finger.

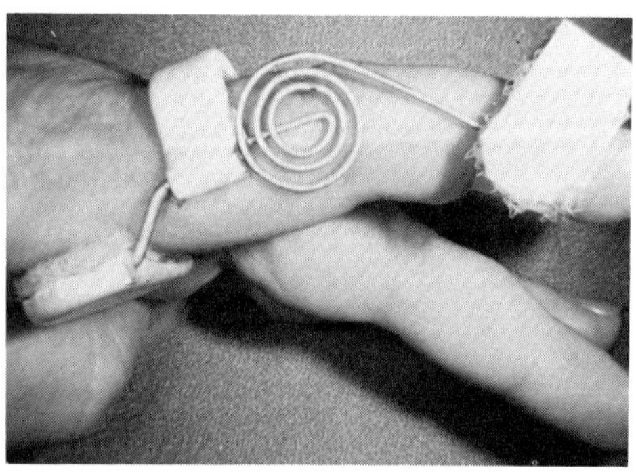

Fig. 28-10. Capener splint for use in the correction of flexion deformities of the interphalangeal joints and for providing resistance for the long flexors.

A B C

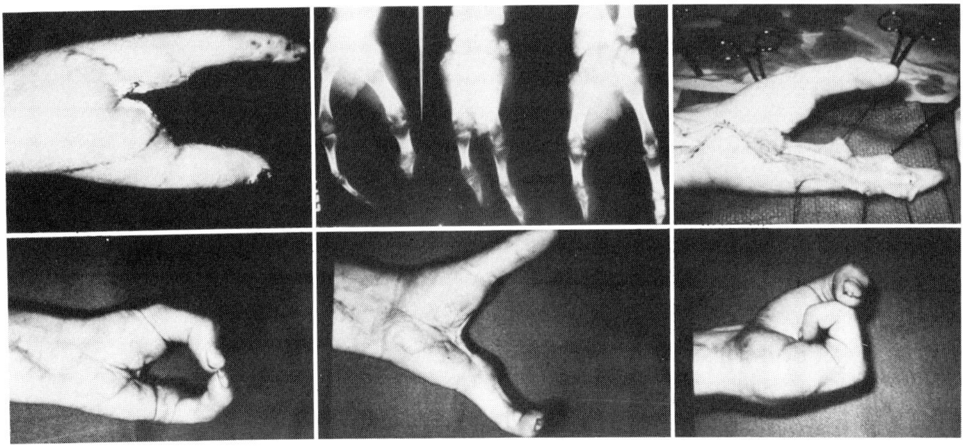

D E F

Fig. 28-11. A 19-year-old voluntary fireman sustained traumatic amputations of his index, long, and ring fingers in an explosion during a July 4th fireworks demonstration. **A,** Skin maceration and drainage deep in cleft in the intervening space between the thumb and little finger. Skin condition was much improved when betadine whirlpool and lanolin massage were instituted. **B,** X-ray film showing amputation of index, long, and ring fingers in their entirety, and the integrity of the remaining joints of the thumb and little finger. **C,** Hunter tendon prosthesis inserted into little finger during Stage I. **D, E,** and **F,** Apposition, extension, and flexion 10 weeks after Stage II procedure.

He had thumb function but limited motion due to stiffness. He completely destroyed the flexor mechanism in his little finger and we did a staged tendon reconstruction. The induration of the hand was greatly helped through physical therapy with whirlpool and massage softening. He had no passive motion at all in his little finger when we started. This is where the whole therapy concept shows results—the careful attention given to the patient's hand preoperatively. We improved the skin condition and passive range of motion. Now he is able to flex his little finger to the distal palmar crease (Fig. 28-11). He is able to oppose; to extend. He returned to his job as an auto mechanic and also to being a volunteer fireman.

The team approach to hand surgery is much more than a method to accomplish hand restoration. It is also geared to improve patient morale, to shorten the period of disability, and to rehabilitate patients as useful members of their community.

Acknowledgment

Photographs of hand rehabilitation techniques by Earl Spangenberg, Audiovisual Department, Jefferson Medical College of Thomas Jefferson University.

29. Occupational therapy following hand tendon surgery

Josephine Cohen, M.A., O.T.R.

Occupational therapy offers the hand surgeon an approach to rehabilitation based on a fourfold concept consisting of: (1) splinting with custom fit, (2) evaluation, (3) sensibility retraining, and (4) treatment utilizing purposeful graded activities.

SPLINTING

A 46-year-old right-handed woman sustained a deep laceration to the left volar wrist resulting in injury to the median and ulnar nerves. The nerves were repaired and a metacarpophalangeal joint arthrodesis of the thumb and two-stage opponensplasty, utilizing an implant, were performed in three surgical procedures.

Approximately 1 week to 10 days after the third operation, a gauntlet was fabricated out of orthoplast, a low temperature material, utilizing a bridge on the volar surface that allowed for the pull of the dynamic opponens cuff to be altered by adding several holes as needed. Its purpose was to support the wrist, abduct the thumb, and stretch the web space, giving resistance to extension. By adding an outrigger of the same material, the splint could function as an exerciser for specific finger joints (Fig. 29-1). As the wrist heals and is able to tolerate resistance, a variation of the splint designed by Dr. J. William Littler of New York can be applied. This device provides passive abduction and extension and gives resistance to flexion and opposition (Fig. 29-2). Splints of this nature are easy to construct, light in weight, and can be kept clean by the patient.

EVALUATION

In the evaluation phase of occupational therapy, which is the determinant of the treatment program, hand prints are used to supply pictorial information concerning the volar aspect of the hand. The outline of the spread hand gives visual data pertaining to the mediolateral alignment of the hands and wrists, to finger abduction, and thumb extension.[1] Prints can be done on a regular

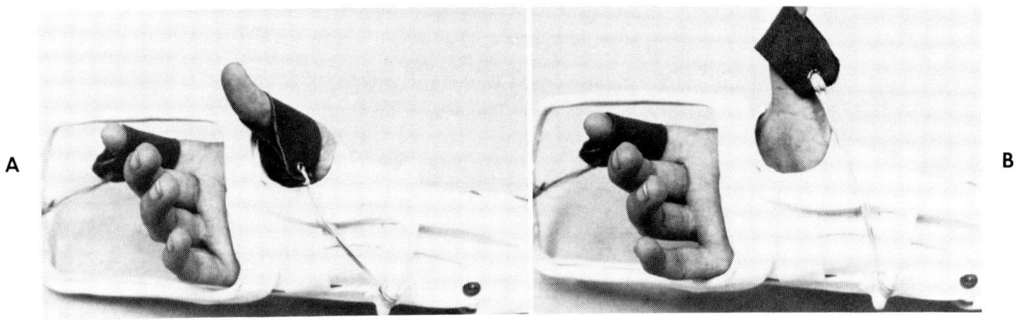

Fig. 29-1. Placement of holes on volar bridge to which rubber band is attached allows for **A**, resistance to thumb extension, and **B**, resistance to thumb abduction and stretch of web space.

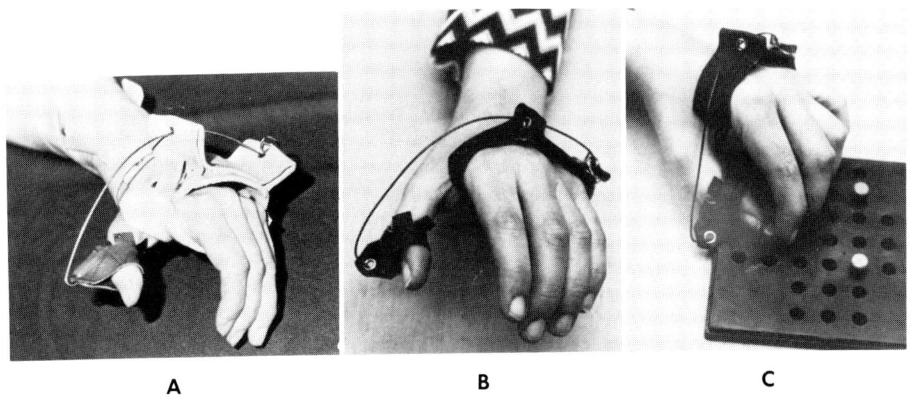

Fig. 29-2. Splint that is simple in design can be fabricated in either **A**, rigid material (Prenyl) or **B**, leather and piano wire. It is important to align raised tab of splint with midpoint of index and long finger metacarpal in order to give proper tension to thumb cuff. **C**, Practical application of splint to training activity.

basis as a method of patient incentive that provides them with a visual record of their progress.

Fingerpaint is the medium used on the volar surface. The patient abducts the fingers as much as possible and then places the hand *lightly* on the paper and a tracing is made by the therapist, marking off the joints as a frame of reference. Areas indicative of muscle tightness and/or joint stiffness or contracture will not make an impression on the paper (Fig. 29-3).

The functional motor evaluation utilizes the Jamar dynamometer with its five levels of grip. The first level requires metacarpophalangeal flexion, indicating the presence of precision grip. Because interphalangeal motion of the fingers and rotation of the thumb are indispensable to power grip, a validation of the patient's problem will emerge with each successive level (Fig. 29-4).

The pinch gauge gives another objective measurement of tip-to-tip prehen-

A

B

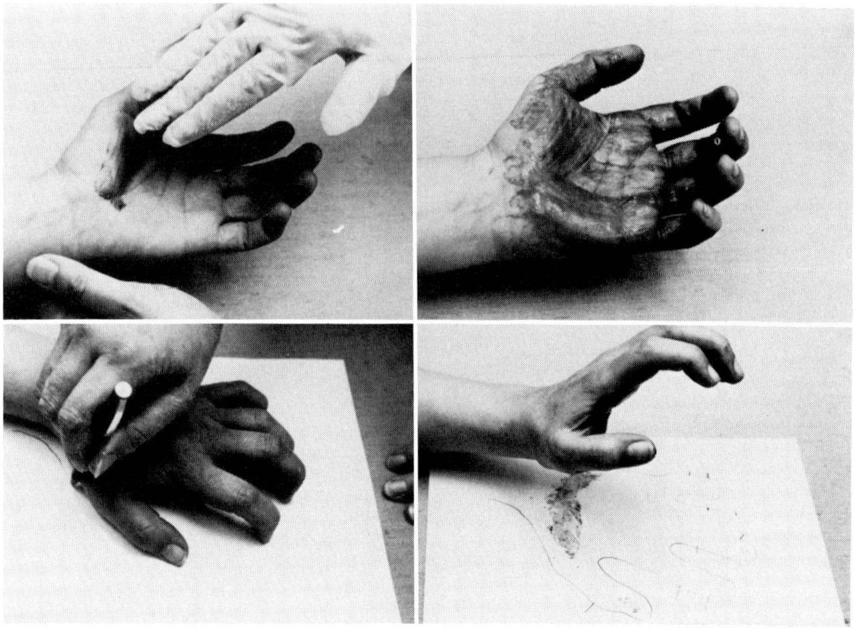

C

D

Fig. 29-3. **A** and **B,** Therapist wears rubber glove to apply finger paint to volar surface of hand. **C,** Forearm and hand should rest on working surface. **D,** Tightness of metacarpophalangeal and interphalangeal joints is immediately visible by lack of color representation.

sion and lateral pinch of thumb to fingers. It is important to position and isolate the individual finger being tested so as not to use the other fingers as a supportive base (Fig. 29-5).

A hand with mobility, strength, and stability of grasp is ultimately dependent on sensory feedback in order to be a functional unit. Moberg states that loss of sensibility means loss of more than 50% of the prehensive function of the part in question.[2] Prior to administering the von Frey hair test, a subjective sensory account of the hand is elicited verbally from the patient and recorded in colors or broken, dotted, or heavy lines. It can be described as drawing a map of the hand, indicating areas that are normal, have a pins and needles sensation, and so forth (Fig. 29-6).

In the von Frey hair test, the filaments are a graduated series of hairs mounted on a handle, which exert different pressures when they begin to bend. Both hands are tested and the eyes are closed. The exam can be given on an intensive basis in which the hand is divided into segments and each tested separately or it can be administered by examining individual fingers for specific nerve involvement, progressing distal to proximal. If there is a question in the therapist's mind, the patient is asked to open the eyes and localize the area touched. It is important that the digit be as extended and flat on the table as possible or else proprioception is being employed.

The numbered filaments have a corresponding value such as diminished

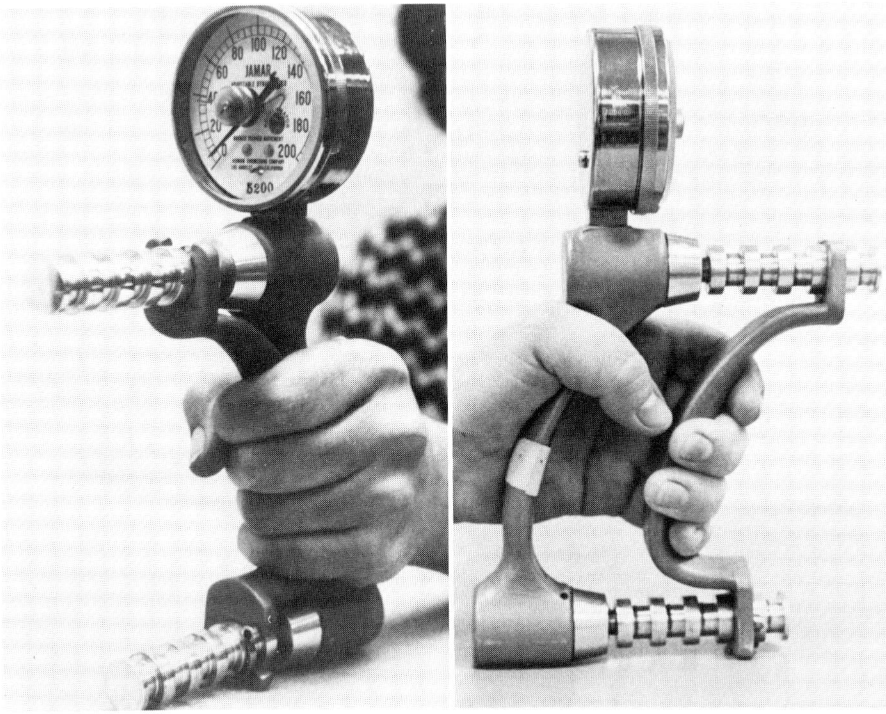

Fig. 29-4. A, Metacarpophalangeal flexion and thumb rotation are necessary for first level of dynamometer. **B,** Metacarpophalangeal extension is seen on fourth level. Results would correspond with hook grasp.

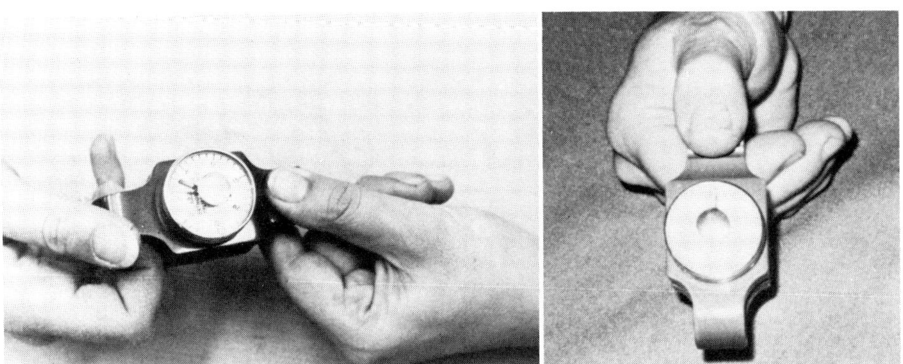

Fig. 29-5. A, Tip-to-tip prehension and **B,** lateral pinch should be measured at regular intervals with pinch gauge.

A

B

C

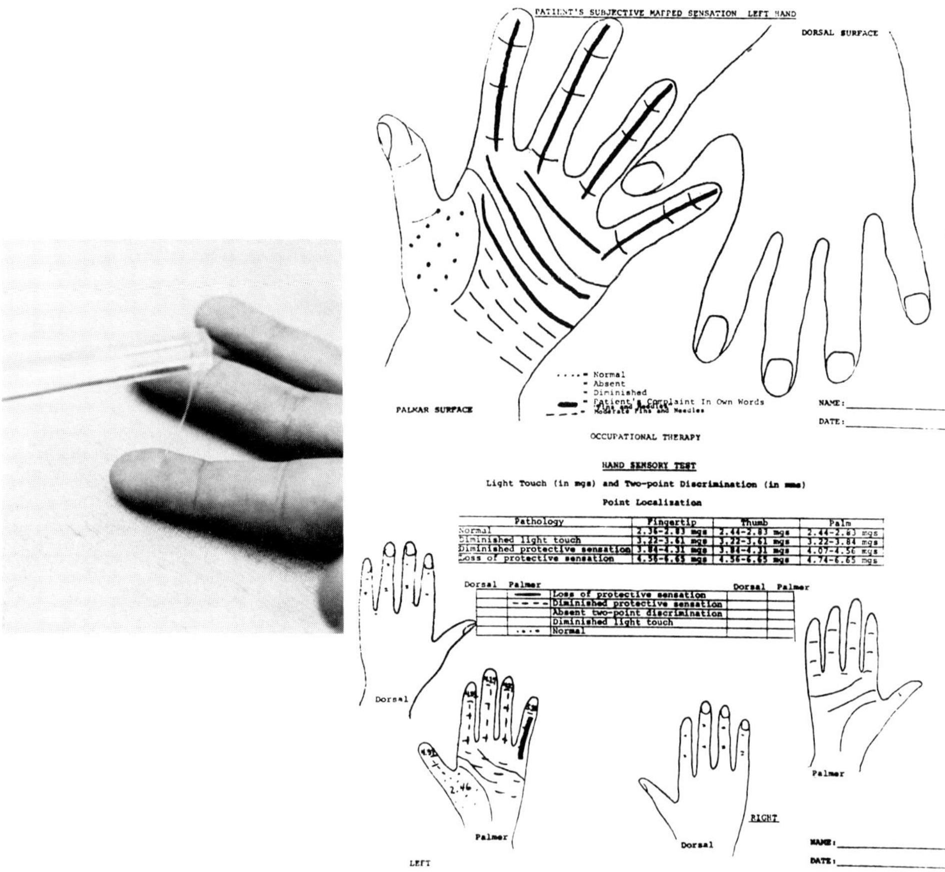

Fig. 29-6. **A,** Patient's verbal subjective description of hand sensation is recorded. **B,** Tested with graduated filament, fingers should be flat on surface to eliminate proprioception. **C,** Charted on sheet that converts numbered filaments to levels such as normal, diminished light touch, diminished protective sensation, and loss of protective sensation.

light touch, loss of protective sensation, and so forth. Here again, colors or variations of a straight line can be used for facilitating results in determining the patient's status. A test of this nature is helpful in pointing out to the patient the extent of the sensory deficit and the precautions involved. For example, loss of protective sensation on a digit or the palm would mean that the patient would not be aware of being burned.

Two point discrimination can be demonstrated with a calibrated millimeter instrument having three blunt ends. It is administered with the patient's eyes closed. The pressure with one or two of the blunt ends of the instrument should not produce a blanching of the skin and should be placed on the skin simultaneously. It is important that the direction of the line through the points be constant, preferably parallel to the finger.[3] Caution is again advised against

A

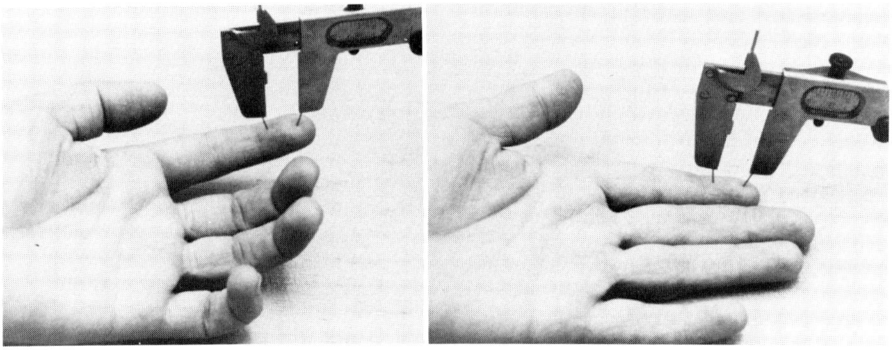

B

Fig. 29-7. **A,** Incorrect and, **B,** proper positioning of fingers for two-point discrimination test.

a raised or flexed digit during the test. If this occurs the reading is not a totally accurate one for pressure alone (Fig. 29-7).

It is important to be thorough in the selection and administration of the evaluation procedures employed. It should be possible to measure the responses objectively and one test should show some correlation with another. This validation provides an understanding of the patient's present methods of functioning and deficits, and localizes areas necessary for treatment.

Functional motor testing and sensory examination results may show a correlation with a form of the Moberg "picking up" test.[2] Seven objects, four of different types of material, a wood dowel ⅛″ thick, two different size hex nuts, a box, and stop watch are used as the testing materials (Fig. 29-8). The patient is first timed taking out and putting back the objects with the eyes open. It is important to observe whether the patient is using a normal prehension pattern, namely the thumb and index and long finger. The object that gives the most difficulty is the dowel or stick. At a point when it is obvious that it cannot be accomplished in the same manner as the others, tell the patient "Do it any way that you can." It is then taken to the edge of the table, picked up, and placed in the box.

In the next part of the test, the patient is asked to perform exactly as before but this time with eyes closed. A different picture of grasp emerges and the timing has more than doubled. As the patient progresses, the fingers will be used on the outside of the box as a guideline. The dorsum of the thumb will be heavily depended upon to give feedback of the object because of the intact radial nerve. The volar surface of the forearm will also be employed to provide the information that some objects are still remaining on the table. In this section, the pattern of approach and grasp are dramatically different from the previous part of the test. The test results in a picture of the patient's functional sensation or tactile gnosis.

It is felt that by administering sensory testing both preoperatively and postoperatively a guide will be provided for both the patient and the surgeon.

A

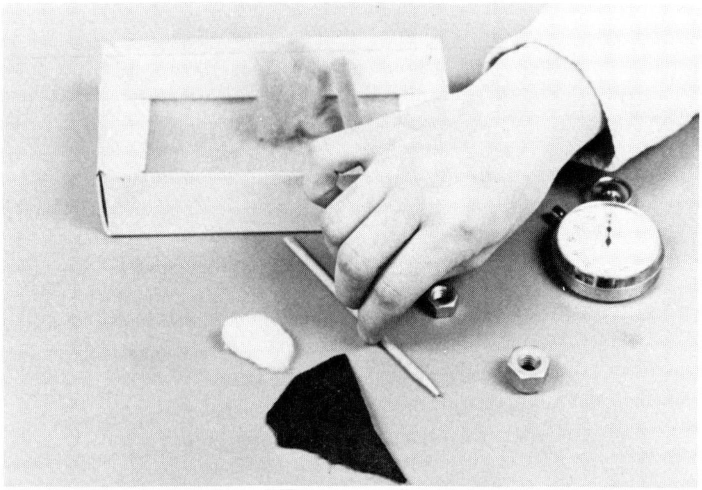

B

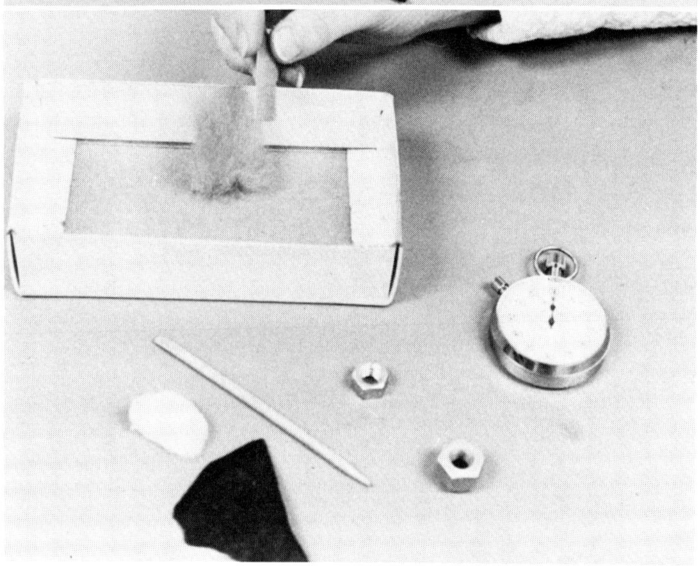

Fig. 29-8. A, Picking up test is simple to assemble and easy to administer. Same objects should be used each time. **B,** With patient's eyes open, test is performed with normal prehension pattern of thumb, index, and long fingers in three jaw chuck pinch.

Functional motor and sensory testing are repeated at approximately 1-month or 6-week intervals.

SENSIBILITY RETRAINING

Sensibility retraining can be initiated by several methods. I am grateful to Janice Maynard, O.T.R., for her skill and guidance in this area. The patient can begin by using different types and grades of material as a stimulator (Fig. 29-9). It is important that the hand and fingers be flat on the working surface

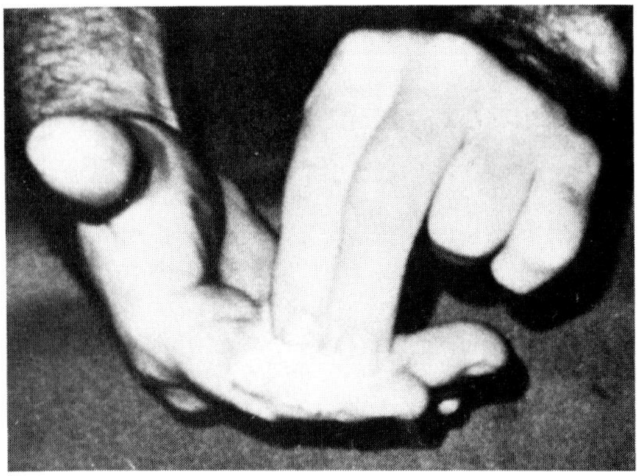

Fig. 29-9. Sensibility retraining begins with material being lightly extended over nerve pathway, always going proximal to distal. Hand and fingers should be flat on surface to eliminate proprioception and not slightly raised as in this picture.

A

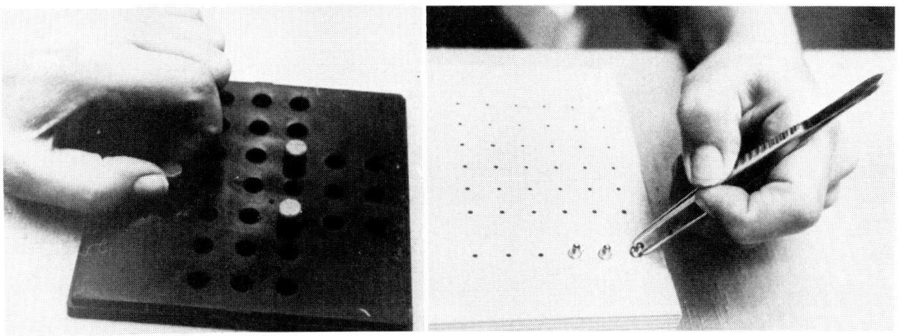

B

Fig. 29-10. A, Graded activities encourage thumb and individual finger prehension. **B,** Resistance is applied through use of tweezers in performing fine eye-to-hand coordinated activity. These types of training activities serve the dual purposes of exercise and assessment of function.

in order to eliminate proprioception. As improvement is noted, activities can be used in conjunction or as a progression of the initial part of the program. String art is an excellent purposeful activity to use in perceiving and gripping. Activities given to the patient are graded according to regeneration as charted at regular intervals through the various evaluation tests described previously.

GRADED ACTIVITIES

At the same time that the patient is engaged in sensibility retraining, the occupational therapist is instituting a program for specific treatment of the surgical procedures.

A successful opponensplasty is dependent upon the rotation of the carpometacarpal joint of the thumb. Therefore, the patient is started with a light activity of picking up plastic pegs, alternating the thumb to the individual fingers. Emphasis is placed on tip prehension (Fig. 29-10).

Using tweezers to pick up collars and pins provides resistance to prehension and utilizes lateral pinch. It is a fine eye-to-hand coordination activity that provides assessment of function in addition to being a training activity.

The patient's program should be a graded and meaningful one and should be custom designed for specific needs. This is one of the exciting challenges of hand therapy.

Grateful acknowledgment for photography to Earl Spangenberg of Jefferson Medical College.

References

1. Dworecka, F., Challenor, Y., Spector, P., Kaplan, L., and Wisham, L.: A practical approach to the evaluation of rheumatoid hand deformity, Am. J. Orth. Surg., April, 1968.
2. Moberg, E.: Methods for examining sensibility of the hand. In Flynn, J. E., editor: Hand surgery, Baltimore, 1966, Williams and Wilkins, pp. 435-449.
3. Önne, L.: Recovery of sensibility and sudomotor activity in the hand after nerve suture, Acta Chir. Scand. (Suppl.) Stockholm, **300**:5-69, 1962.

Appendix

Repair of tendons in the fingers

Sterling Bunnell, M.D.

One of the most baffling problems in surgery is to restore normal function to a finger in which the tendons have been injured. When we consider that the majority of industrial disabilities are from injuries of the hands, and that a successful repair of an injured finger tendon is a rarity, it is apparent that there are especial attendant difficulties, which cannot be overcome by the ordinary surgical procedure.

Before considering these difficulties and formulating methods of overcoming them, let us think of the hand as a marvelously functionating piece of live machinery and regard it with due respect. Though its tissues are tough and compact, its tendons, tendon sheaths, pulleys, joint surfaces and flexible joint capsules all glide on each other so easily and smoothly that there is little in the refinement of motion that the hand cannot do. If infection or trauma insults these perfected parts, a tissue reaction will occur, which will bind the gliding surfaces together, thicken and stiffen the joint capsules, congeal the tissues of the finger, strangulate the nerves and vessels, and loss of function will result.

Atraumatic technique essential. Surgical trauma so brutalizes the tissues and lowers their vitality that they are an easy prey for the few bacteria that even in spite of careful asepsis are unavoidably present. In most repairs of finger tendons free grafts are put in and as these have such a low resistance to infection, it is imperative that in these cases we use not only superasepsis, but also an atraumatic technique. If we are to avoid binding adhesions, we must not have infection even in its milder form of inflammation, in which no pus is formed, nor must we have aseptic traumatic inflammation, as this reaction to pure trauma is almost as binding to movable parts as is the fibrosis of infection.

As binding fibrosis is our arch enemy and trauma is both its direct and by predisposing to infection its indirect cause, we must if we are to achieve success in repairing tendons of the fingers adopt an atraumatic technique.

Handling of the tissues should be reduced to a minimum and really to do this is surprisingly difficult. Every time the tissue is touched a traumatism results. If we keep the delicate histological structure always in mind, we will realize the necessity of never pinching or pulling the tissues to the degree of even microscopic tissue strain. The most gentle retraction and sharpest knife-edge dissection is not showing too great a respect for tissues, even if they are at some distance from the tendon. When handling a tendon or sheath, never should even a tiny scratch be made in the delicate membrane covering their surfaces, as here adhesions will form and prevent gliding. If we operate in a field rendered bloodless by the use of a blood-pressure band as a tourniquet, we may avoid the unnecessary trauma of sponging and can by clearly seeing the tissues dissect with exactness and a minimum of traumatism.

In a former paper[1] I have endeavored to formulate the methods and principles whereby we will meet with better success in reconstructing damaged movable parts.

Reconstruction of gliding mechanism. A tendon alone in the tissues cannot functionate as it will be bound by adhesions. To permit movement back and forth a tendon must have in addition a gliding mechanism. To Dr. Leo Mayer[2] and to Professor Biesalski is due the credit of giving us the exact anatomy of tendons and their gliding mechanisms, and the physiological method of transposing tendons, especially in the foot. They have shown how a tendon in the straight part of its course is surrounded by a loose fatty tissue called paratenon which is pulled back and forth in its central zone with the movements of the tendon, and that wherever a tendon turns a corner it runs in a true sheath, in which the surface of the tendon (epitenon) slips freely in contact with the synovial lining surface of the sheath. In other parts of the body a bloodvessel-bearing mesotenon is present throughout the length of the sheath, much like a mesentery, but in the fingers this is absent, being reduced to the two strands of tissue known as ligamentum breve and ligamentum longum.

In repairing an old injury of a flexor tendon of a finger it is not practical to suture the tendon within the finger. In the gap between the tendon ends the sheath will have become obliterated and there is not room in a finger to envelope the suture line with a sufficiently thick free graft of fat to allow motion. The exception to this rule is where the tendon is severed in the less usual site opposite the middle phalanx or distally, where the repaired portion need pull through but one joint, in which case a fair result can be obtained. Where the suture line pulls through two joints, it is necessary to remove entirely the damaged tendon from the finger and to replace it with a free tendon graft. The suturing of the tendon can then be done at its insertion and in the palm or forearm where adhesions will do less harm.

If the sheath of the tendon has been damaged, the new tendon will not slip and it will be necessary to graft not only a tendon but a gliding mechanism complete. This means a tendon plus its sheath or a tendon plus its paratenon.

[1]An essential in reconstructive surgery—atraumatic technique. California St. J. Med., 1921, May.

[2]The physiological method of tendon transplantation. (Extensive bibliography.) Surg., Gynec. & Obst. 1916, xxii, 182.

The placing of both a sublimis and a profundus flexor tendon in the finger is too complicated. It is found sufficient to sacrifice the sublimis and use the profundus tendon only. The prevention of adhesions by the use of foreign bodies, as cargile membrane, etc., has long since been discarded, nor can a silk thread act as a substitute for a tendon in a finger.

Free tendon grafts cause less reaction than foreign bodies. They subsist on the surrounding lymph until they obtain their own blood supply. Often I have uncovered these grafts at short and long periods afterward. At first they show a slight swelling, but later show their original size and appearance and practically are none the worse from the transplanting. Some have even lived through infection. Function keeps a tendon in good condition, just as with bones, and a tendon with all its blood supply, if left without an insertion, will become yellowish and friable.

Sources of free tendon grafts. Grafts are easily obtained from the sublimis tendon, the palmaris longus, the long extensors of the toes, tubularized triceps, fascia lata, and many other sources. If the sublimis tendon of the same finger is used its upper end may be detached through a transverse incision, 1 centimeter long, in the forearm. It is well here to attach the distal end of the sublimis muscle to the profundus tendon for added strength. The incision is short and transverse for cosmetic reasons and to make a shorter distance for adhesions to form along a tendon in the forearm. If the palmaris longus tendon plus its paratenon is used, it will be necessary to make a longitudinal incision the full length of the graft. A long extensor tendon of the toes plus its paratenon in the dorsum of the foot can be taken without getting toe-drop, as the extensor brevis digitorum will serve to extend the toes. If a very long-branched tendon be desired, the extensor tendons to the second, third, and fourth toes can be used. They converge to form the inner tendon of the extensor communis digitorum above the annular ligament and can be severed here and at the toes. The outer tendon of this muscle (to the fifth toe and peroneus tertius) and the tibialis anticus will prevent foot-drop. It is necessary, however, to strip off the paratenon in the foot before these long tendons can be withdrawn.

If the paratenon is not removed intact with the tendon graft, paratenon fat may be gathered from elsewhere and planted sleeve-like about the tendon graft or other tendon to be mobilized. The fat over the triceps tendon is well suited for this purpose. Paratenon fat is specialized fat and differs much from the tough, short-fibered, subcutaneous fat. It is elastic and pliable and can easily be drawn a long distance back and forth from its moorings, as can be seen by comparing the mobility of the skin over the triceps tendon with that over the outer side of the arm.

Method of suture. The suturing of a tendon must be very strong, as it must stand the strain for the 5 weeks necessary for the physiological union to be complete. The stronger the suturing, the more forceful and continuous can be the all-important, postoperative exercise. The suture must be braided into the tendon for quite a distance and as little as possible of it exposed to the surface. The knots should be buried. If sewed well, the tendon will break before the suturing will. Any crude handling of the tendon, such as by grasping it with tissue forceps, will result in fraying of the tendon and in scratching and tearing the delicate covering or epitenon, and binding adhesions will result. Therefore, I use a specially devised fenestrated clamp and sew through the slits, making an even machine-sewed union and inflicting minimum trauma to the tendon. This I have described in a former paper.[1] Short tendon grafts may be threaded longitudinally on the two strands of thread. The suture material should be soft, slender, and strong. Pagenstecher is too harsh and will sometimes be extruded. Turner patent ligature silk Nos. 1 and 2 is satisfactory and often on exposing the union months later the suture line and silk cannot be seen. A good method is to let the suturing embrace only the half of the diameter of the tendon away from the mesotenon, so that at least the other half of the diameter of the tendon may be unhindered by suture material from making a perfect union. If the union be made in a region such as the forearm, where adhesions are not of such importance, it is well to overlap the cut surfaces of the tendon ends, so as to attain earlier and stronger union for early exercise. The proper tension for uniting a tendon has been worked out by Dr. Leo Mayer, as follows: When the origin and insertion of the muscle are approximated as near together as possible the tension of the tendon should be zero. There is an exception to this rule, however, in the case of a muscle which, owing to the severance of its tendon, has long been contracted. If the rule be followed in this case, it will not be possible to extend the muscle sufficiently for full function, and it will be necessary to make our tendon graft a little longer.

Removing and replacing tendons. It is difficult to remove a tendon neatly from a mass of adhesions and especially from beneath the annular ligament and from within a finger. These are the places where infection does the most damage, as here the firm structures prevent swelling and ischaemia results, encouraging the ravages of the infection. For this purpose I use a stripper specially devised from a cork borer (see former paper) that with a sharp edge and twirling motion planes the tendon smoothly from its binding adhesions. Some of the strippers have flexible handles to fit the curve of a finger.

It is difficult also to place a tendon, with its paratenon, through a tunnel in the finger. This can be done with a flexible probe expanding flatly at its center, so as to widen the tunnel, and terminating posteriorly in a funnel to receive the end of the tendon and draw it through. The sutures from the end of the tendon hook over a peg in a slit in the funnel. A thin rubber tube may envelope the paratenon until it is evenly placed in the finger, and then the tube can be withdrawn.

Freeing adherent tendons. Quite often after a tendon repair or an infection,

[1]Repair of tendons in the fingers and description of two new instruments. Surg., Gynec. & Obst., 1918, xxvi, 103.

or even after a general traumatism to the hand or a simple fracture of a phalanx, it is found that the joints can be passively, but not voluntarily, moved because of adhesions between the tendon and the surrounding tissue. If these adhesions are planed off from the tendon by a tendon stripper (mentioned above) and active motion be started at once and persisted in, a great gain or even the normal range of motion will be attained. If the adhesions are light, this may be accomplished through an incision in the forearm. The finger joints are forced into full flexion, and the tendons in the forearm are separately pulled, until suddenly the adhesions yield and full flexion of the finger can be made by pulling the tendon.

Often after a tendon repair it is necessary to do a second operation of freeing the tendon from adhesions. This is best deferred, however, for several months until the original postoperative induration has passed away, otherwise a summation of postoperative induration might defeat our purpose.

Incisions. The selection of the proper incisions is very important. Many fingers are permanently crippled by the median longitudinal incision. This cuts the pulleys, roughens and causes adhesions on the friction surface of both tendon and sheath and leads later to a contraction like that of Dupuytren. If the median longitudinal incision of the finger, whether on the dorsal or palmar surface, through the matrix or in the pulp, whether for infection or repair, be eliminated entirely from the surgeon's activities, many fingers will be saved from being permanently damaged. Even in the palm the longitudinal incision leads to contraction. It is far better to make transverse incisions in the palm in the line of the creases or L-shaped ones than longitudinal. In the finger lateral incisions between the two lateral nerves and arteries should be made. They should be interrupted so as not to cut the pulleys. As the pulleys are located at the center of the segments of the finger, the lateral incisions should be opposite the joints. Distally, near the insertion of the tendon, the incision may be L-shaped, one arm running transversely across the volar surface of the finger. It is very important not to cut the nerves of the finger, either in the finger or in the palm, as trophic changes will result. On the extensor surface, crescent or L-shaped incisions are satisfactory. It is important to have the skin incision remote from the tendon graft and tendon suture, as otherwise adhesions and infection will be encouraged. If the pulleys have been destroyed by former ill-advised incisions, they may be reconstructed by fascial grafts. Otherwise the tendon will bow across the flexed finger and loss of function will result.

Flexion contracture of a finger. Flexion contracture of a finger is quite common, due either to suppurative tenosynovitis, or to the ill-advised median longitudinal incision. Mild forms may be corrected by using slow traction with a splint. A wire splint resembling a large safety pin, with two flat ends is laid longitudinally on the volar surface of the finger and with a web strap and buckle looped around each wire, the convexity of the finger is day by day gradually drawn forward between the wires until the finger is hyperextended. This position is maintained until the tissues of the volar surface of the finger have grown long enough to allow correction to be permanent.

Greater degrees of flexion contracture can be corrected by excising the contracting band of skin and subcutaneous tissue and after forcing the finger into overcorrection closing in the denuded area by a tubularized pedicle flap, prepared 10 days previously. Wolfe grafts may also be used, but they necessitate perfect immobilization. Thiersch grafts do not furnish enough subcutaneous loose tissue to make a bed for the later tendon repair. After straightening the finger hyperextension must be maintained for a month by splinting. If the contracture is too extreme, gangrene may result from sudden forced extension.

Indications and contra-indications. It is a mistake to attempt to mend a bone, correct a contracture, or mobilize a stiffened joint in a finger at the same time that a tendon is repaired, as failure is sure to result. The added trauma will create adhesions to the tendon and also we will have the impossible double indication both to immobilize and move the finger. Unless the joints are freely movable, it is useless to repair the tendon, as it will not be able to move a stiff joint. The adhesions will then catch the tendon at rest and bind it in its bed.

If the joints of a finger are permanently stiffened, it is better to amputate the finger than to try to reconstruct it. Such joints have adhesions between their articular surfaces that will not allow movement, even after all the tissues, including the capsule of the joint, are cut away. If the stiffened joints are not permanently damaged, they may be drawn into the position of flexion by slow, mild, continuous traction on the ends of the gloved fingers. They will then become more easily mobilized, and the new tendon to be put in will have a chance to functionate. Intermittent strong forcing of the joints only results in straining them, which stiffens them all the more. Traction must be mild and kept up for a long time, so that the tissues will have time to grow enough to be relaxed in the new position, not merely stretched.

When the storm of an infection has passed through a finger and destroyed the flexor tendon, there often results a thin, red, shiny finger, with stiffened joints and firm congealed tissue. The contracted scar tissue throughout the finger has strangled the nerves and vessels, so that great trophic changes have resulted. Such a finger is unfit for repair of the tendons, and amputation is to be preferred. For a tendon repair to be worth while, the bed through which the tendon is to be placed must be soft and succulent. It may first be advisible to excise the damaged firm tissue and replace it by means of a tubularized pedicle skin-graft before tendon repair is done. To avoid latent infection and to await the softening up of the tissues, at least 4 months from the time of infection should elapse before a repair is attempted. A freshly cut tendon may be repaired primarily if an excision of the damaged tissue is done, but if over 24 hours have elapsed since the injury, infection will probably result if the tendon is operated on. One had better treat it conservatively and later do a secondary repair.

It is well to beware of an annular scar, or the too close proximity of another scar, as in such a case necrosis is prone to occur from the diminished nerve and blood supply.

There are certain people, and not always old ones, whose joints and tissues have a tendency to stiffen if traumatized or immobilized and these make poor subjects for tendon repair. The presence of osteo-arthritis suggests this type. There are others who have not enough character to withstand the pain of moving their fingers after the tendon repair. With them an otherwise good result may be prevented. Before attempting a tendon repair, one must weigh well the gain of function to be expected with the amount of inconvenience and trouble to the patient.

After-treatment. The after-treatment is all important. It is best to avoid splinting the fingers, as too much immobilization allows adhesions to form. Instead, the wrist can be strongly flexed for a flexor tendon and held so by a check-rein of adhesive plaster running up and around the forearm. The muscles that pull the tendons are thus robbed of their power of too much traction and still they can keep the tendon actively moving. Motion should be encouraged from the first, but too much or too vigorous early motion causes haematoma and the opening of incisions. Later, a ball, a rounded match box, or a piece of rubber hose can be carried in the pocket and used for exercise in grasping. The restricting check-rein should not be removed for 5 weeks when union will be firm. Later the galvanic current may be used to contract the muscles sharply, thus snapping tiny adhesions. If the hand is soaked in hot water previous to exercising, it helps considerably. Actual hard work and the lapse of several months finally complete the loosening-up process. Co-operation by the patient is essential, and he must be willing to take some punishment in exchange for a good result.

It is well to give a guarded prognosis in these cases, but it is usually possible to restore from 80 to 95 per cent of lost function.

Index